For Reference

Blood and Circulatory Disorders

SOURCEBOOK

FIFTH EDITION

Health Reference Series

Blood and Circulatory Disorders
SOURCEBOOK

FIFTH EDITION

Basic Consumer Health Information about Blood and Circulatory System Disorders, Such as Anemia, Leukemia, Lymphoma, Rh Disease, Hemophilia, Thrombophilia, Other Bleeding and Clotting Deficiencies, and Artery, Vascular, and Venous Diseases, Including Facts about Blood Types, Blood Donation, Bone Marrow and Stem Cell Transplants, Tests and Medications, and Tips for Maintaining Healthy Circulatory System

Along with a Glossary of Related Terms and a List of Resources for Additional Help and Information

OMNIGRAPHICS

615 Griswold, Ste. 520, Detroit, MI 48226

Bibliographic Note

Because this page cannot legibly accommodate all the copyright notices, the Bibliographic Note portion of the Preface constitutes an extension of the copyright notice.

* * *

OMNIGRAPHICS

Angela L. Williams, *Managing Editor*

* * *

Copyright © 2019 Omnigraphics

ISBN 978-0-7808-1715-9
E-ISBN 978-0-7808-1716-6

Library of Congress Cataloging-in-Publication Data

Names: Omnigraphics, Inc., issuing body.

Title: Blood and circulatory disorders sourcebook: basic consumer health information about blood and circulatory system disorders, such as anemia, leukemia, lymphoma, rh disease, hemophilia, thrombophilia, other bleeding and clotting deficiencies, and artery, vascular, and venous diseases, including facts about blood types, blood donation, bone marrow and stem cell transplants, tests and medications, and tips for maintaining circulatory health; along with a glossary of related terms and a list of resources for additional help and information.

Description: Fifth edition. | Detroit, MI: Omnigraphics, Inc., [2019] | Includes bibliographical references and index.

Identifiers: LCCN 2019021354 (print) | LCCN 2019022009 (ebook) | ISBN 9780780817159 (ebook) | ISBN 9780780817159 (hard cover: alk. paper) | ISBN 9780780817166 (e-isbn)

Subjects: LCSH: Blood--Diseases--Popular works. | Blood-vessels--Diseases--Popular works.

Classification: LCC RC636 (ebook) | LCC RC636.B556 2019 (print) | DDC 616.1/3--dc23

LC record available at https://lccn.loc.gov/2019021354

Table of Contents

Part III: Bleeding and Clotting Disorders

Part IV: Circulatory Disorders

Part V: Diagnosing and Treating Blood and Circulatory Disorders

Part VI: Additional Help and Information

Preface

About This Book

Blood plays many important roles in the human body. It carries oxygen and nutrients to the body's cells, helps fight infection, and works to heal wounds. When a disorder inhibits its ability to meet the body's needs or prevents blood from flowing or coagulating properly, a myriad of problems can result. According to the Centers for Disease Control and Prevention (CDC), millions of people across the United States of all ages, races, sexes, and socioecomonic statuses are affected by blood disorders, such as anemia, sickle cell disease, and hemophilia.

Blood and Circulatory Disorders Sourcebook, Fifth Edition offers facts about blood function and composition, the maintenance of a healthy circulatory system, and the types of concerns that arise when processes go awry. It discusses the diagnosis and treatment of many common blood cell disorders, bleeding disorders, and circulatory disorders, including anemia, hemochromatosis, leukemia, lymphoma, hemophilia, hypercoagulation, thrombophilia, atherosclerosis, blood pressure irregularities, coronary artery and heart disease, and peripheral vascular disease. Blood donation, cord blood banking, blood transfusions, and bone marrow and stem cell transplants are also discussed. The book concludes with a glossary of related terms and a list of resources for further help and information.

How to Use This Book

This book is divided into parts and chapters. Parts focus on broad areas of interest. Chapters are devoted to single topics within a part.

Part I: Understanding the Blood and Circulatory System explains the composition and types of blood and how it functions in the body. It describes blood donation and cord blood banking procedures, and it also discusses how aging affects the heart and blood vessels.

Part II: Blood Disorders describes ailments that affect the composition of the blood itself. These include anemia and other hemoglobin disorders, cancers of the blood, plasma cell disorders, and white blood cell disorders. Information about the causes of these disorders is provided, and treatment strategies are discussed.

Part III: Bleeding and Clotting Disorders provides information about bleeding disorders resulting from insufficient clotting, such as hemophilia and von Willebrand disease, and those resulting from excess clotting, including deep vein thrombosis and pulmonary embolism. Methods of diagnosis and treatment options are included.

Part IV: Circulatory Disorders describes disorders affecting the veins, arteries, and heart. It includes information about aneurysms; stroke; blood pressure irregularities; atherosclerosis; carotid artery disease; coronary artery disease; heart disease; peripheral vascular disease; and venous disorders, such as thrombophlebitis and varicose and spider veins. Information about causes and diagnosis, as well as treatment options, is provided.

Part V: Diagnosing and Treating Blood and Circulatory Disorders provides information about medical tests commonly used to identify and monitor blood and circulatory disorders. It offers facts about many of the medications often used in the treatment of these disorders and discusses such procedures as blood transfusion and bone marrow transplants.

Part VI: Additional Help and Information includes a glossary of terms related to blood and circulatory disorders and a directory of resources offering additional help and support.

Bibliographic Note

This volume contains documents and excerpts from publications issued by the following U.S. government agencies: Agency for Healthcare Research and Quality (AHRQ); Centers for Disease Control and

Prevention (CDC); *Eunice Kennedy Shriver* National Institute of Child Health and Human Development (NICHD); Genetic and Rare Diseases Information Center (GARD); Genetics Home Reference (GHR); National Cancer Institute (NCI); National Center for Biotechnology Information (NCBI); National Heart, Lung, and Blood Institute (NHLBI); National Institute of Arthritis and Musculoskeletal and Skin Diseases (NIAMS); National Institute of Diabetes and Digestive and Kidney Diseases (NIDDK); National Institute of General Medical Sciences (NIGMS); National Institute of Neurological Disorders and Stroke (NINDS); National Institute on Aging (NIA); National Institute on Alcohol Abuse and Alcoholism (NIAAA); National Institutes of Health (NIH); Office of Dietary Supplements (ODS); Office of Disease Prevention and Health Promotion (ODPHP); Office on Women's Health (OWH); and U.S. Food and Drug Administration (FDA).

It may also contain original material produced by Omnigraphics and reviewed by medical consultants.

About the Health Reference Series

The *Health Reference Series* is designed to provide basic medical information for patients, families, caregivers, and the general public. Each volume takes a particular topic and provides comprehensive coverage. This is especially important for people who may be dealing with a newly diagnosed disease or a chronic disorder in themselves or in a family member. People looking for preventive guidance, information about disease warning signs, medical statistics, and risk factors for health problems will also find answers to their questions in the *Health Reference Series*. The *Series*, however, is not intended to serve as a tool for diagnosing illness, in prescribing treatments, or as a substitute for the physician/patient relationship. All people concerned about medical symptoms or the possibility of disease are encouraged to seek professional care from an appropriate healthcare provider.

A Note about Spelling and Style

Health Reference Series editors use *Stedman's Medical Dictionary* as an authority for questions related to the spelling of medical terms and the *Chicago Manual of Style* for questions related to grammatical structures, punctuation, and other editorial concerns. Consistent adherence is not always possible, however, because the individual volumes within the *Series* include many documents from a wide variety of different producers, and the editor's primary goal is to present material from each source as accurately as is possible. This sometimes means that information in different chapters or sections may follow other guidelines and alternate spelling authorities. For example, occasionally a copyright holder may require that eponymous terms be shown in possessive forms (Crohn's disease vs. Crohn disease) or that British spelling norms be retained (leukaemia vs. leukemia).

Medical Review

Omnigraphics contracts with a team of qualified, senior medical professionals who serve as medical consultants for the *Health Reference Series*. As necessary, medical consultants review reprinted and originally written material for currency and accuracy. Citations including the phrase "Reviewed (month, year)" indicate material reviewed by this team. Medical consultation services are provided to the *Health Reference Series* editors by:

Dr. Vijayalakshmi, MBBS, DGO, MD
Dr. Senthil Selvan, MBBS, DCH, MD
Dr. K. Sivanandham, MBBS, DCH, MS (Research), PhD

Our Advisory Board

We would like to thank the following board members for providing initial guidance on the development of this series:

- Dr. Lynda Baker, Associate Professor of Library and Information Science, Wayne State University, Detroit, MI
- Nancy Bulgarelli, William Beaumont Hospital Library, Royal Oak, MI
- Karen Imarisio, Bloomfield Township Public Library, Bloomfield Township, MI
- Karen Morgan, Mardigian Library, University of Michigan-Dearborn, Dearborn, MI
- Rosemary Orlando, St. Clair Shores Public Library, St. Clair Shores, MI

Health Reference Series *Update Policy*

The inaugural book in the *Health Reference Series* was the first edition of *Cancer Sourcebook* published in 1989. Since then, the *Series* has been enthusiastically received by librarians and in the medical community. In order to maintain the standard of providing high-quality health information for the layperson the editorial staff at Omnigraphics felt it was necessary to implement a policy of updating volumes when warranted.

Medical researchers have been making tremendous strides, and it is the purpose of the *Health Reference Series* to stay current with the most recent advances. Each decision to update a volume is made on an individual basis. Some of the considerations include how much new information is available and the feedback we receive from people who use the books. If there is a topic you would like to see added to the update list, or an area of medical concern you feel has not been adequately addressed, please write to:

Managing Editor
Health Reference Series
Omnigraphics
615 Griswold, Ste. 520
Detroit, MI 48226

Part One

Understanding the Blood and Circulatory System

Chapter 1

Blood Function and Composition

Blood is a connective tissue, and as a connective tissue, it consists of cells and cell fragments (formed elements) that are suspended in an intercellular matrix (plasma). Blood is the only liquid tissue in the body that measures about five liters in the adult human and accounts for eight percent of body weight.

The body consists of metabolically active cells that need a continuous supply of nutrients and oxygen. Metabolic waste products need to be removed from the cells to maintain a stable cellular environment. Blood is the primary transport medium that is responsible for meeting these cellular demands.

Blood cells are formed in the bone marrow, the soft, spongy center of bones. New (immature) blood cells are called "blasts." Some blasts stay in the marrow to mature. Some travel to other parts of the body to mature.

The activities of the blood may be categorized as transportation, regulation, and protection.

These functional categories overlap and interact as the blood carries out its role in providing suitable conditions for cellular functions.

This chapter includes text excerpted from "Anatomy," Surveillance, Epidemiology, and End Results Program (SEER), National Cancer Institute (NCI), April 28, 2009. Reviewed June 2019.

The transport functions include:

- Carrying oxygen and nutrients to the cells

- Transporting carbon dioxide and nitrogenous wastes from the tissues to the lungs and kidneys where these wastes can be removed from the body

- Carrying hormones from the endocrine glands to the target tissues

The regulation functions include:

- Helping regulate body temperature by removing heat from active areas, such as skeletal muscles, and transporting it to other regions or to the skin where it can be dissipated

- Playing a significant role in fluid and electrolyte balance because the salts and plasma proteins contribute to the osmotic pressure

- Functioning in pH regulation through the action of buffers in the blood

The protection functions include:

- Preventing fluid loss through hemorrhage when blood vessels are damaged due to its clotting mechanisms

- Helping (phagocytic white blood cells (WBCs)) to protect the body against microorganisms that cause disease by engulfing and destroying the agent

- Protecting (antibodies in the plasma) against disease by their reactions with offending agents

Composition of the Blood

When a sample of blood is spun in a centrifuge, the cells and cell fragments are separated from the liquid intercellular matrix. Because the formed elements are heavier than the liquid matrix, they are packed in the bottom of the tube by the centrifugal force. The light yellow colored liquid on the top is the plasma, which accounts for about 55 percent of the blood volume and red blood cells (RBCs), is called the "hematocrit," or "packed cell volume" (PCV). The white blood cells and platelets form a thin white layer, called the "buffy coat," between the plasma and red blood cells.

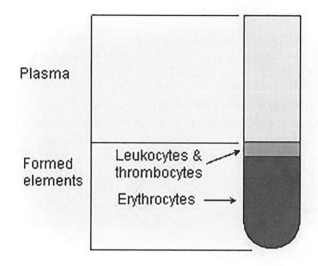

Figure 1.1. *Blood and Its Composition*

Plasma

Plasma is the watery fluid portion of blood (90 percent water) in which the corpuscular elements are suspended. It transports nutrients, as well as waste, throughout the body. Various compounds, including proteins, electrolytes, carbohydrates, minerals, and fats, are dissolved in it.

Formed Elements

The formed elements are cells and cell fragments that are suspended in the plasma. The three classes of formed elements are the erythrocytes (red blood cells), leukocytes (white blood cells), and the thrombocytes (platelets).

Erythrocytes

Erythrocytes, or red blood cells, are the most numerous of the formed elements. Erythrocytes are tiny biconcave disks; they are thin in the middle and thicker around the periphery. The shape provides a combination of flexibility for moving through tiny capillaries with a maximum surface area for the diffusion of gases. The primary function of erythrocytes is to transport oxygen and, to a lesser extent, carbon dioxide.

Leukocytes

Leukocytes, or white blood cells, are generally larger than erythrocytes, but they are fewer in number. Even though they are considered to be blood cells, leukocytes do most of their work in the tissues. They use the blood as a transport medium. Some are phagocytic, others produce antibodies; some secrete histamine and heparin, and others neutralize histamine. Leukocytes are able to move through the capillary walls into the tissue spaces, a process called "diapedesis." In the tissue spaces, they provide a defense against organisms that cause disease and either promote or inhibit inflammatory responses.

There are two main groups of leukocytes in the blood. The cells that develop granules in the cytoplasm are called "granulocytes," and those that do not have granules are called "agranulocytes." Neutrophils, eosinophils, and basophils are granulocytes. Monocytes and lymphocytes are agranulocytes.

Neutrophils, the most numerous leukocytes, are phagocytic and have light-colored granules. Eosinophils have granules and help counteract the effects of histamine. Basophils secrete histamine and heparin, and have blue granules. In the tissues, they are called "mast cells." Lymphocytes are agranulocytes that have a special role in immune processes. Some attack bacteria directly; others produce antibodies.

Thrombocytes

Thrombocytes, or platelets, are not complete cells but are small fragments of very large cells called "megakaryocytes." Megakaryocytes develop from hemocytoblasts in the red bone marrow. Thrombocytes become sticky and clump together to form platelet plugs that close breaks and tears in blood vessels. They also initiate the formation of blood clots.

Blood Cell Lineage

The production of formed elements, or blood cells, is called "hemopoiesis." Before birth, hemopoiesis occurs primarily in the liver and spleen, but some cells develop in the thymus, lymph nodes, and red bone marrow. After birth, most production is limited to red bone marrow in specific regions, but some white blood cells are produced in lymphoid tissue.

All types of formed elements develop from a single cell type—stem cell (pluripotential cells or hemocytoblasts). Seven different cell lines, each controlled by a specific growth factor, develop from the hemocyto-blast. When a stem cell divides, one of the "daughters" remains a stem cell, and the other becomes a precursor cell, either a lymphoid cell or a myeloid cell. These cells continue to mature into various blood cells.

Leukemia can develop at any point in cell differentiation. The figure below shows the development of the formed elements of the blood.

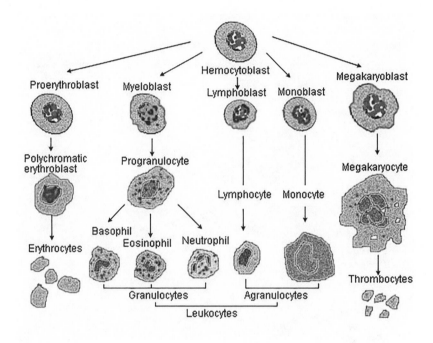

Figure 1.2. *Development of the Formed Elements of the Blood*

Chapter 2

Blood Groups

Characteristics

There are four common blood groups in the ABO system: O, A, B, and AB. The blood groups are defined by the presence of specific carbohydrate sugars on the surface of red blood cells, N-acetylgalactosamine for the A antigen, and D-galactose for the B antigen. Both of these sugars are built upon the H antigen—if the H antigen is left unmodified, the resulting blood group is O because neither the A nor the B antigen can attach to the red blood cells.

Individuals will naturally develop antibodies against the ABO antigens they do not have. For example, individuals with blood group A will have anti-B antibodies, and individuals with blood group O will have both anti-A and anti-B. Before a blood transfusion takes place, routine serological testing checks the compatibility of the ABO (and Rh) blood groups. An ABO incompatible blood transfusion can be fatal, due to the highly immunogenic nature of the A and B antigens, and the corresponding strongly hemolytic antibodies.

Over 80 ABO alleles have been reported. The common alleles include A1, A2, B1, O1, O1v, and O2. Whereas the A and B alleles each encode a specific glycosyl-transferring enzyme, the O allele appears to have no function. A single-base deletion in the O allele means that individuals with blood group O do not produce either the A or B antigens. Blood

---

This chapter includes text excerpted from "Medical Genetics Summaries," National Center for Biotechnology Information (NCBI), July 27, 2015. Reviewed June 2019.

type frequencies vary in different racial/ethnic groups. In the United States, in Caucasians, the ratio of blood group O, A, B, and AB is 45%, 40%, 11%, and 4%, respectively. In Hispanics, the distribution is 57%, 31%, 10%, and 3%; and in Blacks, 50%, 26%, 20%, and 4%.

Diagnosis and Testing

Serological testing is sufficient to determine an individual's blood type (e.g., blood group A) for the purposes of blood donation and transfusion. Molecular genetic testing can be used to determine an individual's ABO genotype (e.g., genotype AO or AA). This may be useful in the research setting, for example, to investigate the link between ABO blood groups and particular diseases, and also in the forensic setting.

Management

Determining an individual's blood group is important prior to blood transfusion and prior to the donation or receiving of a organ transplant.

Occasionally, a person's blood type may appear to change. For example, the ABO antigens can act as tumor markers. Their presence may be decreased in particular diseases, such as acute myeloid leukemia (AML). In contrast, occasionally the B antigen may be acquired in certain infectious diseases. A bacterial infection with specific strains of *Escherichia coli (E. coli)* or *Clostridium tertium* can generate a B-like antigen from an individual who has the A1 allele.

Genetic Counseling

The ABO blood type is inherited in an autosomal codominant fashion. The A and B alleles are codominant, and the O allele is recessive.

Chapter 3

Donating and Preserving Blood

Chapter Contents

11

Section 3.1

Blood Donation Overview

Blood Donation

Blood donation is a voluntary procedure in which one person gives some of their blood to help another person. People need to receive blood donations if they are having surgery; if they lost blood from an injury; or if they have certain illnesses, such as hemophilia, sickle cell disease, anemia, or some types of cancer.

Blood Donors

A blood donor is a person who volunteers to give some of their blood through blood donation. Certain requirements must be met in order to become a blood donor. Blood donors must be healthy adults between the ages of 17 and 70 who weigh at least 110 pounds and have normal blood pressure and body temperature. Donors are eligible to give blood once every 56 days.

Certain restrictions exist to protect both blood donors and blood donation recipients. People who are not able to donate blood include pregnant women, people who have recently had a tattoo or piercing, people who are ill, and those taking specific medications. People who have recently traveled to certain countries may also be disqualified from donating blood.

Blood Donation Process

Blood donations are typically collected at blood drives, blood banks, or at a medical facility. The process usually begins with a donor screening interview, which is conducted in private. During this interview, a healthcare professional asks a series of questions to determine whether a person is able to donate blood. Questions may focus on past and present health conditions and personal behaviors, such as drug use or sexually transmitted diseases (STDs). These questions are asked every time a person donates blood so that any changes in the donor's health can be identified.

After the initial screening interview, the blood donation process takes about 10 minutes. About 1 pint (480 ml) of blood is collected from each blood donor. This amount is equal to about 8 percent of the average adult's total blood volume. The donor's body will replace the volume of donated blood within 24 to 48 hours. The amount of red blood cells in that volume of blood will be replaced by the donor's body in 10 to 12 weeks.

Blood donations are tested and screened to ensure the blood is safe to give to another person. These tests usually screen for blood-borne diseases, such as hepatitis, human immunodeficiency virus (HIV), West Nile virus, and other viruses. Blood that tests positive for any of the screened diseases is discarded as medical waste, and the donor is notified of the test results so that they may seek treatment if needed. Donated blood is also checked to identify the blood type (A, B, AB, O).

Types of Donated Blood

Most donated blood is processed to separate the whole blood into the different components that make up human blood, such as platelets, plasma, and red blood cells. This is done because most blood donation recipients only need to receive a certain component of blood.

The different types of blood donation are:

- Whole blood that contains red and white blood cells, plasma, platelets, antibodies, and other components. This type of blood donation is called "homologous."

- Plasma that is extracted from donated blood with a centrifuge, which is a machine that spins at a high rate of speed to separate the blood into its components. The plasma is then drawn out of the blood, and the red blood cells are returned to the donor. This type of blood donation is called "apheresis."

- Platelets are extracted from blood using a different centrifuge process, and both red blood cells and the plasma are returned to the donor. This type of blood donation is called "pheresis."

- Autologous donation refers to blood that is donated by a person for their own use. This type of blood donation is rare and is usually done in special cases.

- Directed or designated donation refers to blood that is donated for use by a specific person. This type of blood donation is also rare and done only in special cases.

Risks of Donating Blood

The blood donation process is safe, and there are no health risks associated with donating blood. Sterile, prepackaged equipment is used to collect blood donations, and new equipment is used for each donor. The blood donor may develop a small bruise on their arm at the site from which blood was drawn. Some blood donors feel light-headed or slightly dizzy after giving blood. For this reason, most blood donors are given water, fruit juice, and a small snack and asked to sit for a few minutes after their blood is collected. For the first few hours after donating blood, it is recommended that blood donors refrain from physical activity and drink plenty of fluids.

References

1. "Donating Blood: Topic Overview," WebMD, March 12, 2014.

2. "Blood Donation," Better Health, March 2013.

Section 3.2

Apheresis

This section includes text excerpted from "NIH Clinical Center Patient Education Materials—Apheresis for Transfusion," Clinical Center, National Institutes of Health (NIH), December 2015. Reviewed June 2019.

Apheresis is a type of procedure in which a machine draws whole blood from a patient, removes one type of cell (such as white blood cells (WBCs) or stem cells), then returns the rest of the blood to the patient.

Various types of machines are used to do apheresis. These machines use sterile, disposable parts to prevent bloodborne infections. The needs of your protocol will determine the type of machine used for your apheresis and how long the procedure will last.

Preparation
Eat Well

You may eat your usual foods, but avoid fatty foods (such as bacon, sausage, and hamburger) the night before and the morning of your procedure. Be sure to eat breakfast before arriving for your apheresis appointment unless your nurse coordinator has told you otherwise.

Drink Enough Liquid

Drink at least 64 ounces of water, sports drinks, juice, or decaffeinated drinks per day for the 2 days prior to your procedure.

Wear Comfortable Clothing

Wear short sleeves and loose-fitting clothing. If you prefer to wear a hospital gown, the clinic staff can give you one.

Arrive Promptly

Please arrive at the apheresis clinic at your appointed time. Since there is no waiting room in the apheresis clinic, it is not advisable to arrive more than 10 minutes early.

Procedure
Before the Procedure

When you arrive in the clinic, a nurse will take your vital signs (temperature, pulse, and blood pressure), prick your finger to test your hemoglobin level, and ask you to sign a consent form that gives them permission to do apheresis. If you are donating cells for someone other than yourself, you will be asked a series of questions that help to make sure it is both safe for you to have the procedure and safe to give your cells to another person. It is important that you answer all of the questions honestly. Feel free to ask any questions at that time. All of this will take about one hour to an hour and a half.

Starting the Procedure

A nurse will examine your arms for the best sites to insert a steel needle and an intravenous (IV) catheter (a small, flexible plastic tube that stays inside of your vein). These sites will be cleansed thoroughly, the needle and IV catheter will be inserted, a set of labs will be drawn, and tubing from the apheresis machine will be attached to the needle and the catheter.

Some people's veins are too small for the size of needles used during the procedure. If this is the case for you, your nurse coordinator will arrange for you to have a temporary central venous catheter (central line) placed just before you go to the clinic. You will be asked not to eat or drink anything after midnight, the night prior to your procedure. After your central line has been placed, you will be allowed to eat your breakfast.

Answers to Common Questions
How Long Does Apheresis Take?

Depending on how much blood the apheresis machine needs to process, your procedure should take between three and a half to eight hours.

May I Bring Visitors to My Apheresis Procedure?

Because of limited space, only one person can stay with you during the entire procedure. Children may visit for a short time, but they must be supervised by an adult other than you at all times.

What If I Need to Use the Bathroom? Will I Be Able to Come off the Machine?

Before you start apheresis, the staff will ask you to empty your bladder. If you need to urinate while on the machine, the staff will provide you with a bedpan or urinal. Avoid drinking coffee or tea before coming to the clinic because they may cause you to need to urinate more often.

Will I Be Able to Eat and Drink during My Procedure?

Yes, you will. The clinic has juices and snacks, and your nurse can order a bag lunch for you.

Will I Be Able to Read a Book or Newspaper While on the Apheresis Machine?

Because both your arms are needed during the procedure, it is recommended to watch television.

Section 3.3

Ensuring Safe Blood Donation

This section includes text excerpted from "Have You Given Blood Lately?" U.S. Food and Drug Administration (FDA), September 7, 2016.

Every day, hospitals throughout the United States transfuse blood or blood components, such as platelets, to save the lives of people who are in motor vehicle accidents and victims of fires and other emergencies.

Blood is also required for many people with life-threatening illnesses and others undergoing routine surgeries. According to the Centers for Disease Control and Prevention (CDC), an estimated five million patients receive blood annually.

In fact, every two seconds, someone in America needs blood, according to the American Red Cross (ARC). This may include:

- Cancer patients undergoing chemotherapy

- People with sickle cell disease (SCD) or other types of inherited anemia

- Organ transplant recipients

- People undergoing elective surgery

- Women during and following labor and delivery

- Premature babies

- Trauma victims

Blood products from healthy donors are often lifesaving or life-enhancing.

U.S. Food and Drug Administration Oversight

The U.S. Food and Drug Administration (FDA), through the Center for Biologics and Research (CBER), is responsible for ensuring the safety of the more than the approximate 19 million units of whole blood donated each year in the United States. These donations can be further processed into blood components, such as red blood cells (RBCs), platelets, and plasma. The FDA's standards and regulations regarding blood donor selection, blood donation, and processing help protect the health of both the donor and the recipient.

The FDA's oversight of the blood industry includes:

- Approving licenses for blood products

- Approving devices used for blood collection, infectious disease testing, and pathogen reduction technologies

- Developing and enforcing quality standards

- Providing guidance on emerging infectious diseases

- Inspecting all blood facilities at least every two years

- Inspecting "problem" facilities more often

- Monitoring reports of errors and adverse events associated with blood donation or transfusion

- Taking regulatory or legal actions if problems are found

Five Layers of Safety

The FDA's blood safety efforts focus on minimizing the risk of transmitting infectious diseases while maintaining an adequate supply of blood for the nation.

Blood safety is based on five layers of overlapping safeguards:

1. **Donor screening.** Donors are provided with educational material and asked to self-defer if they have risk factors that may affect blood safety. Donors are then asked specific questions about their medical history and other risk factors that may affect the safety of their donation. This "up-front" screening identifies ineligible donors.

2. **Donor deferral lists.** Blood establishments must keep current a list of deferred donors. They must also check all potential donors against that list to prevent the collection or use of blood from deferred donors.

3. **Blood testing.** After donation, blood establishments are required to test each unit of donated blood for the following transfusion-transmitted infections (TTIs):

   - Hepatitis B

   - Hepatitis C

   - Human immunodeficiency viruses (HIV) 1 and 2

   - Human T-cell lymphotropic viruses (HTLV) I and II

- Treponema pallidum, which causes syphilis
- West Nile virus (WNV)
- Trypanosoma cruzi (Chagas disease)
- And most recently, Zika virus

4. **Quarantine.** Donated blood must be quarantined until it is tested and shown to be free of infectious agents.

5. **Problems and deficiencies.** Blood establishments must investigate manufacturing problems, correct all deficiencies, and notify the FDA when product deviations occur in distributed products.

If a violation of any one of these safeguards occurs, the blood product is considered unsuitable for transfusion and may be subject to recall.

Ongoing Safety Efforts

Emerging threats to the blood supply and other potential risks mean that the FDA's Blood Safety Team never stops looking for ways to ensure and preserve the safety of blood and blood products.

The FDA scientists are working to develop sensitive donor screening tests to detect emerging diseases and potential bioterrorism agents in blood donations. They are also working to improve blood donor screening tests to detect variant strains of HIV, West Nile virus, and hepatitis viruses. In addition, the FDA's Office of Blood Research and Review addresses donor deferral issues and updates eligibility requirements when appropriate.

Also, the FDA is a member of the American Association of Blood Banks (AABB) Interorganizational Task Force on Domestic Disasters and Acts of Terrorism that includes other blood organizations, government agencies, and device manufacturers. As such, it works with others to help assure that blood facilities maintain adequate blood inventories at all times in case of a disaster.

Section 3.4

Cord Blood Banking

This section includes text excerpted from "Cord Blood: What You Need to Know," U.S. Food and Drug Administration (FDA), July 30, 2014. Reviewed June 2019.

Found in the blood vessels of the placenta and the umbilical cord, cord blood—a biological product regulated by the U.S. Food and Drug Administration (FDA)—is collected after a baby is born and after the umbilical cord is cut.

"Because cord blood is typically collected after the baby is delivered and the cord is cut, the procedure is generally safe for the mother and baby," explains Keith Wonnacott, Ph.D., Chief of the Cellular Therapies Branch in the FDA's Office of Cellular, Tissue, and Gene Therapies.

Approved Uses

Cord blood is approved only for use in hematopoietic stem cell transplantation (HPSCT) procedures, which are done in patients with disorders affecting the hematopoietic (blood-forming) system. Cord blood contains blood-forming stem cells that can be used in the treatment of patients with blood cancers, such as leukemias and lymphomas, as well as certain disorders of the blood and immune systems, such as sickle cell disease (SCD) and Wiskott-Aldrich syndrome (WAS).

"Cord blood is useful because it is a source of stem cells that form into blood cells. Cord blood can be used for transplantation in people who need regeneration, that is, 'regrowth,' of these blood-forming cells," Wonnacott says.

For instance, in many cancer patients, the disease is found in the blood cells. Chemotherapy treatment of these patients kills both cancer cells and the healthy blood-forming stem cells. Transplanted stem cells from cord blood can help regrow the healthy blood cells after chemotherapy.

However, cord blood is not a cure-all.

"Because cord blood contains stem cells, there have been stem cell fraud cases related to cord blood," says Wonnacott. "Consumers may think that stem cells can cure any disease, but science does not show this to be the case. Patients should be skeptical if the cord blood is being promoted for uses other than blood stem cell regeneration."

About Cord Blood Banking

After cord blood is collected, it is frozen and can be safely stored for many years. "The method of freezing, called 'cryopreservation,' is very important to maintain the integrity of the cells," Wonnacott says. "Cord blood needs to be stored carefully."

You may choose to store your baby's cord blood in a private bank, so it can be available if needed in the future by your child or first- or second-degree relatives. Private cord banks typically charge fees for blood collection and storage. Or, you may donate the cord blood to a public bank so that doctors can use it for a patient who needs a hematopoietic stem cell transplant.

The FDA regulates cord blood in different ways, depending on the source, level of processing, and intended use.

Cord blood stored for personal use, for use in first- or second-degree relatives, and that also meets other criteria in the FDA's regulations, does not require the agency's approval before use. Private cord banks must still comply with other FDA requirements, including establishment registration and listing, current good tissue practice regulations, and donor screening and testing for infectious diseases (except when cord blood is used for the original donor). These FDA requirements ensure the safety of these products by minimizing the risk of contamination and transmission of infectious diseases.

Cord blood stored for use by a patient unrelated to the donor meets the legal definitions of both a drug and a biological product. Cord blood in this category must meet additional requirements and be licensed under a biologics license application or be the subject of an investigational new drug application before use. The FDA requirements help to ensure that these products are safe and effective for their intended use.

Not every cord blood unit will meet requirements for public banking, adds Safa Karandish, M.T., an FDA consumer safety officer. If that happens, some of the donated cord blood may be used for nonclinical research.

Tips for Consumers

If you are considering donating to a cord blood bank, you should look into your options during your pregnancy to have enough time to decide before your baby is born. For public banking, ask whether your delivery hospital participates in a cord blood banking program.

If you have questions about collection procedures and risks, or about the donation process, ask your healthcare provider.

The FDA also offers a searchable database that maintains information on registered cord blood banks.

Be skeptical of claims that cord blood is a miracle cure—it is not. Some parents may consider using a private bank as a form of "insurance" against future illness. But remember that, currently, the only approved use of cord blood is for treatment of blood-related illnesses.

Also, know that in some cases, your stored cord blood may not be suitable for use in the child who donated it. "For instance, you cannot cure some diseases or genetic defects with cord blood that contains the same disease or defect," Karandish says.

Parents from minority ethnic groups may especially want to consider a donation to a public bank, says Wonnacott, because more donations from these populations will help more minority patients who need a stem cell transplant (SCT). The recipients must be matched to donors, so doctors are more likely to find a good match among donors from the recipient's ethnic group.

"When it comes to public banking, there is a proven need for cord blood," Wonnacott says. "And there is a need especially among minorities to have stem cell transplants available. Cord blood is an excellent source for stem cell transplants."

And these transplants can be life-changing for patients.

Chapter 4

Blood Circulatory System

Chapter Contents

Section 4.1

Classification and Structure of Blood Vessels

This section includes text excerpted from "Classification and Structure of Blood Vessels," Surveillance, Epidemiology, and End Results Program (SEER), National Cancer Institute (NCI), July 1, 2002. Reviewed June 2019.

Classification of Blood Vessels

Blood vessels are the channels or conduits through which blood is distributed to body tissues. The vessels make up two closed systems of tubes that begin and end at the heart. One system, the pulmonary vessels, transports blood from the right ventricle to the lungs and back to the left atrium. The other system, the systemic vessels, carries blood from the left ventricle to the tissues in all parts of the body and then returns the blood to the right atrium. Based on their structure and function, blood vessels are classified as either arteries, capillaries, or veins.

Arteries

Arteries carry blood away from the heart. Pulmonary arteries transport blood that has a low-oxygen content from the right ventricle to the lungs. Systemic arteries transport oxygenated blood from the left ventricle to the body tissues. Blood is pumped from the ventricles into large elastic arteries that branch repeatedly into smaller and smaller arteries until the branching results in microscopic arteries called "arterioles." The arterioles play a key role in regulating blood flow into the tissue capillaries. About 10 percent of the total blood volume is in the systemic arterial system at any given time.

The wall of an artery consists of three layers. The innermost layer, the tunica intima (also called the "tunica interna"), is a simple squamous epithelium surrounded by a connective tissue basement membrane with elastic fibers. The middle layer, the tunica media, is primarily smooth muscle and is usually the thickest layer. It not only provides support for the vessel but, also changes vessel diameter to regulate blood flow and blood pressure. The outermost layer, which attaches the vessel to the surrounding tissue, is the tunica externa or tunica adventitia. This layer is connective tissue with varying amounts of elastic and collagenous fibers. The connective tissue in this layer is quite dense where it is adjacent to the tunica media, but it changes to loose connective tissue near the periphery of the vessel.

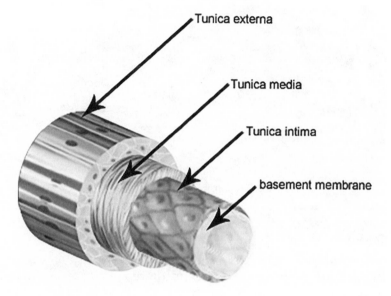

Figure 4.1. *Artery Wall*

Capillaries

Capillaries, the smallest and most numerous of the blood vessels, form the connection between the vessels that carry blood away from the heart (arteries) and the vessels that return blood to the heart (veins). The primary function of capillaries is the exchange of materials between the blood and tissue cells.

Veins

Veins carry blood toward the heart. After blood passes through the capillaries, it enters the smallest veins, called the "venules." From the venules, it flows into progressively larger and larger veins until it reaches the heart. In the pulmonary circuit, the pulmonary veins transport blood from the lungs to the left atrium of the heart. This blood has a high oxygen content because it has just been oxygenated in the lungs. Systemic veins transport blood from the body tissue to the right atrium of the heart. This blood has reduced oxygen content because the oxygen has been used for metabolic activities in the tissue cells.

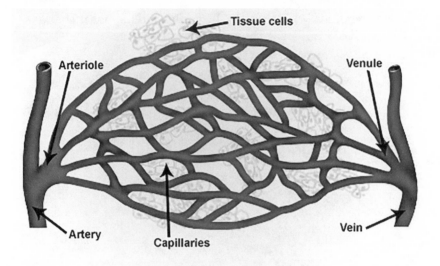

Figure 4.2. *Capillaries*

The walls of veins have the same three layers as the arteries. Although all the layers are present, there is less smooth muscle and connective tissue. This makes the walls of veins thinner than those of arteries, which is related to the fact that blood in the veins has less pressure than in the arteries. Because the walls of the veins are thinner and less rigid than arteries, veins can hold more blood. Almost 70 percent of the total blood volume is in the veins at any given time. Medium and large veins have venous valves, similar to the semilunar valves associated with the heart, that help keep the blood flowing toward the heart. Venous valves are especially important in the arms and legs, where they prevent the backflow of blood in response to the pull of gravity.

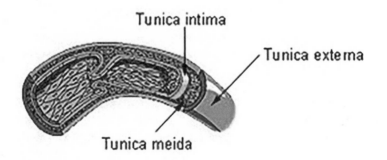

Figure 4.3. *Vein*

Section 4.2

Physiology of Circulation

This section includes text excerpted from "Physiology of Circulation,"
Surveillance, Epidemiology, and End Results Program (SEER),
National Cancer Institute (NCI), July 1, 2002. Reviewed June 2019.

Roles of Capillaries

In addition to forming the connection between the arteries and
veins, capillaries have a vital role in the exchange of gases, nutrients,
and metabolic waste products between the blood and tissue cells. Substances pass through the capillary wall by diffusion, filtration, and
osmosis. Oxygen and carbon dioxide move across the capillary wall
by diffusion. Fluid movement across a capillary wall is determined
by a combination of hydrostatic and osmotic pressure. The net result
of the capillary microcirculation created by hydrostatic and osmotic
pressure is that substances leave the blood at one end of the capillary
and return at the other end.

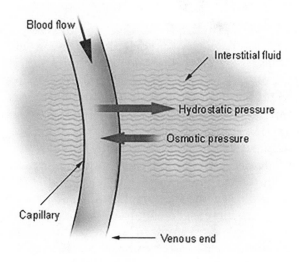

Figure 4.4. *Capillaries Microcirculation*

Blood Flow

Blood flow refers to the movement of blood through the vessels from
the arteries to the capillaries and then into the veins. The pressure is

a measure of the force that the blood exerts against the vessel walls as it moves the blood through the vessels. As with all fluids, blood flows from a high-pressure area to a region with lower pressure. Blood flows in the same direction as the decreasing pressure gradient: arteries to capillaries to veins.

The rate, or velocity, of blood flow varies inversely with the total cross-sectional area of the blood vessels. As the total cross-sectional area of the vessels increases, the velocity of flow decreases. Blood flow is slowest in the capillaries, which allows time for exchange of gases and nutrients.

Resistance is a force that opposes the flow of a fluid. In blood vessels, most of the resistance is due to vessel diameter. As vessel diameter decreases, the resistance increases and blood flow decreases.

Very little pressure remains by the time blood leaves the capillaries and enters the venules. Blood flow through the veins is not the direct result of ventricular contraction. Instead, venous return depends on skeletal muscle action, respiratory movements, and constriction of smooth muscle in venous walls.

Pulse and Blood Pressure

Pulse refers to the rhythmic expansion of an artery that is caused by ejection of blood from the ventricle. It can be felt where an artery is close to the surface and rests on something firm.

In common usage, the term "blood pressure" refers to arterial blood pressure, the pressure in the aorta and its branches. Systolic pressure is due to ventricular contraction. Diastolic pressure occurs during cardiac relaxation. Pulse pressure is the difference between systolic pressure and diastolic pressure. Blood pressure is measured with a sphygmomanometer and is recorded as the systolic pressure over the diastolic pressure. Four major factors interact to affect blood pressure: cardiac output, blood volume, peripheral resistance, and viscosity. When these factors increase, blood pressure also increases.

Arterial blood pressure is maintained within normal ranges by changes in cardiac output and peripheral resistance. Pressure receptors (baroreceptors), located in the walls of the large arteries in the thorax and neck, are important for short-term blood pressure regulation.

Section 4.3

Circulatory Pathways

This section includes text excerpted from "Circulatory Pathways," Surveillance, Epidemiology, and End Results Program (SEER), National Cancer Institute (NCI), July 1, 2002. Reviewed June 2019.

The blood vessels of the body are functionally divided into two distinctive circuits: pulmonary circuit and systemic circuit. The pump for the pulmonary circuit, which circulates blood through the lungs, is the right ventricle. The left ventricle is the pump for the systemic circuit, which provides the blood supply for the tissue cells of the body.

Pulmonary Circuit

Pulmonary circulation transports oxygen-poor blood from the right ventricle to the lungs, where the blood picks up a new blood supply. Then, it returns the oxygen-rich blood to the left atrium.

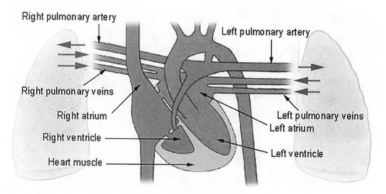

Figure 4.5. *Pulmonary Circuit*

Systemic Circuit

The systemic circulation provides the functional blood supply to all body tissue. It carries oxygen and nutrients to the cells and picks up carbon dioxide and waste products. Systemic circulation carries oxygenated blood from the left ventricle, through the arteries, to the capillaries in the tissues of the body. From the tissue capillaries, the deoxygenated blood returns through a system of veins to the right atrium of the heart.

The coronary arteries are the only vessels that branch from the ascending aorta. The brachiocephalic, left common carotid, and left subclavian arteries branch from the aortic arch. The blood supply for the brain is provided by the internal carotid and vertebral arteries. The subclavian arteries provide the blood supply for the upper extremity. The celiac, superior mesenteric, suprarenal, renal, gonadal, and inferior mesenteric arteries branch from the abdominal aorta to supply the abdominal viscera. Lumbar arteries provide blood for the muscles and spinal cord. Branches of the external iliac artery provide the blood supply for the lower extremity. The internal iliac artery supplies the pelvic viscera.

Major Systemic Arteries

All systemic arteries are branches, either directly or indirectly, from the aorta. The aorta ascends from the left ventricle, curves posteriorly and to the left, then descends through the thorax and abdomen. This geography divides the aorta into three portions: ascending aorta, aortic arch, and descending aorta. The descending aorta is further subdivided into the thoracic aorta and abdominal aorta.

Major Systemic Veins

After blood delivers oxygen to the tissues and picks up carbon dioxide, it returns to the heart through a system of veins. The capillaries, where the gaseous exchange occurs, merge into venules and these converge to form larger and larger veins until the blood reaches either the superior vena cava (SVC) or inferior vena cava (IVC), which drain into the right atrium.

Fetal Circulation

Most circulatory pathways in a fetus are similar to those in an adult, but there are some notable differences because the lungs, the gastrointestinal tract (GI), and the kidneys are not functioning before birth. The fetus obtains its oxygen and nutrients from the mother and also depends on maternal circulation to carry away the carbon dioxide and waste products.

The umbilical cord contains two umbilical arteries to carry fetal blood to the placenta and one umbilical vein to carry oxygen-and-nutrient-rich blood from the placenta to the fetus. The ductus venosus allows blood to bypass the immature liver in fetal circulation. The foramen ovale and ductus arteriosus are modifications that permit blood to bypass the lungs in fetal circulation.

Chapter 5

Maintaining a Healthy Circulatory System

Keeping Your Arteries Healthy

The well-being of your arteries depends on a healthy endothelium, the inner lining of your blood vessels.

"Endothelial cells are the prima donnas within the blood vessels. They control almost every activity that occurs in the vessels, and they're fundamentally altered with age," says Dr. Edward Lakatta, M.D., chief of the Laboratory of Cardiovascular Science at the National Institutes of Health (NIH). "People who maintain a healthy endothelium as they get older and those who make an effort to do things that promote the repair of injured endothelium can reduce the risk of heart attacks and strokes caused by atherosclerosis or hypertension."

Although scientists still have much to learn about the endothelium and what can be done to keep it healthy, a number of studies suggest that certain modifiable risk factors can have an important impact on the cardiovascular system. For instance, regular moderate exercise, such as running, walking, or swimming can reduce body fat, increase lean muscle mass, decrease blood pressure, increase high-density lipoprotein (HDL) cholesterol (the "good" cholesterol) levels, and lessen

This chapter includes text excerpted from "Blood Vessels and Aging: The Rest of the Journey," National Institute on Aging (NIA), National Institutes of Health (NIH), July 2014. Reviewed June 2019.

33

the extent of arterial stiffening. All of these exercise-induced changes can have a positive influence on endothelial cells.

In addition, scientists have long known that tobacco smoke contains numerous toxic compounds, such as carbon monoxide, that promote endothelial cell damage. Smoking also increases blood pressure and heart rate. Free radicals in smoke slash the amount of nitric oxide available in the bloodstream. Nitric oxide is a signaling molecule that helps keep arteries pliable. Because nicotine causes narrowing of blood vessels, less oxygen is transported to the heart. If you smoke, blood platelets become stickier and are more apt to form clots in your arteries.

High blood pressure—hypertension—causes blood vessels to thicken, diminishes the production of nitric oxide, promotes blood clotting, and contributes to the development of atherosclerotic plaques in the arteries. Blood pressure is considered high when systolic pressure exceeds 140 mmHg and when diastolic blood pressure is higher than 90mmHg.

Excessive weight increases the risk of high blood pressure and can increase the likelihood that you will have high blood triglycerides and low HDL cholesterol, Dr. Lakatta says. Being overweight can also increase the probability you will develop insulin resistance, a precursor of diabetes.

Diabetes, a disease in which the body does not produce or properly use insulin, becomes more common as we age. In fact, nearly half of all cases are diagnosed after the age of 55. Atherosclerosis develops earlier and is more aggressive in people who have diabetes. In part, this occurs because diabetes causes the endothelium to produce excessive amounts of superoxide anion, a free radical that destroys nitric oxide. People 65 years of age and older who have diabetes are nearly 4 times more likely than those who do not to develop the peripheral vascular disease, a condition that clogs the arteries that carry blood to the legs or arms. And, cardiovascular diseases and stroke are leading causes of diabetes-related deaths. If you suspect you have or are at risk for diabetes, check with your doctor. Symptoms include increased thirst, increased hunger, fatigue, increased urination—especially at night, unexplained weight loss, blurred vision, and slow healing of wounds and sores.

Researchers have also found that stress reduction techniques, such as taking a walk, practicing yoga, or deep breathing, are important to cardiovascular health. Emotional stress triggers the release of adrenaline from the adrenal gland and noradrenaline from the nerve endings in your heart and blood vessels. These hormones make the heart beat faster and adversely affect blood vessels. Under stress, an older person's blood pressure rises more rapidly and stays higher longer than a younger person's because the older person's blood vessels are stiffer and have lost much of their elasticity.

Exercise: Your Heart's Best Friend

Regular physical exercise is no joke. In fact, it may be the most important thing a person can do to fend off heart disease, stroke, and other age-associated diseases. Emerging scientific evidence suggests that people who exercise regularly not only live longer, they live better.

Scientists have long known that regular exercise causes certain changes in the hearts of younger people: resting heart rate is lower, heart mass is higher, and stroke volume is higher than in their sedentary counterparts. These differences make the heart a better pump. Evidence now suggests these changes occur even when exercise training begins later in life, at age 60 or 70, for instance. In other words, you do not lose the ability to become better physically conditioned. In addition, several studies have shown that exercise not only helps reduce debilitating symptoms, such as breathlessness and fatigue, in people who have heart failure, it also prolongs life.

Exercise training may be effective because it appears to improve the function of virtually every cell in the cardiovascular system. Animal studies, for instance, suggest that regular aerobic workouts help heart muscle cells remove calcium from their inner fluid at a faster rate after a contraction. This improved calcium cycling allows the heart to relax more and fill with more blood between beats.

Exercise also improves blood vessel elasticity and endothelial function, in part, by blocking the production of damaging free radicals and maintaining the production of nitric oxide, an important signaling molecule that helps protect the inner layer of the arteries. Together, these changes can slow the progression of atherosclerosis and other age-related cardiovascular conditions.

Endurance exercises, such as brisk walking, increase your stamina and improve the health of your heart, lungs, and circulatory system. But other exercises are equally important to maintaining health and self-reliance as you get older. Strength exercises, for instance, build muscles and reduce your risk of osteoporosis. Balance exercises help prevent a major cause of disability in older adults: falls. Flexibility or stretching exercises help keep your body limber. As part of a daily routine, these exercises and other physical activities you enjoy can make a difference in your life as you get older.

Metabolic Syndrome Accelerates Aging of Arteries

Many older Americans have high blood pressure or high blood sugar or just a bit too much fat on the belly. While each of these conditions alone is bad enough, having all of these conditions at once—a cluster called "metabolic syndrome"—magnifies the risk of developing heart disease and stroke. And the National Institute on Aging (NIA) scientists may have discovered a reason why: metabolic syndrome appears to accelerate stiffening and thickening of the arteries.

Metabolic syndrome—also known as "syndrome X" or "insulin resistance syndrome"—may affect as many as 47 million Americans, according to the Centers for Disease Control and Prevention (CDC). After age 50, a person has a better than one in three chance of developing this group of medical conditions characterized by insulin resistance and the presence of obesity, abdominal fat, high blood sugar and triglycerides, low HDL (good) blood cholesterol, and high blood pressure.

To determine the effects of metabolic syndrome on aging arteries, NIA researchers studied 471 participants—with an average age of 59—in the Baltimore Longitudinal Study of Aging (BLSA). None of these participants had any detectable signs of cardiovascular disease when initially examined. But those who had 3 or more conditions associated with metabolic syndrome developed stiffer and thicker arteries at earlier ages than those who didn't have the syndrome.

"It's as if the metabolic syndrome makes your blood vessels older," says Angelo Scuteri, M.D., Ph.D., an investigator at the NIA's Laboratory of Cardiovascular Science. "If you have metabolic syndrome when you are 40 your arteries look like they are 55 or 60."

As this work moves forward, scientists hope they can determine how metabolic syndrome promotes accelerated aging in the arteries and perhaps discover ways to prevent or treat it.

Healthy Foods, Healthy Arteries: Is There a Connection?

What you eat can help keep your heart and arteries healthy—or lead to excessive weight, high blood pressure, and high blood cholesterol—three key factors that increase the risk of developing cardiovascular disease, according to the National Heart, Lung, and Blood Institute (NHLBI). Based on the best available scientific evidence, the American Heart Association (AHA) recommends a diet that includes a variety of fruits, vegetables, and grains, while limiting consumption of saturated fat and sodium.

Fruits and vegetables have lots of antioxidants, such as vitamin C and vitamin A, that neutralize free radicals and may prevent oxidation in the arteries, dietary experts say. Fruits and vegetables also contain plenty of soluble fiber, a substance that has been shown to reduce blood cholesterol levels, which is healthy for the endothelium.

Bread, cereals, and other grain foods, which provide complex carbohydrates, vitamins, minerals, and fiber, are associated with a decreased risk of cardiovascular disease, according to the AHA Dietary Guidelines. However, some studies suggest eating less sugar, bread, and other simple and complex carbohydrates can lower blood insulin levels and decrease body fat and weight—three factors that are linked to an increased risk of heart disease and stroke. In recent years, a number of dietary recommendations based on these findings have become popular and are currently catching the public's awareness. While contentious, these are important issues and long-term studies are required to determine the risks and benefits of such diets, Dr. Lakatta says.

Saturated fats are usually solid at room temperature. These fats are primarily found in animal foods, such as meat; poultry; and dairy products, such as butter. Saturated fats tend to raise levels of "bad" low-density lipoprotein (LDL) and increase the risk of atherosclerosis. In fact, within 2 hours of eating a high saturated fat meal, endothelial cells do not work as well. Such meals can cause a temporary 50 percent dip in endothelial function, even in healthy young people who have no risk factors for atherosclerosis, Dr. Lakatta says.

In addition to saturated fats, some scientists are concerned about trans-fatty acids—unsaturated fats that have been artificially solidified by food manufacturers in a process called "hydrogenation" to make products such as margarine and vegetable shortenings. These scientists suspect that trans-fatty acids, which are often described as hydrogenated or partially hydrogenated fats on many food labels, are more damaging to the heart and arteries than saturated fats.

But researchers have found other types of fats may be beneficial. Monounsaturated fats, found mainly in plant foods such as peanuts and olives, help lower LDL cholesterol. Like polyunsaturated fats, monounsaturated fats are usually liquid at room temperature. Polyunsaturated fats, found in fish, nuts, and dark leafy vegetables, have been getting a lot of attention from scientists in the past few years. They have concluded that one type of polyunsaturated fat—omega-3 fatty acid—found in fish may promote several things that improve endothelial function, including increasing nitric oxide production, slashing the production of free radicals and other substances that cause inflammation, and boosting HDL cholesterol levels. Fish such as salmon, herring, and mackerel are good sources of omega-3.

Control over the condition of our arteries may also lie in how much salt we consume. In cultures where little sodium (in the form of salt) is consumed, blood pressures do not rise with age. Cultural differences have also been found in arterial stiffness. One study compared rural and urban populations in China. The urban population consumed much higher levels of sodium than rural groups. And they had stiffer arteries. Other researchers found that sodium appears to accelerate age-associated stiffening of arteries. In particular, sodium promotes thickening of aging arterial walls, reduces the amount of nitric oxide available to endothelial cells, and promotes the formation of oxygen free radicals. But shifting to a low sodium diet, research suggests, can begin to diminish arterial stiffness in as little as 2 weeks.

Most of the sodium in your diet comes from processed foods. The remaining is added at the table and while cooking. Scientists who study this issue suggest limiting the amount of sodium that you consume from all these sources to no more than 1,500 milligrams (mg) each day (an average American adult consumes about 3,300 milligrams daily). They recommend reading food labels carefully and buying foods that say "reduced sodium," "low in sodium," "sodium free," or "no salt added." Some dietitians suggest seasoning foods with herbs and spices, such as oregano, onion powder, or garlic instead of sodium.

Scientists suspect the more lifestyle changes, including diet and exercise, you can incorporate into your life, the better off your arteries will be, because these interventions work independently as well as in unison to promote the vitality of endothelial cells and contribute to reducing the risk of cardiovascular disease.

Chapter 6

How Aging Affects the Heart

How Does the Heart Work?

Your heart is a strong muscle that pumps blood to your body. A normal, healthy adult heart is about the size of your clenched fist. Just like an engine makes a car go, the heart keeps your body running. The heart has two sides, each with a top chamber (atrium) and a bottom chamber (ventricle). The right side pumps blood to the lungs to pick up oxygen. The left side receives blood rich with oxygen from the lungs and pumps it through arteries throughout the body. An electrical system in the heart controls the heart rate (heartbeat or pulse) and coordinates the contraction of the heart's top and bottom chambers.

How Your Heart Changes with Age

People 65 years of age and older are much more likely than younger people to suffer a heart attack, have a stroke, or develop coronary heart disease (commonly called "heart disease") and heart failure. Heart disease is also a major cause of disability, limiting the activity and eroding the quality of life of millions of older people.

Aging can cause changes in the heart and blood vessels. For example, as you get older, your heart cannot beat as fast during physical activity or times of stress as it did when you were younger. However,

---

This chapter includes text excerpted from "Heart Health and Aging," National Institute on Aging (NIA), National Institutes of Health (NIH), June 1, 2018.

the number of heartbeats per minute (heart rate) at rest does not change significantly with normal aging.

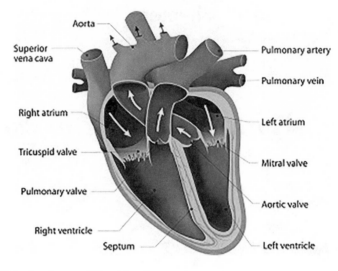

Figure 6.1. *Anatomy of the Heart*

Changes that happen with age may increase a person's risk of heart disease. A major cause of heart disease is the buildup of fatty deposits in the walls of arteries over many years. The good news is there are things you can do to delay, lower, or possibly avoid or reverse your risk.

The most common aging change is increased stiffness of the large arteries, called "arteriosclerosis," or hardening of the arteries. This causes high blood pressure, or hypertension, which becomes more common as we age.

High blood pressure and other risk factors, including advancing age, increase the risk of developing atherosclerosis. Because there are several modifiable risk factors for atherosclerosis, it is not necessarily a normal part of aging. Plaque builds up inside the walls of your arteries and, over time, hardens and narrows your arteries, which limits the flow of oxygen-rich blood to your organs and other parts of your body. Oxygen and blood nutrients are supplied to the heart muscle through the coronary arteries. Heart disease develops when plaque builds up in the coronary arteries, reducing blood flow to your heart muscle. Over time, the heart muscle can become weakened and/or damaged, resulting in heart failure. Heart damage can be caused by heart attacks, long-standing hypertension and diabetes, and chronic heavy alcohol use.

Age can cause other changes to the heart. For example:

- There are age-related changes in the electrical system that can lead to arrhythmias—a rapid, slowed, or irregular heartbeat—and/or the need for a pacemaker. Valves—the one-way, door-like parts that open and close to control blood flow between the chambers of your heart—may become thicker and stiffer. Stiffer valves can limit the flow of blood out of the heart and become leaky, both of which can cause fluid to build up in the lungs or in the body (legs, feet, and abdomen).

- The chambers of your heart may increase in size. The heart wall thickens, so the amount of blood that a chamber can hold may decrease despite the increased overall heart size. The heart may fill more slowly. Long-standing hypertension is the main cause of increased thickness of the heart wall, which can increase the risk of atrial fibrillation, a common heart rhythm problem in older people.

- With increasing age, people become more sensitive to salt, which may cause an increase in blood pressure and/or ankle or foot swelling (edema).

Other factors, such as thyroid disease or chemotherapy, may also weaken the heart muscle. Things you cannot control, such as your family history, might increase your risk of heart disease. But, leading a heart-healthy lifestyle might help you avoid or delay serious illness.

What Is Heart Disease?

Heart disease is caused by atherosclerosis, which is the buildup of fatty deposits, or plaques, in the walls of the coronary arteries over many years. The coronary arteries surround the outside of the heart and supply blood nutrients and oxygen to the heart muscle. When plaque builds up inside the arteries, there is less space for blood to flow normally and deliver oxygen to the heart. If the flow of blood to your heart is reduced by plaque buildup or is blocked if a plaque suddenly ruptures, it can cause angina (chest pain or discomfort) or a heart attack. When the heart muscle does not get enough oxygen and blood nutrients, the heart muscle cells will die (heart attack) and weaken the heart, diminishing its ability to pump blood to the rest of the body.

Signs of Heart Disease

Early heart disease often does not have symptoms, or the symptoms may be barely noticeable. That is why regular checkups with your doctor are important.

Contact your doctor right away if you feel any chest pain, pressure, or discomfort. However, chest pain is a less common sign of heart disease as it progresses, so be aware of other symptoms. Tell your doctor if you have:

- Pain, numbness, and/or tingling in the shoulders, arms, neck, jaw, or back
- Shortness of breath when active, at rest, or while lying flat
- Chest pain during physical activity that gets better when you rest
- Light-headedness
- Dizziness
- Confusion
- Headaches
- Cold sweats
- Nausea/vomiting
- Tiredness or fatigue
- Swelling in the ankles, feet, legs, stomach, and/or neck
- Reduced ability to exercise or be physically active
- Problems doing your normal activities

Problems with arrhythmia are much more common in older adults than younger people. Arrhythmia needs to be treated. See a doctor if you feel a fluttering in your chest or have the feeling that your heart is skipping a beat or beating too hard, especially if you are weaker than usual, dizzy, tired, or get short of breath when active.

If you have any signs of heart disease, your doctor may send you to a cardiologist, a doctor who specializes in the heart.

What Can I Do to Prevent Heart Disease?

There are many steps you can take to keep your heart healthy.

Try to be more physically active. Talk with your doctor about the type of activities that would be best for you. If possible, aim to get at least 150 minutes of physical activity each week. Every day is best. It does not have to be done all at once.

Start by doing activities you enjoy—brisk walking, dancing, bowling, bicycling, or gardening, for example. Avoid spending hours every day sitting.

If you smoke, quit. Smoking is the leading cause of preventable death. Smoking adds to the damage to the artery walls. It is never too late to get some benefit from quitting smoking. Quitting, even in later life, can lower your risk of heart disease, stroke, and cancer over time.

Follow a heart-healthy diet. Choose foods that are low in trans and saturated fats, added sugars, and salt. As we get older, we become more sensitive to salt, which can cause swelling in the legs and feet. Eat plenty of fruits, vegetables, and foods high in fiber, such as those made from whole grains.

Keep a healthy weight. Balancing the calories you eat and drink with the calories burned by being physically active helps to maintain a healthy weight. Some ways you can maintain a healthy weight include limiting portion size and being physically active.

Keep your diabetes, high blood pressure, and/or high cholesterol under control. Follow your doctor's advice to manage these conditions, and take medications as directed.

Do not drink a lot of alcohol. Men should not have more than two drinks a day and women only one. One drink is equal to:

- One 12-ounce can or bottle of regular beer, ale, or wine cooler
- One 8- or 9-ounce can or bottle of malt liquor
- One 5-ounce glass of red or white wine
- One 1.5-ounce shot glass of distilled spirits, such as gin, rum, tequila, vodka, or whiskey

Manage stress. Learn how to manage stress, relax, and cope with problems to improve physical and emotional health. Consider activities such as a stress management program, meditation, physical activity, and talking things out with friends or family.

The Future of Research on Aging and the Heart

Adults 65 years of age and older are more likely than younger people to suffer from cardiovascular disease (CVD), which is problems with the heart, blood vessels, or both. Aging can cause changes in the heart and blood vessels that may increase a person's risk of developing cardiovascular disease.

To understand how aging is linked to cardiovascular disease so that we can ultimately develop cures for this group of diseases, we need to first understand what is happening in the healthy but aging heart and blood vessels. This understanding has advanced dramatically in the past 30 years.

At present, more than ever, scientists understand what causes your blood vessels and heart to age, and how your aging cardiovascular system leads to cardiovascular disease. In addition, they have pinpointed risk factors that increase the odds a person will develop cardiovascular disease. They are learning much more about how physical activity, diet, and other lifestyle factors influence the "rate of aging" in the healthy heart and arteries. The aging of other organ systems, including the muscles, kidneys, and lungs, also likely contributes to heart disease. Research is ongoing to unravel how these aging systems influence each other, which may reveal new targets for treatments.

In the future, interventions or treatments that slow accelerated aging of the heart and arteries in young and middle-aged people who seem to be healthy could prevent or delay the onset of heart disease, stroke, and other cardiovascular disorders in later life. Some interventions that we already know slow the rate of aging in the heart and arteries include healthy eating, exercise, reducing stress, and quitting smoking. The more we understand the changes that take place in cells and molecules during aging, for example, the closer we get to the possibility of designing drugs that target those changes. Gene therapies can also target specific cellular changes and could potentially be a way to intervene in the aging process. While waiting for these new therapies to be developed, you can still enjoy activities, such as exercise and a healthy diet, that can benefit your heart.

Part Two

Blood Disorders

Chapter 7

Anemia

Chapter Contents

Section 7.1

What Is Anemia?

This section includes text excerpted from "Anemia,"
National Heart, Lung, and Blood Institute (NHLBI),
January 18, 2019.

Anemia is a condition in which your blood has a lower-than-normal amount of red blood cells or hemoglobin.

Hemoglobin is an iron-rich protein that helps red blood cells carry oxygen from the lungs to the rest of the body. If you have anemia, your body does not get enough oxygen-rich blood. This can cause you to feel tired or weak. You may also have shortness of breath, dizziness, headaches, or an irregular heartbeat.

There are many types and causes of anemia. Mild anemia is a common and treatable condition that can occur in anyone. Some people—including women during their menstrual periods and pregnancy, and people who donate blood frequently; do not get enough iron or certain vitamins; or take certain medicines or treatments, such as chemotherapy for cancer—are at a higher risk for anemia.

Anemia may also be a sign of a more serious condition. It may result from chronic bleeding in the stomach. Chronic inflammation from an infection, kidney disease, cancer, or autoimmune diseases can also cause the body to make fewer red blood cells.

Your doctor will consider your medical history and physical exam and test results when diagnosing and treating anemia. She or he will use a simple blood test to confirm that you have low amounts of red blood cells or hemoglobin. For some types of mild to moderate anemia, your doctor may recommend over-the-counter (OTC) or prescription iron supplements, certain vitamins, intravenous iron therapy, or medicines that make your body produce more red blood cells. To prevent anemia in the future, your doctor may also suggest healthy eating changes. If you have severe anemia, your doctor may recommend red blood cell transfusions.

Section 7.2

Anemia of Chronic Disease

This section includes text excerpted from "Anemia of Inflammation or Chronic Disease," National Institute of Diabetes and Digestive and Kidney Diseases (NIDDK), March 2019.

What Is Anemia of Inflammation?

Anemia of inflammation, also called "anemia of chronic disease" or "ACD," is a type of anemia that affects people who have conditions that cause inflammation, such as infections; autoimmune diseases; cancer; and chronic kidney disease (CKD).

Anemia is a condition in which your blood has fewer red blood cells (RBCs) than normal. Your red blood cells may also have less hemoglobin than normal. Hemoglobin is the iron-rich protein that allows red blood cells to carry oxygen from your lungs to the rest of your body. Your body needs oxygen to work properly. With fewer red blood cells or less hemoglobin, your body may not get enough oxygen.

In anemia of inflammation, you may have a normal or sometimes increased amount of iron stored in your body tissues, but you have a low level of iron in your blood. Inflammation may prevent your body from using stored iron to make enough healthy red blood cells, leading to anemia.

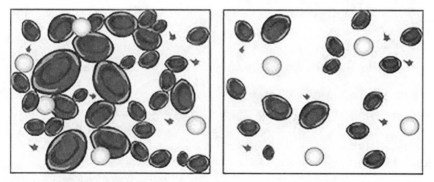

Normal blood   **Anemia**

Figure 7.1. *Normal Blood and Anemic Blood*

Anemia is a condition in which your blood has fewer red blood cells or less hemoglobin than normal.

Why Is Anemia of Inflammation Also Called "Anemia of Chronic Disease?"

Anemia of inflammation is also called "anemia of chronic disease" because this type of anemia commonly occurs in people who have chronic conditions that may be associated with inflammation.

Are There Other Types of Anemia?

There are many types of anemia. Common types include:

- **Iron-deficiency anemia,** a condition in which the body's stored iron is used up, causing the body to make fewer healthy red blood cells. In people with iron-deficiency anemia, iron levels are low in both body tissues and the blood. This is the most common type of anemia.

- **Pernicious anemia,** which is caused by a lack of vitamin B_{12}

- **Aplastic anemia**, a condition in which the bone marrow does not make enough new red blood cells, white blood cells (WBCs), and platelets because the bone marrow's stem cells are damaged

- **Hemolytic anemia,** a condition in which red blood cells are destroyed earlier than normal

How Common Is Anemia of Inflammation?

Anemia of inflammation is the second-most common type of anemia, after iron-deficiency anemia.

Who Is More Likely to Have Anemia of Inflammation?

While anemia of inflammation can affect people of any age, older adults are more likely to have this type of anemia because they are more likely to have chronic diseases that cause inflammation. In the United States, about 1 million people older than the age of 65 have anemia of inflammation.

Does Anemia of Inflammation Lead to Other Health Problems?

Anemia of inflammation is typically mild or moderate, meaning that hemoglobin levels in your blood are lower than normal but not severely low. If your anemia becomes severe, the lack of oxygen in your blood can cause symptoms, such as feeling tired or short of breath. Severe anemia can become life-threatening.

In people who have CKD, severe anemia can increase the chance of developing heart problems.

What Are the Symptoms of Anemia of Inflammation?

Anemia of inflammation typically develops slowly and may cause few or no symptoms. In fact, you may only experience symptoms of the disease that is causing anemia and not notice additional symptoms.

Symptoms of anemia of inflammation are the same as in any type of anemia and include:

- A fast heartbeat

- Body aches

- Fainting or feeling dizzy or light-headed

- Feeling tired or weak

- Getting tired easily during or after physical activity

- Pale skin

- Shortness of breath

What Causes Anemia of Inflammation

Experts think that when you have an infection or disease that causes inflammation, your immune system causes changes in how your body works that may lead to anemia of inflammation.

- Your body may not store and use iron normally.

- Your kidneys may produce less erythropoietin (EPO), a hormone that signals your bone marrow—the spongy tissue inside most of your bones—to make red blood cells.

- Your bone marrow may not respond normally to EPO, making fewer red blood cells than needed.

- Your red blood cells may live for a shorter time than normal, causing them to die faster than they can be replaced.

51

Chronic Conditions That Cause Anemia of Inflammation

Many different chronic conditions can cause inflammation that leads to anemia, including:

- Autoimmune diseases, such as rheumatoid arthritis (RA) or lupus
- Cancer
- Chronic infections, such as human immunodeficiency virus/ acquired immunodeficiency syndrome (HIV/AIDS) and tuberculosis (TB)
- Chronic kidney disease
- Inflammatory bowel diseases (IBDs), such as Crohn disease or ulcerative colitis (UC)
- Other chronic diseases that involve inflammation, such as diabetes and heart failure

In people with certain chronic conditions, anemia may have more than one cause. For example:

- Causes of anemia in CKD may include inflammation, low levels of EPO due to kidney damage, or low levels of the nutrients needed to make red blood cells. Hemodialysis to treat CKD may also lead to iron-deficiency anemia.
- People with IBD may have both iron-deficiency anemias, due to blood loss, and anemia of inflammation.
- In people who have cancer, anemia may be caused by inflammation, blood loss, and cancers that affect or spread to the bone marrow. Cancer treatments, such as chemotherapy and radiation therapy (RT), may also cause or worsen anemia.

Other Causes of Inflammation That May Lead to Anemia

While anemia of inflammation typically develops slowly, anemia of critical illness is a type of anemia of inflammation that develops quickly in patients who are hospitalized for severe acute infections, trauma, or other conditions that cause inflammation.

In some cases, older adults develop anemia of inflammation that is not related to an underlying infection or chronic disease. Experts think that the aging process may cause inflammation and anemia.

How Do Healthcare Professionals Diagnose Anemia of Inflammation?

Healthcare professionals use a medical history and blood tests to diagnose anemia of inflammation.

Medical History

A healthcare professional will ask about your history of infections or chronic diseases that may lead to anemia of inflammation.

Blood Tests

Healthcare professionals use blood tests to check for signs of anemia of inflammation, other types of anemia, or other health problems. A healthcare professional will take a blood sample from you and send the sample to a lab to test.

Blood count tests can check many parts and features of your blood, including:

- The number of red blood cells

- The average size of red blood cells

- The amount of hemoglobin in your blood and in your red blood cells

- The number of developing red blood cells, called "reticulocytes," in your blood

Some of these blood count tests and others may be combined in a test called a "complete blood count." A blood smear may be used to examine the size, shape, and number of red blood cells in your blood.

A healthcare professional may also use blood tests to check the amount of iron in your blood and stored in your body. These tests may measure:

- Iron in your blood

- Transferrin, a protein in your blood that carries iron

- Ferritin, the protein that stores iron in your body's cells

A healthcare professional may diagnose anemia of inflammation if blood test results suggest that you have anemia, a low level of iron in your blood, and a normal level of iron stored in your body tissues.

If blood test results suggest you have anemia of inflammation but the cause is unknown, a healthcare professional may perform additional tests to look for the cause.

How Do Healthcare Professionals Treat Anemia of Inflammation?

Healthcare professionals treat anemia of inflammation by treating the underlying condition and by treating the anemia with medicines and occasionally with blood transfusions.

Treating the Underlying Condition

Healthcare professionals typically treat anemia of inflammation by treating the underlying condition that is causing the inflammation. If treatments are available that can reduce the inflammation, the treatments may cause the anemia to improve or go away. For example, taking medicines to treat inflammation in rheumatoid arthritis can improve anemia.

Medicines

A healthcare professional may prescribe the erythropoiesis-stimulating agents (ESAs) epoetin alpha or darbepoetin alpha to treat anemia related to CKD, chemotherapy treatments for cancer, or certain treatments for HIV. ESAs cause the bone marrow to make more red blood cells. Healthcare professionals typically give ESAs as shots and may teach you how to give yourself these shots at home. A healthcare professional may prescribe iron supplements, given as pills or shots, to help ESAs work.

If you are on hemodialysis, you may be able to receive intravenous (IV) ESAs and iron supplements during hemodialysis.

Blood Transfusions

In some cases, healthcare professionals may use blood transfusions to treat severe anemia of inflammation. A blood transfusion can quickly increase the amount of hemoglobin in your blood and boost oxygen.

Can I Prevent Anemia of Inflammation?

Experts have not yet found a way to prevent anemia of inflammation. For some chronic conditions that cause inflammation, treatments may be available to reduce or prevent the inflammation that can lead to anemia. Talk with your doctor about treatments and follow the treatment plan your doctor recommends.

How Does Eating, Diet, and Nutrition Affect Anemia of Inflammation?

If you have a chronic condition that is causing anemia of inflammation, follow the advice of your doctor or dietitian about healthy eating and nutrition.

Section 7.3

Aplastic Anemia

This section includes text excerpted from "Aplastic Anemia," Genetic and Rare Diseases Information Center (GARD), National Center for Advancing Translational Sciences (NCATS), July 5, 2017.

What Is Aplastic Anemia?

Aplastic anemia is a blood disorder caused by the failure of the bone marrow to make enough new blood cells. Bone marrow is a sponge-like tissue inside the bones that makes stem cells that develop into red blood cells (RBCs), white blood cells (WBCs), and platelets. Symptoms may include fatigue, weakness, dizziness, shortness of breath, frequent infections, and bleeding. Aplastic anemia can lead to other health concerns, such as an irregular heartbeat, an enlarged heart, and heart failure. It can be caused by injury to blood stem cells due to exposure to certain drugs; chemotherapy; congenital disorders; drug therapy to suppress the immune system; pregnancy; radiation therapy (RT); or toxins, such as benzene or arsenic. When the cause is unknown, it is referred to as "idiopathic aplastic anemia." In about half of all cases, no cause can be found. A blood disorder can be acute or chronic. Treatment may consist of supportive care only, blood transfusions, medicines to suppress the immune system, or hematopoietic cell transplantation (HCT).

Symptoms of Aplastic Anemia

The symptoms of aplastic anemia vary depending on how severe it is and how low blood counts are. Signs and symptoms may include:

- **Low numbers of red blood cells (anemia):** may cause paleness (pallor), headache, palpitations, rapid heart rate, feeling out of breath, fatigue, or foot swelling

- **Low numbers of platelets (thrombocytopenia):** may result in gum bleeding, nosebleeds or bleeding in the internal organs and skin bruises

- **Low white blood cells (neutropenia):** may present infections, recurrent infections, mouth sores

Diagnosis of Aplastic Anemia

Making a diagnosis for a genetic or rare disease can often be challenging. Healthcare professionals typically look at a person's medical history, symptoms, physical exam, and laboratory test results in order to make a diagnosis. If you have questions about getting a diagnosis, you should contact a healthcare professional.

Treatment of Aplastic Anemia

Treatment for aplastic anemia varies depending on the severity. While some individuals with mild to moderate aplastic anemia may not require treatment, for others, treatment may include:

- Blood transfusions to keep blood cell counts at acceptable levels

- Blood and marrow stem cell transplants to replace damaged stem cells with healthy ones from a donor (another person)

- Medications to stimulate the bone marrow, suppress the immune system, and prevent and treat infections

Blood and marrow stem cell transplants may cure aplastic anemia in some instances. This treatment option works best in children and young adults with severe aplastic anemia who are otherwise in good health.

For patients with severe aplastic anemia who are under the age of 20 and for those between 20 and 50 years of age who are otherwise in good health, the first option is the transplant when a sibling donor is available. For those who do not have an available sibling donor, the medication eltrombopag or eltrombopag plus immunosuppressive therapy can be used.

For patients over 50 years of age, the decision is based on the patient's overall health and preferences, and treatment may include eltrombopag or eltrombopag plus immunosuppressive therapy (horse antithymocyte globulin (ATG), cyclosporin A (CSA), and glucocorticoids). People older than 50 years of age have more risks of having rejection with the transplant and have greater risks of treatment toxicity and early mortality.

Prognosis of Aplastic Anemia

A small number of people with aplastic anemia may spontaneously recover with supportive care; however, for most individuals, the condition worsens without identification and treatment of the underlying cause and/or treatment of the disease. Bone marrow transplant may cure the disease in children and young patients and has a 10-year survival rate of approximately 73 percent. For many, bone marrow transplant is not an option due to the risks and potential long-term side effects.

Section 7.4

Fanconi Anemia

This section includes text excerpted from "Fanconi Anemia," National Heart, Lung, and Blood Institute (NHLBI), January 18, 2019.

What Is Fanconi Anemia?

Fanconi anemia (FA) is a rare but serious blood disorder that prevents your bone marrow from making enough new blood cells for your body to work normally. It can also cause your bone marrow, the sponge-like tissue inside your bones, to make abnormal blood cells.

Fanconi anemia is an inherited disease caused by mutations in certain genes, known as "FA genes." These genes provide instructions to help the body repair certain types of deoxyribonucleic acid (DNA) damage. The cells of healthy people often repair DNA damage, but cells affected by Fanconi anemia cannot make these repairs. In people who have Fanconi anemia, certain cells may die or stop working properly.

Symptoms of Fanconi Anemia

You may be screened for Fanconi anemia based on your signs and symptoms, or if you have a close relative who has Fanconi anemia. Most often, signs and symptoms of Fanconi anemia appear at birth or early in childhood, between 5 and 10 years of age. Children may have delayed growth and development, including delayed puberty or anemia symptoms, such as fatigue, shortness of breath, and bruising easily.

Risk Factors of Fanconi Anemia

Fanconi anemia can lead to serious complications, such as bone marrow failure, which happens when the bone marrow stops making as many blood cells. This can lead to low blood cell counts or severe aplastic anemia. Cancers, such as acute myeloid leukemia (AML) and myelodysplastic syndromes (MDS), are other possible complications of Fanconi anemia.

Diagnosis of Fanconi Anemia

To diagnose Fanconi anemia, you or your child's doctor may look for dark spots on the skin called "café au lait spots." The most common test for Fanconi anemia is a blood test called a "chromosomal breakage test."

Treatment of Fanconi Anemia

Treatment for Fanconi anemia depends on your age and how well your bone marrow is making new blood cells. Treatment may include a blood and bone marrow transplant, blood transfusions, or medicine to help your body make more red blood cells (RBCs). Researchers are also studying new and promising treatments for Fanconi anemia, including genetic therapies. If diagnosed with Fanconi anemia, you or your child will benefit from lifelong monitoring, which may include regular blood and bone marrow tests and making healthy lifestyle changes to manage complications.

Section 7.5

Glucose-6-Phosphate Dehydrogenase Deficiency

This section includes text excerpted from "Glucose-6-Phosphate Dehydrogenase Deficiency," Genetic and Rare Diseases Information Center (GARD), National Center for Advancing Translational Sciences (NCATS), May 8, 2017.

What Is Glucose-6-Phosphate Dehydrogenase Deficiency?

Glucose-6-phosphate dehydrogenase (G6PD) deficiency is a hereditary condition in which red blood cells (RBCs) break down (hemolysis) when the body is exposed to certain foods, drugs, infections, or stress. It occurs when a person is missing or has low levels of the enzyme glucose-6-phosphate dehydrogenase. This enzyme helps red blood cells work properly. Symptoms during a hemolytic episode may include dark urine, fatigue, paleness, rapid heart rate, shortness of breath, and yellowing of the skin (jaundice). G6PD deficiency is inherited in an X-linked recessive manner, and symptoms are more common in males (particularly African Americans and those from certain parts of Africa, Asia, and the Mediterranean). It is caused by mutations in the *G6PD* gene. Treatment may involve medicines to treat infection, stopping drugs that are causing red blood cell (RBC) destruction, and/or transfusions, in some cases.

Symptoms of Glucose-6-Phosphate Dehydrogenase Deficiency

People with glucose-6-phosphate dehydrogenase deficiency generally do not have symptoms unless their red blood cells are exposed to certain chemicals in food or medicine, certain bacterial or viral infections, or to stress. Many people with this condition never experience symptoms. The most common medical problem associated with G6PD deficiency is hemolytic anemia, which occurs when red blood cells are destroyed faster than the body can replace them. This type of anemia leads to paleness, jaundice, dark urine, fatigue, shortness of breath, an enlarged spleen, and a rapid heart rate. Some patients have a history of chronic hemolytic anemia. Skin ulcers are uncommon but may occur in people with severe G6PD deficiency.

Because glucose-6-phosphate dehydrogenase deficiency is inherited in an X-linked recessive manner, it is more common for males to have symptoms. This is because males have only one copy of the *G6PD* gene. If this one copy has a mutation, they will definitely have G6PD deficiency. However, while females have two copies of the *G6PD* gene, some females are as severely affected as males. This can be the case in females who have a mutation in both copies of the *G6PD* gene or even in females who have only one mutation. Females with one mutation may have lower G6PD activity than would normally be expected due to a phenomenon called "skewed lyonization."

Causes of Glucose-6-Phosphate Dehydrogenase Deficiency

Glucose-6-phosphate dehydrogenase deficiency is caused by mutations in the *G6PD* gene. This gene gives the body instructions to make an enzyme called "G6PD," which is involved in processing carbohydrates. This enzyme also protects red blood cells from potentially harmful molecules called "reactive oxygen species." Chemical reactions involving G6PD produce compounds that prevent reactive oxygen species from building up to toxic levels within red blood cells.

Mutations in the *G6PD* gene lower the amount of G6PD or alter its structure, lessening its ability to play its protective role. As a result, reactive oxygen species can accumulate and damage red blood cells. Factors such as infections, certain drugs, or eating fava beans can increase the levels of reactive oxygen species, causing red blood cells to be destroyed faster than the body can replace them. This reduction of red blood cells causes the signs and symptoms of hemolytic anemia in people with G6PD deficiency.

Inheritance of Glucose-6-Phosphate Dehydrogenase Deficiency

Glucose-6-phosphate dehydrogenase deficiency is inherited in an X-linked recessive manner. X-linked recessive conditions are much more common in males, who have only one X chromosome (and one Y chromosome). Females have two X chromosomes, so if they have a mutation on one of them, they still have one X chromosome without the mutation. Females with one X chromosome mutation are known as "carriers" and are usually unaffected. However, females can be affected if they have a mutation in both copies of the *G6PD* gene, or in some cases if they have only one mutation.

If a mother is a carrier of an X-linked recessive condition and the father is not, the risk to each child depends on whether the child is male or female.

Each son has a 50 percent chance to be unaffected, and a 50 percent chance to be affected

Each daughter has a 50 percent chance to be unaffected, and a 50 percent chance to be a carrier.

If a father has the condition and the mother is not a carrier, all sons will be unaffected, and all daughters will be carriers.

There is nothing either parent can do, before or during pregnancy, to cause a child to have this condition.

Diagnosis of Glucose-6-Phosphate Dehydrogenase Deficiency

Making a diagnosis for a genetic or rare disease can often be challenging. Healthcare professionals typically look at a person's medical history, symptoms, physical exam, and laboratory test results in order to make a diagnosis. The following resources provide information relating to diagnosis and testing for this condition. If you have questions about getting a diagnosis, you should contact a healthcare professional.

Newborn Screening

- Baby's First Test is the nation's newborn screening education center for families and providers. Their website provides information and resources about screening at the local, state, and national levels and serves as the clearinghouse for newborn screening information.

- The Newborn Screening Coding and Terminology Guide has information on the standard codes used for newborn screening tests. Using these standards helps compare data across different laboratories. This resource was created by the U.S. National Library of Medicine (NLM).

- The National Newborn Screening and Global Resource Center (NNSGRC) provides information and resources in the area of newborn screening and genetics to benefit health professionals, the public health community, consumers, and government officials.

Treatment of Glucose-6-Phosphate Dehydrogenase Deficiency

The most important aspect of management for G6PD deficiency is to avoid agents that might trigger an attack. In cases of acute hemolytic anemia, a blood transfusion or even an exchange transfusion may be required.

The G6PD Deficiency Association, which is an advocacy group that provides information and supportive resources to individuals and families affected by G6PD deficiency, provides a list of drugs and food ingredients that individuals with this condition should avoid. They also maintain a list of low-risk drugs that are generally safe to take in low doses.

Section 7.6

Hemoglobin E Disease

This section includes text excerpted from "Hemoglobin E Disease," Genetic and Rare Diseases Information Center (GARD), National Center for Advancing Translational Sciences (NCATS), March 22, 2017.

What Is Hemoglobin E Disease?

Hemoglobin E (HbE) disease is a mild, inherited blood disorder characterized by an abnormal form of hemoglobin, called "hemoglobin E." People with this condition may have very mild anemia, but the condition typically does not cause any symptoms. It is inherited in an autosomal recessive manner and is caused by a mutation in the HBB gene. The mutation that causes hemoglobin E disease primarily occurs in Southeast Asian populations and occurs rarely in Chinese populations. Most people with HbE disease do not need any treatment.

Symptoms of Hemoglobin E Disease

Most people with HbE disease do not have any symptoms. Some people may have mild anemia and microcytosis (a red blood cell (RBC) size smaller than the normal range).

Diagnosis of Hemoglobin E Disease

Many babies with HbE disease are first picked up through state newborn screening programs. A diagnosis is usually made by looking at the red blood cells (RBCs) by doing a mean corpuscular volume (MCV) test, which is commonly part of a complete blood count (CBC) test. More specialized tests, such as a hemoglobin electrophoresis and iron studies, might be done. These tests indicate whether a person has different types of hemoglobin. Genetic testing of the *HBB* gene can also be done to confirm a diagnosis, if needed.

Newborn Screening

- An ACTion (ACT) sheet is available for this condition that describes the short-term actions a health professional should follow when an infant has a positive newborn screening result. ACT sheets were developed by experts in collaboration with the American College of Medical Genetics (ACMG).

- An algorithm flowchart is available for this condition for determining the final diagnosis in an infant with a positive newborn screening result. Algorithms are developed by experts in collaboration with the ACMG.

- The Newborn Screening Coding and Terminology Guide has information on the standard codes used for newborn screening tests. Using these standards helps compare data across different laboratories. This resource was created by the U.S. National Library of Medicine (NLM).

Treatment of Hemoglobin E Disease

Treatment for hemoglobin E disease is typically not needed. Folic acid supplements may be prescribed to help the body produce normal red blood cells if mild anemia causes symptoms. Most people do not have any symptoms. People with hemoglobin E disease can expect to lead a normal life.

Section 7.7

Iron-Deficiency Anemia

This section includes text excerpted from "Iron-Deficiency Anemia," Office on Women's Health (OWH), U.S. Department of Health and Human Services (HHS), April 1, 2019.

What Is Iron-Deficiency Anemia?

Iron-deficiency anemia is the most common type of anemia, a condition that happens when your body does not make enough healthy red blood cells (RBCs) or the blood cells do not work correctly.

Iron-deficiency anemia happens when you do not have enough iron in your body. Your body needs iron to make hemoglobin, the part of the red blood cell (RBC) that carries oxygen through your blood to all parts of your body.

Who Gets Iron-Deficiency Anemia

Iron-deficiency anemia affects more women than men. The risk of iron-deficiency anemia is highest for women who:

- Are pregnant. Iron-deficiency anemia affects one in six pregnant women. You need more iron during pregnancy to support your unborn baby's development.

- Have heavy menstrual periods. Up to five percent of women of childbearing age develop iron-deficiency anemia because of heavy bleeding during their periods.

Infants, small children, and teens are also at high risk for iron-deficiency anemia.

What Are the Symptoms of Iron-Deficiency Anemia?

Iron-deficiency anemia often develops slowly. In the beginning, you may not have any symptoms, or they may be mild. As it gets worse, you may notice one or more of these symptoms:

- Fatigue (very common)

- Weakness (very common)

- Dizziness

- Headaches

- Low body temperature
- Pale or yellow "sallow" skin
- Rapid or irregular heartbeat
- Shortness of breath or chest pain, especially with physical activity
- Brittle nails
- Pica (unusual cravings for ice; very cold drinks; or nonfood items, such as dirt or paper)

If you think you may have iron-deficiency anemia, talk to your doctor or nurse.

What Causes Iron-Deficiency Anemia

Women can have low iron levels for several reasons:

- Iron lost through bleeding. Bleeding can cause you to lose more blood cells and iron than your body can replace. Women may have low iron levels from bleeding caused by:
  - Digestive system problems, such as ulcers, colon polyps, or colon cancer
  - Regular, long-term use of aspirin and other over-the-counter (OTC) pain relievers
  - Donating blood too often or without enough time in between donations for your body to recover
  - Heavier or longer than normal menstrual periods
  - Uterine fibroids, which are noncancerous growths in the uterus that can cause heavy bleeding
- Increased need for iron during pregnancy. During pregnancy, your body needs more iron than normal to support the fetus.
- Not eating enough food that contains iron. Your body absorbs the iron in animal-based foods, such as meat, chicken, and fish, two to three times better than the iron in plant-based foods. Vegetarians or vegans, who eat little or no animal-based foods, need to choose other good sources of iron to make sure they get enough. Your body also absorbs iron from plant-based foods better when you eat them with foods that have vitamin C, such

as oranges and tomatoes. But, most people in the United States get enough iron from food.

- Problems absorbing iron. Certain health conditions, such as Crohn disease or celiac disease, or gastric bypass surgery for weight loss, can make it harder for your body to absorb iron from food.

How Is Iron-Deficiency Anemia Diagnosed?

Talk to your doctor if you think you might have iron-deficiency anemia. Your doctor may:

- Ask you questions about your health history, including how regular or heavy your menstrual periods are. Your doctor may also ask you about any digestive system problems you may have, such as blood in your stool.

- Do a physical exam

- Talk to you about the foods you eat, the medicines you take, and your family health history

- Do blood tests. Your doctor will do a complete blood count (CBC). The CBC measures many parts of your blood. If the CBC test shows that you have anemia, your doctor will likely do another blood test to measure the iron levels in your blood and confirm that you have iron-deficiency anemia.

If you have iron-deficiency anemia, your doctor may want to do other tests to find out what is causing it.

Do I Need to Be Tested for Iron-Deficiency Anemia?

Maybe. Talk to your doctor about getting tested as part of your regular health exam if you have heavy menstrual periods or a health problem, such as Crohn disease or celiac disease.

How Is Iron-Deficiency Anemia Treated?

Treatment for iron-deficiency anemia depends on the cause:

- Blood loss from a digestive system problem. If you have an ulcer, your doctor may give you antibiotics or other medicine to treat the ulcer. If your bleeding is caused by a polyp or cancerous tumor, you may need surgery to remove it.

- Blood loss from heavy menstrual periods. Your doctor may give you hormonal birth control to help relieve heavy periods. If your heavy bleeding does not get better, your doctor may recommend surgery. Types of surgery to control heavy bleeding include endometrial ablation, which removes or destroys your uterine lining, and a hysterectomy, which removes all or parts of your uterus.

- Increased need for iron. If you have problems absorbing iron or have lower iron levels but do not have severe anemia, your doctor may recommend:

  - Iron pills to build up your iron levels as quickly as possible. Do not take any iron pills without first talking to your doctor or nurse.

  - Eating more foods that contain iron. Good sources of iron include meat, fish, eggs, beans, peas, and fortified foods (look for cereals fortified with 100% of the daily value for iron).

  - Eating more foods with vitamin C. Vitamin C helps your body absorb iron. Good sources of vitamin C include oranges, broccoli, and tomatoes.

If you have severe bleeding or symptoms of chest pain or shortness of breath, your doctor may recommend iron or red blood cell transfusions. Transfusions are only for severe iron deficiencies, and they are much less common.

What Do I Need to Know about Iron Pills?

Your doctor may recommend iron pills to help build up your iron levels. Do not take these pills without talking to your doctor or nurse first. Taking iron pills can cause side effects, including an upset stomach, constipation, and diarrhea. If taken as a liquid, iron supplements may stain your teeth.

You can reduce side effects from iron pills by taking these steps:

- Start with half of the recommended dose. Gradually increase to the full dose.

- Take iron in divided doses. For example, if you take two pills daily, take one in the morning with breakfast and the other after dinner.

- Take iron with food (especially something with vitamin C, such as a glass of orange juice, to help your body absorb the iron).

- If one type of iron pill causes side effects, ask your doctor for another type.

- If you take iron as a liquid instead of as a pill, aim it toward the back of your mouth. This will prevent the liquid from staining your teeth. You can also brush your teeth after taking the medicine to help prevent staining.

What Can Happen If Iron-Deficiency Anemia Is Not Treated?

If left untreated, iron-deficiency anemia can cause serious health problems. Having too little oxygen in the body can damage organs. With anemia, the heart must work harder to make up for the lack of red blood cells or hemoglobin. This extra work can harm the heart.

Iron-deficiency anemia can also cause problems during pregnancy.

How Can I Prevent Iron-Deficiency Anemia?

You can help prevent iron-deficiency anemia with the following steps:

- Treat the cause of blood loss. Talk to your doctor if you have heavy menstrual periods or if you have digestive system problems, such as frequent diarrhea or blood in your stool.

- Eat foods with iron. Good sources of iron include lean meat and chicken; dark, leafy vegetables; and beans.

- Eat and drink foods that help your body absorb iron, such as orange juice, strawberries, broccoli, or other fruits and vegetables with vitamin C.

- Make healthy food choices. Most people who make healthy, balanced food choices get the iron and vitamins their bodies need from the foods they eat.

- Avoid drinking coffee or tea with meals. These drinks make it harder for your body to absorb iron.

- Talk to your doctor if you take calcium pills. Calcium can make it harder for your body to absorb iron. If you have a hard time getting enough iron, talk to your doctor about the best way to also get enough calcium.

How Much Iron Do I Need Every Day?

Table 7.1 below lists how much iron you need every day. The recommended amounts are listed in milligrams (mg).

Table 7.1. Recommended Amounts of Iron per Day

Age	Women	Pregnant Women	Breastfeeding Women	Vegetarian Women*
14 to 18 years	15 mg	27 mg	10 mg	27 mg
19 to 50 years	18 mg	27 mg	9 mg	32 mg
51+ years	8 mg	n/a	n/a	14 mg

(Source: Adapted from Institute of Medicine (IOM), Food and Nutrition Board (FNB).)
* Vegetarians need more iron from food than people who eat meat do. This is because the body can absorb iron from meat better than from plant-based foods.

What Foods Contain Iron

Food sources of iron include:

- Fortified breakfast cereals (18 milligrams per serving)
- Oysters (8 milligrams per 3-ounce serving)
- Canned white beans (8 milligrams per cup)
- Dark chocolate (7 milligrams per 3-ounce serving)
- Beef liver (5 milligrams per 3-ounce serving)
- Spinach (3 milligrams per ½ cup)
- Tofu, firm (3 milligrams per ½ cup)
- Kidney beans (2 milligrams per ½ cup)
- Canned tomatoes (2 milligrams per ½ cup)
- Lean beef (2 milligrams for a 3-ounce serving)
- Baked potato (2 milligrams for a medium potato)

Section 7.8

Pernicious Anemia

This section includes text excerpted from "Pernicious Anemia," National Heart, Lung, and Blood Institute (NHLBI), October 30, 2011. Reviewed June 2019.

What Is Pernicious Anemia?

Pernicious anemia is a condition in which the body cannot make enough healthy red blood cells (RBCs) because it does not have enough vitamin B_{12}.

Vitamin B_{12} is a nutrient found in some foods. The body needs this nutrient to make healthy red blood cells and to keep its nervous system working properly.

People who have pernicious anemia cannot absorb enough vitamin B_{12} from food. This is because they lack intrinsic factor, a protein made in the stomach. A lack of this protein leads to vitamin B_{12} deficiency.

Other conditions and factors also can cause vitamin B_{12} deficiency. Examples include infections, surgery, medicines, and diet. Technically, the term "pernicious anemia" refers to vitamin B_{12} deficiency due to a lack of intrinsic factor. Often though, vitamin B_{12} deficiency due to other causes also is called "pernicious anemia."

Causes of Pernicious Anemia

Pernicious anemia is caused by a lack of intrinsic factor or other causes, such as infections, surgery, medicines, or diet.

Lack of Intrinsic Factor

Intrinsic factor is a protein made in the stomach. It helps your body absorb vitamin B_{12}. In some people, an autoimmune response causes a lack of intrinsic factor.

An autoimmune response occurs if the body's immune system makes antibodies (proteins) that mistakenly attack and damage the body's tissues or cells.

In pernicious anemia, the body makes antibodies that attack and destroy the parietal cells. These cells line the stomach and make intrinsic factor. Why this autoimmune response occurs is not known.

As a result of this attack, the stomach stops making intrinsic factor. Without intrinsic factor, your body cannot move vitamin B_{12} through the small intestine, where it is absorbed. This leads to vitamin B_{12} deficiency.

A lack of intrinsic factor also can occur if you have had part or all of your stomach surgically removed. This type of surgery reduces the number of parietal cells available to make intrinsic factor.

Rarely, children are born with an inherited disorder that prevents their bodies from making intrinsic factor. This disorder is called "congenital pernicious anemia."

Other Causes

Pernicious anemia also has other causes, besides a lack of intrinsic factor. Malabsorption in the small intestine and a diet lacking vitamin B_{12} both can lead to pernicious anemia.

Malabsorption in the Small Intestine

Sometimes, pernicious anemia occurs because the body's small intestine cannot properly absorb vitamin B_{12}. This may be the result of:

- Too much of the wrong kind of bacteria in the small intestine. This is a common cause of pernicious anemia in older adults. The bacteria use up the available vitamin B_{12} before the small intestine can absorb it.

- Diseases that interfere with vitamin B_{12} absorption. One example is celiac disease. This is a genetic disorder in which your body cannot tolerate a protein called "gluten." Another example is Crohn disease, an inflammatory bowel disease (IBD). Human immunodeficiency virus (HIV) also may interfere with vitamin B_{12} absorption.

- Certain medicines that alter bacterial growth or prevent the small intestine from properly absorbing vitamin B_{12}. Examples include antibiotics and certain diabetes and seizure medicines.

- Surgical removal of part or all of the small intestine

- A tapeworm infection. The tapeworm feeds off of the vitamin B_{12}. Eating undercooked, infected fish may cause this type of infection.

Diet Lacking Vitamin B$_{12}$

Some people get pernicious anemia because they do not have enough vitamin B$_{12}$ in their diets. This cause of pernicious anemia is less common than other causes.

Good food sources of vitamin B$_{12}$ include:

- Breakfast cereals with added vitamin B$_{12}$

- Meats, such as beef, liver, poultry, and fish

- Eggs and dairy products (such as milk, yogurt, and cheese)

- Foods fortified with vitamin B$_{12}$, such as soy-based beverages and vegetarian burgers

Strict vegetarians who do not eat any animal or dairy products and do not take a vitamin B$_{12}$ supplement are at risk for pernicious anemia.

Breastfed infants of strict vegetarian mothers also are at risk for pernicious anemia. These infants can develop anemia within months of being born. This is because they have not had enough time to store vitamin B$_{12}$ in their bodies. Doctors treat these infants with vitamin B$_{12}$ supplements.

Other groups, such as the elderly and people who suffer from alcoholism, also may be at risk for pernicious anemia. These people may not get the proper nutrients in their diets.

Risk Factors of Pernicious Anemia

Pernicious anemia is more common in people of Northern European and African descent than in other ethnic groups.

Older people also are at higher risk for the condition. This is mainly due to a lack of stomach acid and intrinsic factor, which prevents the small intestine from absorbing vitamin B$_{12}$. As people grow older, they tend to make less stomach acid.

Pernicious anemia also can occur in younger people and other populations. You are at higher risk for pernicious anemia if you:

- Have a family history of the condition

- Have had part or all of your stomach surgically removed. The stomach makes intrinsic factor. This protein helps your body absorb vitamin B$_{12}$.

- Have an autoimmune disorder that involves the endocrine glands, such as Addison disease, type 1 diabetes, Graves disease, or vitiligo. Research suggests that a link may exist between these autoimmune disorders and pernicious anemia that is caused by an autoimmune response.

- Have had part or all of your small intestine surgically removed. The small intestine is where vitamin B_{12} is absorbed.

- Have certain intestinal diseases or other disorders that may prevent your body from properly absorbing vitamin B_{12}. Examples include Crohn disease, intestinal infections, and HIV.

- Take medicines that prevent your body from properly absorbing vitamin B_{12}. Examples of such medicines include antibiotics and certain seizure medicines.

- Are a strict vegetarian who does not eat any animal or dairy products and does not take a vitamin B_{12} supplement, or if you eat poorly overall

Screening and Prevention of Pernicious Anemia

You cannot prevent pernicious anemia caused by a lack of intrinsic factor. Without intrinsic factor, you would not be able to absorb vitamin B_{12} and will develop pernicious anemia.

Although uncommon, some people develop pernicious anemia because they do not get enough vitamin B_{12} in their diets. You can take steps to prevent pernicious anemia caused by dietary factors.

Eating foods high in vitamin B_{12} can help prevent low vitamin B_{12} levels. Good food sources of vitamin B_{12} include:

- Breakfast cereals with added vitamin B_{12}

- Meats, such as beef, liver, poultry, and fish

- Eggs and dairy products (such as milk, yogurt, and cheese)

- Foods fortified with vitamin B_{12}, such as soy-based beverages and vegetarian burgers

If you are a strict vegetarian, talk with your doctor about having your vitamin B_{12} level checked regularly.

Vitamin B_{12} also is found in multivitamins and B-complex vitamin supplements. Doctors may recommend supplements for people at risk for vitamin B_{12} deficiency, such as strict vegetarians or people who have had stomach surgery.

Older adults may have trouble absorbing vitamin B_{12}. Thus, doctors may recommend that older adults eat foods fortified with vitamin B_{12} or take vitamin B_{12} supplements.

Signs, Symptoms, and Complications of Pernicious Anemia

A lack of vitamin B_{12} (vitamin B_{12} deficiency) causes the signs and symptoms of pernicious anemia. Without enough vitamin B_{12}, your body cannot make enough healthy red blood cells, which causes anemia.

Some of the signs and symptoms of pernicious anemia apply to all types of anemia. Other signs and symptoms are specific to a lack of vitamin B_{12}.

Signs and Symptoms of Anemia

The most common symptom of all types of anemia is fatigue (tiredness). Fatigue occurs because your body does not have enough red blood cells to carry oxygen to its various parts.

A low red blood cell count also can cause shortness of breath, dizziness, headache, coldness in your hands and feet, pale or yellowish skin, and chest pain.

A lack of red blood cells also means that your heart has to work harder to move oxygen-rich blood through your body. This can lead to irregular heartbeats called "arrhythmias," heart murmur, an enlarged heart, or even heart failure.

Signs and Symptoms of Vitamin B_{12} Deficiency

Vitamin B_{12} deficiency may lead to nerve damage. This can cause tingling and numbness in your hands and feet, muscle weakness, and loss of reflexes. You also may feel unsteady, lose your balance, and have trouble walking. Vitamin B_{12} deficiency can cause weakened bones and may lead to hip fractures.

Severe vitamin B_{12} deficiency can cause neurological problems, such as confusion, dementia, depression, and memory loss.

Other symptoms of vitamin B_{12} deficiency involve the digestive tract. These symptoms include nausea (feeling sick to your stomach) and vomiting, heartburn, abdominal bloating and gas, constipation or diarrhea, loss of appetite, and weight loss. An enlarged liver is another symptom.

A smooth, thick, red tongue also is a sign of vitamin B_{12} deficiency and pernicious anemia.

Infants who have vitamin B_{12} deficiency may have poor reflexes or unusual movements, such as face tremors. They may have trouble feeding due to tongue and throat problems. They also may be irritable. If vitamin B_{12} deficiency is not treated, these infants may have permanent growth problems.

Living with Pernicious Anemia

With proper treatment, people who have pernicious anemia can recover, feel well, and live normal lives. If you have complications of pernicious anemia, such as nerve damage, early treatment may help reverse the damage.

Ongoing Care

If you have pernicious anemia, you may need lifelong treatment. See your doctor regularly for checkups and ongoing care. Take vitamin B_{12} supplements as your doctor advises. This may help prevent symptoms and complications.

During your follow-up visits, your doctor may check for signs of vitamin B_{12} deficiency. She or he also may adjust your treatment as needed.

If you have pernicious anemia, you are at a higher risk for stomach cancer. See your doctor regularly so she or he can check for this complication.

Also, tell your family members, especially your children and brothers and sisters, that you have pernicious anemia. Pernicious anemia can run in families, so they may have a higher risk for the condition.

Section 7.9

Sickle Cell Disease

This section includes text excerpted from "Sickle Cell Disease," National Heart, Lung, and Blood Institute (NHLBI), December 3, 2018.

What Is Sickle Cell Disease?

Sickle cell disease (SCD) is a group of inherited red blood cell (RBC) disorders. People who have sickle cell disease have an abnormal protein in their red blood cells. In the United States, most people who have sickle cell disease are of African ancestry, but the condition is also common in people with a Hispanic background. Because the disease runs in families, couples planning to have children can have genetic testing.

Early signs and symptoms of sickle cell disease include swelling of the hands and feet; symptoms of anemia include fatigue (extreme tiredness) and jaundice. Over time, sickle cell disease can lead to complications, such as infections; delayed growth; and episodes of pain, called "pain crises." Most children who have sickle cell disease are pain-free between crises, but adolescents and adults may also suffer with chronic, ongoing pain. Over a lifetime, sickle cell disease can harm a patient's spleen, brain, eyes, lungs, liver, heart, kidneys, penis, joints, bones, or skin.

A blood and bone marrow transplant is currently the only cure for sickle cell disease, and only a small number of people who have sickle disease are able to have the transplant. There are effective treatments that can reduce symptoms and prolong life. Early diagnosis and regular medical care to prevent complications also contribute to an improved well-being. Sickle cell disease is a lifelong illness. The severity of the disease varies widely from person to person.

Causes of Sickle Cell Disease

Abnormal hemoglobin, called "hemoglobin S," causes sickle cell disease.

Hemoglobin S *Gene*

Sickle cell disease is an inherited disease caused by defects, called "mutations," in the beta globin gene that helps make hemoglobin.

Normally, hemoglobin in red blood cells takes up oxygen in the lungs and carries it through the arteries to all the cells in the tissues of the body. Red blood cells that contain normal hemoglobin are disc-shaped and flexible so that they can move easily through large and small blood vessels to deliver oxygen.

Sickle hemoglobin is not similar to normal hemoglobin. The mutations in the gene cause a problem when oxygen levels in the blood are lower, which occurs once the hemoglobin has delivered oxygen to the cells in the body's tissues. With less oxygen, the abnormal *hemoglobin S* gene can cause rigid, nonliquid protein strands to form within the red blood cell. These rigid strands can change the shape of the cell, causing the sickled red blood cell that gives the disease its name.

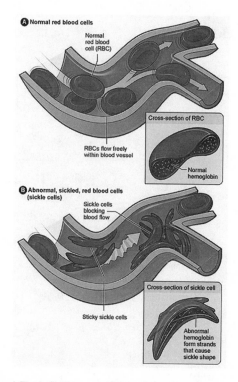

Figure 7.2. *Normal Red Cells and Sickle Red Cells*

Figure A shows normal red blood cells flowing freely in a blood vessel. The inset image shows a cross-section of a normal red blood cell with normal hemoglobin. Figure B shows abnormal, sickled red blood cells blocking blood flow in a blood vessel. The inset image shows a cross-section of a sickle cell with abnormal (sickle) hemoglobin forming rigid strands.

Sickle-shaped cells are not flexible and can stick to vessel walls, causing a blockage that slows or stops the flow of blood. When this happens, oxygen is unable to reach nearby tissues. The lack of oxygen in tissue can cause attacks of sudden, severe pain. These pain attacks can occur without warning, and a person who has them often needs to go to the hospital for effective treatment.

Because sickle cells cannot change shape easily, they tend to burst apart. Normal red blood cells live about 90 to 120 days, but sickle cells last only 10 to 20 days. The body is always making new red blood cells to replace the old cells. However, in sickle cell disease, the body may have trouble keeping up with how fast the cells are being destroyed. Because of this, the number of red blood cells is usually lower than normal. This condition, called "anemia," can cause a person to have less energy.

How Is the Hemoglobin S *Gene Inherited?*

When the *hemoglobin S* gene is inherited from only one parent, and a normal hemoglobin gene—*hemoglobin A*—is inherited from the other, a person will have sickle cell trait. People with sickle cell trait are generally healthy.

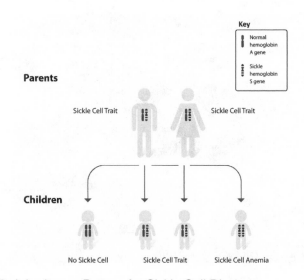

Figure 7.3. *Inheritance Pattern for Sickle Cell Disease*

The figure shows how hemoglobin S genes are inherited. A person inherits two hemoglobin genes—one from each parent. A normal hemoglobin A gene will make normal hemoglobin. A hemoglobin S gene will make abnormal hemoglobin.

Only rarely do people who have sickle cell trait have complications similar to those seen in people who have sickle cell disease. But, people with sickle cell trait are carriers of a defective *hemoglobin S* gene, so they can pass it on when they have a child.

If the child's other parent also has sickle cell trait or another abnormal hemoglobin gene, such as *thalassemia, hemoglobin C, hemoglobin D,* or *hemoglobin E,* that child has a chance of having sickle cell disease.

In figure 7.3, each parent has one normal *hemoglobin A* gene and one *hemoglobin S* gene, which means each of their children has:

- A 25 percent chance of inheriting two normal *hemoglobin A* genes. In this case, the child does not have sickle cell trait or disease.

- A 50 percent chance of inheriting one normal *hemoglobin A* gene and one *hemoglobin S* gene. This child has sickle cell trait.

- A 25 percent chance of inheriting two *hemoglobin S* genes. This child has sickle cell disease.

It is important to keep in mind that each time this couple has a child, the chances of that child having sickle cell disease remain the same. In other words, if the firstborn child has sickle cell disease, there is still a 25 percent chance that the second child will also have the disease. Both boys and girls can inherit sickle cell trait, sickle cell disease, or normal hemoglobin.

If a person wants to know whether she or he carries a sickle hemoglobin gene, a doctor can order a blood test to find out.

Risk Factors of Sickle Cell Disease

In the United States, most people with sickle cell disease are of African ancestry or identify themselves as black.

- About one in 13 Black babies is born with sickle cell trait.

- About one in every 365 Black babies is born with sickle cell disease.

- There are also many people with this disease who come from Hispanic, Southern European, Middle Eastern, or Asian Indian backgrounds.

About 100,000 Americans have sickle cell disease.

Screening and Prevention of Sickle Cell Disease

People who do not know whether they carry an abnormal hemoglobin gene can ask their doctor to have their blood tested.

Couples who are planning to have children and know that they are at risk of having a child with sickle cell disease may want to meet with a genetic counselor. A genetic counselor can answer questions about the risk and explain the choices that are available.

Signs, Symptoms, and Complications of Sickle Cell Disease

Sickle cell disease is a lifelong illness. The severity of the disease varies widely from person to person. People with sickle cell disease can experience both acute and chronic signs, symptoms, and complications.

Early Signs and Symptoms

If a person has sickle cell disease, it is present at birth. But, most infants do not have any problems from the disease until they are about five or six months of age. Every state in the United States, the District of Columbia, and the U.S. territories require that all newborn babies receive screening for sickle cell disease. When a child has sickle cell disease, parents are notified before the child has symptoms.

Some children with sickle cell disease will start to have problems early on, and some later. Early symptoms of sickle cell disease may include:

- A yellowish color of the skin, known as "jaundice," or whites of the eyes, known as "icterus," that occurs when a large number of red cells undergo hemolysis

- Fatigue or fussiness from anemia

- Painful swelling of the hands and feet, known as "dactylitis"

The signs and symptoms of sickle cell disease will vary from person to person and can change over time. Most of the signs and symptoms of sickle cell disease are related to complications of the disease.

Complications
Acute Pain (Sickle Cell or Vaso-Occlusive) Crisis

Acute pain episodes, or crises, can occur without warning when sickle cells block blood flow and decrease oxygen delivery. People describe this pain as sharp, intense, stabbing, or throbbing. Severe crises can be even more uncomfortable than postsurgical pain or childbirth.

Pain can strike almost anywhere in the body and in more than one spot at a time. But, the pain often occurs in several places:

- Abdomen
- Arms
- Chest
- Lower back
- Legs

A crisis can be brought on by various conditions:

- High altitudes
- Dehydration, or not drinking enough fluids
- Illness
- Stress
- Temperature changes

Often, a person does not know what triggers, or causes, the crisis.

Chronic Pain

Many adolescents and adults with sickle cell disease suffer from chronic pain. This kind of pain has been hard for people to describe, but it is usually different from crisis pain or the pain that results from organ damage.

Chronic pain can be severe and can make life difficult. Its cause is not well understood.

Severe Anemia

People with sickle cell disease usually have mild to moderate anemia. At times, however, they can have severe anemia. Severe anemia can be life-threatening. Severe anemia in an infant or child with sickle cell disease may be a result of one of the following events:

- Aplastic crisis. Aplastic crisis is usually caused by a parvovirus B19 infection, also called "fifth disease" or "slapped cheek syndrome." Parvovirus B19 is a very common infection, but in sickle cell disease, it can cause the bone marrow to stop producing new red cells for a while, leading to severe anemia.

- Blood cells getting trapped in the spleen. The spleen is an organ that is located in the upper left side of the belly. The spleen filters your blood and destroys old blood cells. In people who have sickle cell disease, red blood cells may get trapped in the spleen, making it enlarge quickly. With red blood cells trapped in the spleen, fewer are available to circulate in the blood, and this can set off severe anemia. A large spleen may also cause pain in the left side of the belly. A parent can usually feel the enlarged spleen in the belly of her or his child.

Splenic sequestration crisis and aplastic crisis most commonly occur in infants and children who have sickle cell disease. Adults who have sickle cell disease may also experience episodes of severe anemia, but these usually have other causes.

No matter the cause, severe anemia may lead to symptoms that include:

- Fatigue

- Dizziness

- Pale skin

- Shortness of breath

Babies and newborns with severe anemia may not want to eat and may seem very sluggish.

Infections

The spleen is important for protection against certain kinds of infections. Sickle cells can damage the spleen and weaken or destroy its function, even in young patients.

People who have sickle cell disease who have damaged spleens are at-risk for serious bacterial infections in the blood, lung, brain, or bone that can be life-threatening. Some of these bacteria include:

- Chlamydia

- Haemophilus influenzae type B (Hib)

- Meningococcus

- Mycoplasma pneumoniae

- Pneumococcus

- Salmonella

- Staphylococcus

Acute Chest Syndrome

Sickling in blood vessels of the lungs can deprive a person's lungs of oxygen. When this happens, areas of lung tissue are damaged and cannot exchange oxygen properly. This condition is known as "acute chest syndrome" (ACS). In acute chest syndrome, at least one segment of the lung is damaged.

This condition is very serious and should be treated right away at a hospital.

Acute chest syndrome often starts a few days after a painful crisis begins. A lung infection may accompany acute chest syndrome.

Symptoms may include:

- Chest pain

- Cough

- Fever

- Rapid breathing

- Shortness of breath

Brain Complications
Clinical Stroke

A stroke occurs when blood flow is blocked to a part of the brain. When this happens, brain cells can become damaged or die. In sickle cell disease, a clinical stroke means that a person shows outward signs that something is wrong. The symptoms depend upon what part of the brain is affected. Symptoms of stroke may include:

- Loss of balance

- Severe headache

- Trouble speaking, walking, or understanding

- Weakness of an arm or leg on one side of the body

As many as 24 percent of people with hemoglobin SS and 10 percent of people with hemoglobin SC may suffer a clinical stroke by the age of 45.

In children, clinical stroke occurs most commonly between the ages of two and nine, but recent prevention strategies have lowered the risk.

When people who have sickle cell disease show symptoms of stroke, their families or friends should call 911 right away.

Silent Stroke and Thinking Problems

Brain imaging and tests of thinking, or cognitive studies, have shown that children and adults with hemoglobin SS and hemoglobin Sβ0 thalassemia often have signs of silent brain injury, also called "silent stroke." Silent brain injury is damage to the brain without showing outward signs of stroke.

This injury is common. Silent brain injury can lead to difficulty in earning, making decisions, or holding down a job.

Eye Problems

Sickle cell disease can injure blood vessels in the eye. The most common site of damage is the retina, where blood vessels can overgrow, get blocked, or bleed. The retina is the light-sensitive layer of tissue that lines the inside of the eye and sends visual messages through the optic nerve to the brain.

Detachment of the retina can occur. When the retina detaches, it is lifted or pulled from its normal position. These problems can cause visual impairment or loss.

Heart Disease

People who have sickle cell disease can have problems with blood vessels in the heart and with heart function. The heart can become larger than normal. People who have sickle cell disease can also develop pulmonary hypertension.

People who have sickle cell disease and who have received frequent blood transfusions may also have heart damage from iron overload.

Pulmonary Hypertension

In adolescents and adults, injury to blood vessels in the lungs can make it hard for the heart to pump blood through those blood vessels. This causes the pressure in lung blood vessels to rise. High pressure in these blood vessels is called "pulmonary hypertension." Symptoms may include shortness of breath and fatigue.

When this condition is severe, it has been associated with a higher risk of death.

Kidney Problems

The kidneys are sensitive to the effects of red blood cell sickling.

Sickle cell disease causes the kidneys to have trouble making the urine as concentrated as it should be. This may lead to a need to urinate often and to have bedwetting or uncontrolled urination during the night. This often starts in childhood. Other problems may include:

- Blood in the urine

- Decreased kidney function

- Kidney disease

- Protein loss in the urine

Priapism

Males who have sickle cell disease can have unwanted, sometimes prolonged, painful erections. This condition is called "priapism."

Priapism happens when blood flow out of the erect penis is blocked by sickled cells. If it goes on for a long period of time, priapism can cause permanent damage to the penis and lead to impotence.

If priapism lasts for more than four hours, emergency medical care should be sought to avoid complications.

Gallstones

When red cells undergo hemolysis, they release hemoglobin. Hemoglobin gets broken down into a substance called "bilirubin." Bilirubin can form stones that get stuck in the gallbladder. The gallbladder is a small, sac-shaped organ beneath the liver that helps with digestion. Gallstones are a common problem in sickle cell disease.

Gallstones may be formed early on but may not produce symptoms for years. When symptoms develop, they may include:

- Nausea

- Right-side upper belly pain

- Vomiting

If problems continue or recur, a person may need surgery to remove the gallbladder.

Liver Complications

There are a number of ways in which the liver may be injured in sickle cell disease.

Sickle cell intrahepatic cholestasis (SCIC) is an uncommon but severe type of liver damage that occurs when sickled red cells block blood vessels in the liver. This blockage prevents enough oxygen from reaching liver tissue.

These episodes are usually sudden and may recur. Children often recover, but some adults may have chronic problems that lead to liver failure.

People who have sickle cell disease who have received frequent blood transfusions may develop liver damage from iron overload.

Leg Ulcers

Sickle cell ulcers are sores that usually start small and then get larger and larger.

The number of ulcers can vary from one to many. Some ulcers will heal quickly, but others may not heal and may last for long periods of time. Some ulcers come back after healing.

People who have sickle cell disease usually do not get ulcers until after the age of 10.

Joint Complications

Sickling in the bones of the hip and, less commonly, the shoulder joints, knees, and ankles can decrease oxygen flow and result in severe damage. This damage is a condition called "avascular necrosis" or "aseptic necrosis." This disease is usually found in adolescents and adults.

Symptoms include pain and problems with walking and joint movement. A person may need pain medicines, surgery, or joint replacement if symptoms persist.

Delayed Growth and Puberty

Children who have sickle cell disease may grow and develop more slowly than their peers because of anemia. They will reach full sexual maturity, but this may be delayed.

Pregnancy

Pregnancies in women who have sickle cell disease can be risky for both the mother and the fetus.

Mothers may have medical complications that include:

- Blood clots

- High blood pressure

- Increased pain episodes

- Infections

They also are at higher risk for:

- Miscarriages

- Premature births

- Small-for-date or underweight babies

Mental Health

As in other chronic diseases, people who have sickle cell disease may feel sad and frustrated at times. The limitations that sickle cell disease can impose on a person's daily activities may cause them to feel isolated from others. Sometimes, they become depressed.

People who have sickle cell disease may also have trouble coping with pain and fatigue, as well as with frequent medical visits and hospitalizations.

Living with Sickle Cell Disease

If you or your child has sickle cell disease, you should learn as much as you can about the disease. Your healthcare providers are there to help you, and you should feel comfortable asking questions.

Pursue a Healthy Lifestyle

Similar to other people, you and your child should strive to maintain a healthy lifestyle that includes:

- Being physically active. People who have sickle cell disease often tire easily, so be careful to pace yourself and avoid very strenuous activities.

- Getting enough sleep

- Heart-healthy eating, including limiting alcohol. Drink extra water to avoid dehydration.

- Quitting smoking. For free help and support to quit smoking, you can call the National Cancer Institute's (NCI) Smoking Quitline at 877-44U-QUIT (877-448-7848).

Prevent and Control Complications

To prevent and control complications, your doctor may recommend the following:

- Avoid overexertion and dehydration. Take time out to rest, and drink plenty of fluids.

- Avoid situations that may set off a crisis. Extreme heat or cold, as well as abrupt changes in temperature, are often triggers. When going swimming, ease into the water rather than jumping right in.

- Do not travel in an aircraft cabin that is unpressurized.

- Take your medicines as your doctor prescribes. Get any medical and lab tests or immunizations that your doctor orders.

See a doctor right away if you have any of the following danger signs:

- Fever

- Problems breathing

- Stroke symptoms

- Sudden loss of vision

- Symptoms of a spleen that is larger than normal

- Symptoms of severe anemia

If your child attends day care, preschool, or school, speak to her or his teacher about the disease. Teachers need to know what to watch for and how to accommodate your child.

Get Ongoing Care

Make and keep regular appointments with your doctor or medical team. These visits will help to reduce the number of acute problems that need immediate care. Your medical team can help prevent complications and improve your quality of life (QOL).

Learn Ways to Manage Pain

Every patient experiences pain differently. Work with your doctor to develop a pain management plan that works for you. This often includes over-the-counter (OTC) medicines, as well as stronger medicines that you get with a prescription.

You may find other methods that help your pain, such as:

- Using a heating pad

- Taking a warm bath

- Engaging in distracting and relaxing activities, such as listening to music, talking on the phone, or watching TV

- Massage therapy

- Physical therapy

- Acupuncture

Take Care of Your Mental Health

Living with sickle cell disease can be very stressful. At times, you may feel sad or depressed. Talk to your doctor or medical team if you or your child is having any emotional problems. Tell your doctor right away if you or your child is feeling very depressed. Some people find counseling or antidepressant medicines helpful.

You may find that speaking to a counselor or psychiatrist or participating in a support group is helpful. When they provide love and support to people who have sickle cell disease, friends and families can help to relieve stress and sadness. Let your loved ones know how you feel and what you need.

Section 7.10

Thalassemia

This section includes text excerpted from "What Is Thalassemia?" Centers for Disease Control and Prevention (CDC), April 23, 2019.

What Is Thalassemia?

Thalassemia is an inherited (i.e., passed from parents to children through genes) blood disorder caused by the body not making enough of a protein called "hemoglobin," an important part of red blood cells (RBCs). When there is not enough hemoglobin, the body's red blood cells do not function properly, and they last for shorter periods of time, so there are fewer healthy red blood cells traveling in the bloodstream.

Red blood cells carry oxygen to all the cells of the body. Oxygen is a sort of food that cells use to function. When there are not enough healthy red blood cells, there is also not enough oxygen delivered to all the other cells of the body, which may cause a person to feel tired, weak, or short of breath. This is a condition called "anemia." People with thalassemia may have mild or severe anemia. Severe anemia can damage organs and lead to death.

What Are the Different Types of Thalassemia?

When we talk about different "types" of thalassemia, we might be talking about one of two things: the specific part of hemoglobin that is affected (usually either alpha or beta), or the severity of thalassemia, which is noted by words such as "trait," "carrier," "intermedia," or "major."

Hemoglobin, which carries oxygen to all cells in the body, is made of two different parts, called "alpha" and "beta." When thalassemia is called "alpha" or "beta," this refers to the part of hemoglobin that is not being made. If either the alpha or beta part is not made, there are not enough building blocks to make normal amounts of hemoglobin. Low alpha is called "alpha-thalassemia." Low beta is called "beta-thalassemia."

When the words "trait," "minor," "intermedia," or "major" are used, these words describe how severe the thalassemia is. A person who has thalassemia trait may not have any symptoms at all or may have only mild anemia, while a person with thalassemia major may have severe symptoms and may need regular blood transfusions.

In the same way that traits for hair color and body structure are passed down from parents to children, thalassemia traits are passed from parents to children. The type of thalassemia that a person has depends on how many and what type of traits for thalassemia a person has inherited. For instance, if a person receives a beta-thalassemia trait from his father and another from his mother, he will have beta-thalassemia major. If a person received an alpha-thalassemia trait from her mother and the normal alpha parts from her father, she would have alpha-thalassemia trait (also called "alpha-thalassemia minor"). Having a thalassemia trait means that you may not have any symptoms, but you might pass that trait on to your children and increase their risk for having thalassemia.

Sometimes, thalassemias have other names, such as "Constant Spring," "Cooley anemia," or "hemoglobin Bart hydrops fetalis." These names are specific to certain thalassemias—for instance, Cooley's anemia is the same thing as beta-thalassemia major.

How Do I Know If I Have Thalassemia?

People with moderate and severe forms of thalassemia usually find out about their condition in childhood because they have symptoms of severe anemia early in life. People with less severe forms of thalassemia may only find out because they are having symptoms of anemia or because a doctor finds anemia on a routine blood test or a test done for another reason.

Because thalassemias are inherited, the condition sometimes runs in families. Some people find out about their thalassemia because they have relatives with a similar condition.

People who have family members from certain parts of the world have a higher risk for having thalassemia. Traits for thalassemia are more common in people from Mediterranean countries, such as Greece and Turkey, and in people from Asia, Africa, and the Middle East. If you have anemia and you also have family members from these areas, your doctor might test your blood further to find out if you have thalassemia.

Can I Prevent Thalassemia?

Because thalassemia is passed from parents to children, it is very hard to prevent. However, if you or your partner knows of family members with thalassemia, or if you both have family members from places in the world where thalassemia is common, you can speak to a genetic counselor to determine what your risk would be of passing thalassemia to your children.

Signs, Symptoms, and Complications of Thalassemia

A lack of oxygen in the bloodstream causes the signs and symptoms of thalassemias. The lack of oxygen occurs because the body does not make enough healthy red blood cells and hemoglobin. The severity of symptoms depends on the severity of the disorder.

No Symptoms

Alpha-thalassemia silent carriers generally have no signs or symptoms of the disorder. The lack of the alpha globin protein is so minor that the body's hemoglobin works normally.

Mild Anemia

People who have alpha or beta-thalassemia trait can have mild anemia. However, many people who have these types of thalassemia have no signs or symptoms.

Mild anemia can make you feel tired. Mild anemia caused by alpha-thalassemiab trait might be mistaken for iron-deficiency anemia.

Mild to Moderate Anemia and Other Signs and Symptoms

People who have beta-thalassemia intermedia have mild to moderate anemia. They also may have other health problems, such as:

- **Slowed growth and delayed puberty.** Anemia can slow down a child's growth and development.

- **Bone problems.** Thalassemia may cause bone marrow to expand. Bone marrow is the spongy substance inside bones that makes blood cells. When bone marrow expands, the bones become wider than normal. They may become brittle and break easily.

- **An enlarged spleen.** The spleen is an organ that helps your body fight infection and remove unwanted material. When a person has thalassemia, the spleen has to work very hard. As a result, the spleen becomes larger than normal. This makes anemia worse. If the spleen becomes too large, it must be removed.

Severe Anemia and Other Signs and Symptoms

People who have hemoglobin H disease or beta-thalassemia major (also called "Cooley anemia") have severe thalassemia. Signs and symptoms usually occur within the first two years of life. They may include severe anemia and other health problems, such as:

- A pale and listless appearance
- Poor appetite
- Dark urine (a sign that red blood cells are breaking down)
- Slowed growth and delayed puberty
- Jaundice (a yellowish color of the skin or whites of the eyes)
- An enlarged spleen, liver, or heart
- Bone problems (especially with bones in the face)

Complications of Thalassemias

Better treatments now allow people who have moderate and severe thalassemias to live much longer. As a result, these people must cope with complications of these disorders that occur over time.

Heart and Liver Diseases

Regular blood transfusions are a standard treatment for thalassemias. Transfusions can cause iron to build up in the blood (iron overload). This can damage organs and tissues, especially the heart and liver.

Heart disease caused by iron overload is the main cause of death in people who have thalassemias. Heart disease includes heart failure, arrhythmias (irregular heartbeats), and heart attack.

Infection

Among people who have thalassemias, infections are a key cause of illness and the second most common cause of death. People who have had their spleens removed are at an even higher risk because they no longer have this infection-fighting organ.

Osteoporosis

Many people who have thalassemias have bone problems, including osteoporosis. This is a condition in which bones are weak and brittle and break easily.

Diagnosis of Thalassemia

Doctors diagnose thalassemias using blood tests, including a complete blood count (CBC) and special hemoglobin tests.

- A CBC measures the amount of hemoglobin and the different kinds of blood cells, such as red blood cells, in a sample of blood. People who have thalassemias have fewer healthy red blood cells and less hemoglobin than normal in their blood. People who have alpha or beta-thalassemia trait may have red blood cells that are smaller than normal.

- Hemoglobin tests measure the types of hemoglobin in a blood sample. People who have thalassemias have problems with the alpha or beta globin protein chains of hemoglobin.

Moderate and severe thalassemias usually are diagnosed in early childhood. This is because signs and symptoms, including severe anemia, often occur within the first two years of life.

People who have milder forms of thalassemia might be diagnosed after a routine blood test shows they have anemia. Doctors might suspect thalassemia if a person has anemia and is a member of an ethnic group that is at an increased risk for thalassemias.

Doctors also test the amount of iron in the blood to find out whether the anemia is due to iron deficiency or thalassemia. Iron-deficiency anemia occurs if the body does not have enough iron to make hemoglobin. The anemia in thalassemia occurs because of a problem with either the alpha globin or beta globin chains of hemoglobin, not because of a lack of iron.

Because thalassemias are passed from parents to children through genes, family genetic studies also can help diagnose the disorder. These studies involve taking a family medical history and doing blood tests on family members. The tests will show whether any family members have missing or altered hemoglobin genes.

If you know of family members who have thalassemias and you are thinking of having children, consider talking with your doctor and a genetic counselor. They can help determine your risk for passing the disorder to your children.

If you are expecting a baby and you and your partner are thalassemia carriers, you may want to consider prenatal testing.

Prenatal testing involves taking a sample of amniotic fluid or tissue from the placenta. (Amniotic fluid is the fluid in the sac surrounding a growing embryo. The placenta is the organ that attaches the umbilical cord to the mother's womb.) Tests done on the fluid or tissue can show whether your baby has thalassemia and how severe it might be.

Treatment of Thalassemia

Treatments for thalassemias depend on the type and severity of the disorder. People who are carriers or who have alpha or beta thalassemia trait have mild or no symptoms. They will likely need little or no treatment.

Doctors use three standard treatments for moderate and severe forms of thalassemia. These treatments include blood transfusions, iron chelation therapy, and folic acid supplements. Other treatments have been developed or are being tested, but they are used much less often.

Standard Treatments
Blood Transfusions

Transfusions of red blood cells are the main treatment for people who have moderate or severe thalassemias. This treatment gives you healthy red blood cells with normal hemoglobin.

During a blood transfusion, a needle is used to insert an intravenous (IV) line into one of your blood vessels. Through this line, you receive healthy blood. The procedure usually takes one to four hours.

Red blood cells live only for about 120 days. So, you may need repeated transfusions to maintain a healthy supply of red blood cells.

If you have hemoglobin H disease or beta-thalassemia intermedia, you may need blood transfusions occasionally. For example, you may have transfusions when you have an infection or other illness, or when your anemia is severe enough to cause tiredness.

If you have beta-thalassemia major, you will likely need regular blood transfusions (often every two to four weeks). These transfusions will help you maintain normal hemoglobin and red blood cell levels.

Blood transfusions allow you to feel better, enjoy normal activities, and live into adulthood. This treatment is lifesaving, but it is expensive and carries a risk of transmitting infections and viruses (for example, hepatitis). However, the risk is very low in the United States because of careful blood screening.

Iron Chelation Therapy

The hemoglobin in red blood cells is an iron-rich protein. Thus, regular blood transfusions can lead to a buildup of iron in the blood. This condition is called "iron overload." It damages the liver, heart, and other parts of the body.

To prevent this damage, doctors use iron chelation therapy to remove excess iron from the body. Two medicines are used for iron chelation therapy.

- Deferoxamine is a liquid medicine that is given slowly under the skin, usually with a small portable pump used overnight. This therapy takes time and can be mildly painful. Side effects include problems with vision and hearing.

- Deferasirox is a pill taken once daily. Side effects include headache, nausea (feeling sick to the stomach), vomiting, diarrhea, joint pain, and tiredness.

Folic Acid Supplements

Folic acid is a B vitamin that helps build healthy red blood cells. Your doctor may recommend folic acid supplements in addition to treatment with blood transfusions and/or iron chelation therapy.

Other Treatments

Other treatments for thalassemias have been developed or are being tested, but they are used much less often.

Blood and Marrow Stem Cell Transplant

A blood and marrow stem cell transplant replaces faulty stem cells with healthy ones from another person (a donor). Stem cells are the cells inside bone marrow that make red blood cells and other types of blood cells.

A stem cell transplant is the only treatment that can cure thalassemia. But, only a small number of people who have severe thalassemias are able to find a good donor match and have a risky procedure.

Possible Future Treatments

Researchers are working to find new treatments for thalassemias. For example, it might be possible someday to insert a normal hemoglobin gene into stem cells in bone marrow. This will allow people who have thalassemias to make their own healthy red blood cells and hemoglobin.

Researchers also are studying ways to trigger a person's ability to make fetal hemoglobin after birth. This type of hemoglobin is found in fetuses and newborns. After birth, the body switches to making adult hemoglobin. Making more fetal hemoglobin might make up for the lack of healthy adult hemoglobin.

Treating Complications

Better treatments now allow people who have moderate and severe thalassemias to live longer. As a result, these people must cope with complications that occur over time.

An important part of managing thalassemias is treating complications. Treatment might be needed for heart or liver diseases, infections, osteoporosis, and other health problems.

Living with Thalassemia

Survival and quality of life have improved for people who have moderate or severe thalassemias. This is because:

- More people are able to get blood transfusions now.

- Blood screening has reduced the number of infections from blood transfusions. Also, treatments for other kinds of infections have improved.

- Iron chelation treatments are available that are easier for some people to take.

- Some people have been cured through blood and marrow stem cell transplants.

- Living with thalassemia can be challenging, but several approaches can help you cope.

Follow Your Treatment Plan

Following the treatment plan your doctor gives you is important. For example, get blood transfusions as your doctor recommends, and take your iron chelation medicine as prescribed.

Iron chelation treatment can take time and be mildly painful. However, do not stop taking your medicine. The leading cause of death among people who have thalassemias is heart disease caused by iron overload. Iron buildup can damage your heart, liver, and other organs.

Several chelation treatments are now available, including injections and pills. Your doctor will talk with you about which treatment is best for you.

Take folic acid supplements if your doctor prescribes them. Folic acid is a B vitamin that helps build healthy red blood cells. Also, talk with your doctor about whether you need other vitamin or mineral supplements, such as vitamins A, C, or D or selenium.

Get Ongoing Medical Care

Keep your scheduled medical appointments, and get any tests that your doctor recommends.

These tests may include:

- Monthly CBCs and tests for blood iron levels every three months

- Yearly tests for heart function, liver function, and viral infections (for example, hepatitis B and C and HIV)

- Yearly tests to check for iron buildup in your liver

- Yearly vision and hearing tests

- Regular checkups to make sure blood transfusions are working

- Other tests as needed (such as lung function tests, genetic tests, and tests to match your tissues with a possible donor if a stem cell transplant is being considered)

- Children who have thalassemias should receive yearly checkups to monitor their growth and development. The checkups include a physical exam, including a height and weight check, and any necessary tests.

Take Steps to Stay Healthy

Take steps to stay as healthy as possible. Follow a healthy eating plan and your doctor's instructions for taking iron supplements.

Get vaccinations as needed, especially if you have had your spleen removed. You may need vaccines for the flu, pneumonia, hepatitis B, and meningitis. Your doctor will advise you about which vaccines you need.

- Wash your hands often.

- Avoid crowds during cold and flu season.

- Keep the skin around the site where you get blood transfusions as clean as possible.

- Call your doctor if a fever develops.

Emotional Issues and Support

If you or your child has thalassemia, you may have fear, anxiety, depression, or stress. Talk about how you feel with your healthcare team. Talking to a professional counselor also can help. If you are very depressed, your doctor may recommend medicines or other treatments that can improve your quality of life.

Joining a patient support group may help you adjust to living with thalassemia. You can see how other people who have the same symptoms have coped with them. Talk with your doctor about local support groups or check with an area medical center.

Support from family and friends also can help relieve stress and anxiety. Let your loved ones know how you feel and what they can do to help you.

Some teens and young adults who have thalassemias may have a hard time moving from pediatric care to adult care. Doctors and other health professionals who care for these children might not be familiar with adult issues related to the disorder, such as certain complications.

Also, it might be hard for adults who have thalassemias to find doctors who specialize in treating the disorder. Ask your child's doctor to help you find a doctor who can care for your child when the time comes to make the switch. Planning and good communication can help this move go smoothly.

Chapter 8

Hemochromatosis

What Is Hemochromatosis?

Hemochromatosis is a disease in which too much iron builds up in your body. Your body needs iron, but too much of it is toxic. If you have hemochromatosis, you absorb more iron than you need. Your body has no natural way to get rid of the extra iron. It stores it in body tissues, especially the liver, heart, and pancreas. The extra iron can damage your organs. Without treatment, it can cause your organs to fail.

There are two types of hemochromatosis. Primary hemochromatosis is an inherited disease. Secondary hemochromatosis is usually the result of something else, such as anemia, thalassemia, liver disease, or blood transfusions.

What Causes Hemochromatosis
Primary Hemochromatosis

Inherited genetic defects cause primary hemochromatosis, and mutations in the *HFE* gene are associated with up to 90 percent of cases. The *HFE* gene helps regulate the amount of iron absorbed from

This chapter contains text excerpted from the following sources: Text under the heading "What Is Hemochromatosis?" is excerpted from "Hemochromatosis," MedlinePlus, National Institutes of Health (NIH), February 7, 2019; Text beginning with the heading "What Causes Hemochromatosis" is excerpted from "Hemochromatosis," National Institute of Diabetes and Digestive and Kidney Diseases (NIDDK), March 2014. Reviewed June 2019.

food. The two known mutations of *HFE* are *C282Y* and *H63D*. *C282Y* defects are the most common cause of primary hemochromatosis.

People inherit two copies of the *HFE* gene—one copy from each parent. Most people who inherit two copies of the *HFE* gene with the *C282Y* defect will have higher-than-average iron absorption. However, not all of these people will develop health problems associated with hemochromatosis. One study found that 31 percent of people with 2 copies of the *C282Y* defect developed health problems by their early fifties. Men who develop health problems from *HFE* defects typically develop them after the age of 40. Women who develop health problems from *HFE* defects typically develop them after menopause.

People who inherit two *H63D* defects or one *C282Y* and one *H63D* defect may have higher-than-average iron absorption. However, they are unlikely to develop iron overload and organ damage.

Rare defects in other genes may also cause primary hemochromatosis. Mutations in the hemojuvelin or hepcidin genes cause juvenile hemochromatosis, a type of primary hemochromatosis. People with juvenile hemochromatosis typically develop severe iron overload and liver and heart damage between the ages of 15 and 30.

Secondary Hemochromatosis

Hemochromatosis that is not inherited is called "secondary hemochromatosis." The most common cause of secondary hemochromatosis is frequent blood transfusions in people with severe anemia. Anemia is a condition in which red blood cells (RBCs) are fewer or smaller than normal, which means they carry less oxygen to the body's cells. Types of anemia that may require frequent blood transfusions include:

- Congenital (inherited) anemias, such as sickle cell disease (SCD), thalassemia, and Fanconi syndrome

- Severe acquired anemias, which are not inherited, such as aplastic anemia and autoimmune hemolytic anemia

Liver diseases—such as alcoholic liver disease, nonalcoholic steatohepatitis, and chronic hepatitis C infection—may cause mild iron overload. However, this iron overload causes much less liver damage than the underlying liver disease causes.

Neonatal Hemochromatosis

Neonatal hemochromatosis is a rare disease characterized by liver failure and death in fetuses and newborns. Researchers are studying the causes of neonatal hemochromatosis and believe that more than one factor may lead to the disease.

Experts previously considered neonatal hemochromatosis a type of primary hemochromatosis. However, studies suggest genetic defects that increase iron absorption do not cause this disease. Instead, the mother's immune system may produce antibodies—proteins made by the immune system to protect the body from foreign substances such as bacteria or viruses—that damage the liver of the fetus. Women who have had one child with neonatal hemochromatosis are at risk for having more children with the disease. Treating these women during pregnancy with intravenous (IV) immunoglobulin—a solution of antibodies from healthy people—can prevent fetal liver damage.

Researchers supported by the National Institute of Diabetes and Digestive and Kidney Diseases (NIDDK) found that a combination of exchange transfusion—removing blood and replacing it with donor blood—and IV immunoglobulin is an effective treatment for babies born with neonatal hemochromatosis.

Who Is More Likely to Develop Hemochromatosis?

Primary hemochromatosis mainly affects Caucasians of Northern European descent. This disease is one of the most common genetic disorders in the United States. About 4 to 5 out of every 1,000 Caucasians carry 2 copies of the *C282Y* mutation of the *HFE* gene and are susceptible to developing hemochromatosis. About 1 out of every 10 Caucasians carries 1 copy of *C282Y*.

Hemochromatosis is extremely rare in African Americans, Asian Americans, Hispanics/Latinos, and American Indians. *HFE* mutations are usually not the cause of hemochromatosis in these populations.

Both men and women can inherit the gene defects for hemochromatosis; however, not all will develop the symptoms of hemochromatosis. Men usually develop symptoms at a younger age than women. Women lose blood—which contains iron—regularly during menstruation; therefore, women with the gene defects that cause hemochromatosis may not develop iron overload and related symptoms and complications until after menopause.

What Are the Symptoms of Hemochromatosis?

A person with hemochromatosis may notice one or more of the following symptoms:

- Joint pain

- Fatigue, or feeling tired
- Unexplained weight loss
- Abnormal bronze or gray skin color
- Abdominal pain
- Loss of sex drive

Not everyone with hemochromatosis will develop these symptoms.

What Are the Complications of Hemochromatosis?

Without treatment, iron may build up in the organs and cause complications, including:

- Cirrhosis, or scarring of liver tissue
- Diabetes
- Irregular heart rhythms or weakening of the heart muscle
- Arthritis
- Erectile dysfunction

The complication most often associated with hemochromatosis is liver damage. Iron buildup in the liver causes cirrhosis, which increases the chance of developing liver cancer.

For some people, complications may be the first sign of hemochromatosis. However, not everyone with hemochromatosis will develop complications.

Who Should Be Tested for Hemochromatosis?

Experts recommend testing for hemochromatosis in people who have symptoms, complications, or a family history of the disease.

Some researchers have suggested widespread screening for the *C282Y* mutation in the general population. However, screening is not cost effective. Although the *C282Y* mutation occurs quite frequently, the disease caused by the mutation is rare, and many people with two copies of the mutation never develop iron overload or organ damage.

Researchers and public health officials suggest the following:

- Siblings of people who have hemochromatosis should have their blood tested to see if they have the *C282Y* mutation.

- Parents, children, and other close relatives of people who have hemochromatosis should consider being tested.

- Healthcare providers should consider testing people who have severe and continuing fatigue, unexplained cirrhosis, joint pain or arthritis, heart problems, erectile dysfunction, or diabetes because these health issues may result from hemochromatosis.

Eating, Diet, and Nutrition

Iron is an essential nutrient found in many foods. People with hemochromatosis absorb much more iron from the food they eat compared with healthy people. People with hemochromatosis can help prevent iron overload by:

- Eating only moderate amounts of iron-rich foods, such as red meat and organ meat

- Avoiding supplements that contain iron

- Avoiding supplements that contain vitamin C, which increases iron absorption

People with hemochromatosis can take steps to help prevent liver damage, including:

- Limiting the amount of alcoholic beverages they drink because alcohol increases their chance of cirrhosis and liver cancer

- Avoiding alcoholic beverages entirely if they already have cirrhosis

Chapter 9

Leukemia

Chapter Contents

Section 9.1

Leukemia: An Overview

This section includes text excerpted from "Leukemia," Centers for
Disease Control and Prevention (CDC), May 29, 2018.

What Is Leukemia?

Leukemia is a cancer of the bone marrow (the soft, sponge-like
tissue in the center of most bones that makes blood cells) and blood.
The two main kinds of leukemia are:

- Lymphocytic leukemia (also known as "lymphoblastic leukemia")
  is when the body makes too many of a certain kind of white
  blood cells (WBCs), called "lymphocytes."

- Myelogenous leukemia (also known as "myeloid leukemia" or
  "myelocytic leukemia") is when the body makes too many of a
  certain kind of white blood cells, called "granulocytes."

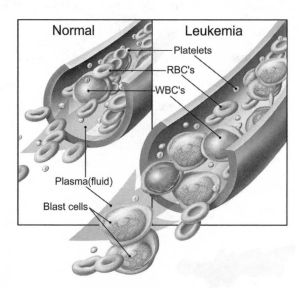

Figure 9.1. *Normal Blood Cells and Blood Cells with Leukemia*

*This image shows normal blood cells and blood cells with leukemia. Platelets, red
blood cells (RBC's), white blood cells (WBC's), plasma (fluid), and blast cells are
labeled.*

Leukemia can be acute or chronic. Acute types of leukemia progress quickly, while chronic types of leukemia progress slowly, leading to different treatments.

Leukemia is the most common kind of cancer among children and teens. Acute lymphocytic leukemia (ALL) is more common among children and teens than among adults. However, because other types of leukemia become more common with age, most leukemia is found in among adults.

What Causes Leukemia

Scientists do not fully understand all of the causes of leukemia, but research has found many links. For example:

- Being exposed to benzene or large doses of ionizing radiation has caused leukemia in some people.

- Tobacco smoke contains cancer-causing chemicals (including benzene), which are linked to acute myeloid leukemia (AML) in adults.

- Family history also has been linked with higher risk of some kinds of leukemia, such as chronic lymphocytic leukemia (CLL).

- Some people with Down syndrome or blood disorders, such as polycythemia vera (a disease in which there are too many red blood cells in the bone marrow and blood, causing the blood to thicken), may be more likely to develop leukemia.

- Most people with chronic myelogenous leukemia (CML) have a gene mutation (change) called the "Philadelphia chromosome" (Ph). It results in the bone marrow making an enzyme that causes too many stem cells to become white blood cells. The Philadelphia chromosome is not passed from parent to child.

- White people are more likely than Black people to develop lymphocytic leukemia, but scientists do not know why. Scientists also do not know why men are more likely than women to develop leukemia.

What Are the Symptoms of Leukemia?

Chronic lymphocytic leukemia usually does not cause any symptoms and is usually found during a routine blood test. If it does cause symptoms, they can include swollen lymph nodes and feeling tired. Symptoms of chronic myelogenous leukemia include fever, night sweats, and feeling tired. Sometimes, chronic myelogenous leukemia does not cause any symptoms.

The early symptoms of acute myelogenous leukemia (AML) and acute lymphocytic leukemia may be like those caused by the flu or other common diseases. Symptoms include fever, night sweats, feeling tired, feeling out of breath, and bruising or bleeding easily.

These symptoms can also come from other conditions. If you have any of them, talk to your doctor.

Section 9.2

Childhood Acute Lymphoblastic Leukemia

This section includes text excerpted from "Childhood Acute Lymphoblastic Leukemia Treatment (PDQ®)—Patient Version," National Cancer Institute (NCI), January 15, 2019.

What Is Childhood Acute Lymphoblastic?

Childhood acute lymphoblastic leukemia (also called "ALL" or "acute lymphocytic leukemia") is a cancer of the blood and bone marrow. This type of cancer usually gets worse quickly if it is not treated.

Acute lymphoblastic leukemia is the most common type of cancer in children.

Leukemia and Blood Stem Cells

In a healthy child, the bone marrow makes blood stem cells (immature cells) that become mature blood cells over time. A blood stem cell may become a myeloid stem cell or a lymphoid stem cell.

A myeloid stem cell becomes one of three types of mature blood cells:

- Red blood cells that carry oxygen and other substances to all tissues of the body

- Platelets that form blood clots to stop bleeding

- White blood cells that fight infection and disease

A lymphoid stem cell becomes a lymphoblast cell and then becomes one of three types of lymphocytes (white blood cells):

- B lymphocytes that make antibodies to help fight infection

- T lymphocytes that help B lymphocytes make the antibodies that help fight infection

- Natural killer cells that attack cancer cells and viruses

In a child with ALL, too many stem cells become lymphoblasts, B lymphocytes, or T lymphocytes. The cells do not work as normal lymphocytes and are not able to fight infection very well. These cells are cancer (leukemia) cells. Also, as the number of leukemia cells increases in the blood and bone marrow, there is less room for healthy white blood cells, red blood cells, and platelets. This may lead to infection, anemia, and easy bleeding.

Risks of Childhood Acute Lymphoblastic Leukemia

Anything that increases your risk of getting a disease is called a "risk factor." Having a risk factor does not mean that you will get cancer; not having risk factors does not mean that you will not get cancer. Talk with your child's doctor if you think your child may be at risk.

Possible risk factors for ALL include the following:

- Being exposed to X-rays before birth

- Being exposed to radiation

- Past treatment with chemotherapy

- Having certain genetic conditions, such as:
  - Down syndrome
  - Neurofibromatosis type 1
  - Bloom syndrome
  - Fanconi anemia
  - Ataxia-telangiectasia
  - Li-Fraumeni syndrome
  - Constitutional mismatch repair deficiency (CMMRD) (mutations in certain genes that stop deoxyribonucleic acid (DNA) from repairing itself, which leads to the growth of cancers at an early age)

- Having certain changes in the chromosomes or genes

Signs of Childhood Acute Lymphoblastic Leukemia

These and other signs and symptoms may be caused by childhood ALL or by other conditions. Check with your child's doctor if your child has any of the following:

- Fever

- Easy bruising or bleeding

- Petechiae (flat, pinpoint, dark-red spots under the skin that are caused by bleeding)

- Bone or joint pain

- Painless lumps in the neck, underarm, stomach, or groin

- Pain or feeling of fullness below the ribs

- Weakness, feeling tired, or looking pale

- Loss of appetite

Diagnosis of Childhood Acute Lymphoblastic Leukemia

The following tests and procedures may be used to diagnose childhood ALL and to find out if leukemia cells have spread to other parts of the body, such as the brain or testicles:

- **Physical exam and history:** An exam of the body to check general signs of health, including checking for signs of disease, such as lumps or anything else that seems unusual. A history of the patient's health habits and past illnesses and treatments will also be taken.

- **A complete blood count (CBC) with differential:** A procedure in which a sample of blood is drawn and checked for the following:

  - The number of red blood cells and platelets

  - The number and type of white blood cells

  - The amount of hemoglobin (the protein that carries oxygen) in the red blood cells

  - The portion of the sample made up of red blood cells

- **Blood chemistry studies:** A procedure in which a blood sample is checked to measure the amounts of certain substances released into the blood by organs and tissues in the body. An unusual (higher or lower than normal) amount of a substance can be a sign of disease.

- **Bone marrow aspiration and biopsy:** The removal of bone marrow and a small piece of bone by inserting a hollow needle into the hipbone or breastbone. A pathologist views the bone marrow and bone under a microscope to look for signs of cancer.

The following tests are done on blood or the bone marrow tissue that is removed:

- **Cytogenetic analysis:** A laboratory test in which the cells in a sample of blood or bone marrow are viewed under a microscope to look for certain changes in the chromosomes of lymphocytes. For example, in Philadelphia chromosome-positive ALL, part of one chromosome switches places with part of another chromosome. This is called the "Philadelphia chromosome" (Ph).

- **Immunophenotyping:** A laboratory test in which the antigens or markers on the surface of a blood or bone marrow cell are checked to see if they are lymphocytes or myeloid cells. If the cells are malignant lymphocytes (cancer), they are checked to see if they are B lymphocytes or T lymphocytes.

- **Lumbar puncture (LP):** A procedure used to collect a sample of cerebrospinal fluid (CSF) from the spinal column. This is done by placing a needle between two bones in the spine and into the CSF around the spinal cord and removing a sample of the fluid. The sample of CSF is checked under a microscope for signs that leukemia cells have spread to the brain and spinal cord. This procedure is also called an "LP" or "spinal tap." This procedure is done after leukemia is diagnosed to find out if leukemia cells have spread to the brain and spinal cord. Intrathecal chemotherapy is given after the sample of fluid is removed to treat any leukemia cells that may have spread to the brain and spinal cord.

- **Chest X-ray:** An X-ray of the organs and bones inside the chest. An X-ray is a type of energy beam that can go through the body and onto film, making a picture of areas inside the body. The chest X-ray is done to see if leukemia cells have formed a mass in the middle of the chest.

Factors Affecting Prognosis and Treatment Options

The prognosis (chance of recovery) depends on:

- How quickly and how low the leukemia cell count drops after the first month of treatment
- Age at the time of diagnosis, sex, race, and ethnic background
- The number of white blood cells in the blood at the time of diagnosis
- Whether the leukemia cells began from B lymphocytes or T lymphocytes
- Whether there are certain changes in the chromosomes or genes of the lymphocytes with cancer
- Whether the child has Down syndrome
- Whether leukemia cells are found in the cerebrospinal fluid
- The child's weight at the time of diagnosis and during treatment

Treatment options depend on:

- Whether the leukemia cells began from B lymphocytes or T lymphocytes
- Whether the child has standard-risk, high-risk, or very high-risk ALL
- The age of the child at the time of diagnosis
- Whether there are certain changes in the chromosomes of lymphocytes, such as the Philadelphia chromosome
- Whether the child was treated with steroids before the start of induction therapy
- How quickly and how low the leukemia cell count drops during treatment

For leukemia that relapses (comes back) after treatment, the prognosis and treatment options depend partly on the following:

- How long it is between the time of diagnosis and when leukemia comes back
- Whether leukemia comes back in the bone marrow or in other parts of the body

Section 9.3

Adult Acute Lymphoblastic Leukemia

This section includes text excerpted from "Adult Acute Lymphoblastic Leukemia Treatment (PDQ®)—Patient Version," National Cancer Institute (NCI), April 12, 2019.

What Is Adult Acute Lymphoblastic Leukemia?

Adult acute lymphoblastic leukemia (ALL, also called "acute lymphocytic leukemia") is a cancer of the blood and bone marrow. This type of cancer usually gets worse quickly if it is not treated.

Leukemia and Blood Stem Cells

Normally, the bone marrow makes blood stem cells (immature cells) that become mature blood cells over time. A blood stem cell may become a myeloid stem cell or a lymphoid stem cell.

A myeloid stem cell becomes one of three types of mature blood cells:

- Red blood cells (RBCs) that carry oxygen and other substances to all tissues of the body

- Platelets that form blood clots to stop bleeding

- Granulocytes (white blood cells (WBCs)) that fight infection and disease

A lymphoid stem cell becomes a lymphoblast cell and then becomes one of three types of lymphocytes (white blood cells):

- B lymphocytes that make antibodies to help fight infection

- T lymphocytes that help B lymphocytes make the antibodies that help fight infection

- Natural killer cells that attack cancer cells and viruses

In acute lymphoblastic leukemia, too many stem cells become lymphoblasts, B lymphocytes, or T lymphocytes. These cells are also called "leukemia cells." These leukemia cells are not able to fight infection very well. Also, as the number of leukemia cells increases in the blood and bone marrow, there is less room for healthy white blood cells, red blood cells, and platelets. This may cause infection, anemia, and easy bleeding. The cancer can also spread to the central nervous system (brain and spinal cord).

Risks of Developing Acute Lymphoblastic Leukemia

Anything that increases your risk of getting a disease is called a "risk factor." Having a risk factor does not mean that you will get cancer; not having risk factors does not mean that you will not get cancer. Talk with your doctor if you think you may be at risk. Possible risk factors for ALL include the following:

- Being male

- Being White

- Being older than 70 years of age

- Having had past treatment with chemotherapy or radiation therapy

- Being exposed to high levels of radiation in the environment (such as nuclear radiation)

- Having certain genetic disorders, such as Down syndrome

Signs and Symptoms of Adult Acute Lymphoblastic Leukemia

The early signs and symptoms of ALL may be similar to the flu or other common diseases. Check with your doctor if you have any of the following:

- Weakness or feeling tired

- Fever or night sweats

- Easy bruising or bleeding

- Petechiae (flat, pinpoint spots under the skin, caused by bleeding)

- Shortness of breath

- Weight loss or loss of appetite

- Pain in the bones or stomach

- Pain or feeling of fullness below the ribs

- Painless lumps in the neck, underarm, stomach, or groin

- Having many infections

These and other signs and symptoms may be caused by adult acute lymphoblastic leukemia or by other conditions.

Diagnosis of Adult Acute Lymphoblastic Leukemia

The following tests and procedures may be used:

- **Physical exam and history:** An exam of the body to check general signs of health, including checking for signs of disease, such as infection or anything else that seems unusual. A history of the patient's health habits and past illnesses and treatments will also be taken.

- **A complete blood count (CBC) with differential:** A procedure in which a sample of blood is drawn and checked for the following:

  - The number of red blood cells and platelets

  - The number and type of white blood cells

  - The amount of hemoglobin (the protein that carries oxygen) in the red blood cells

  - The portion of the blood sample made up of red blood cells

- **Blood chemistry studies:** A procedure in which a blood sample is checked to measure the amounts of certain substances released into the blood by organs and tissues in the body. An unusual (higher or lower than normal) amount of a substance can be a sign of disease.

- **Peripheral blood smear:** A procedure in which a sample of blood is checked for blast cells, the number and kinds of white blood cells, the number of platelets, and changes in the shape of blood cells.

- **Bone marrow aspiration and biopsy:** The removal of bone marrow, blood, and a small piece of bone by inserting a hollow needle into the hipbone or breastbone. A pathologist views the bone marrow, blood, and bone under a microscope to look for abnormal cells.

The following tests may be done on the samples of blood or bone marrow tissue that are removed:

- **Cytogenetic analysis:** A laboratory test in which the cells in a sample of blood or bone marrow are looked at under a microscope to find out if there are certain changes in the chromosomes of lymphocytes. For example, in Philadelphia chromosome-positive ALL, part of one chromosome switches places with part of another chromosome. This is called the "Philadelphia chromosome" (Ph).

- **Immunophenotyping:** A process used to identify cells, based on the types of antigens or markers on the surface of the cell. This process is used to diagnose the subtype of ALL by comparing the cancer cells to normal cells of the immune system. For example, a cytochemistry study may test the cells in a sample of tissue using chemicals (dyes) to look for certain changes in the sample. A chemical may cause a color change in one type of leukemia cell but not in another type of leukemia cell.

Factors Affecting Prognosis and Treatment Options

The prognosis (chance of recovery) and treatment options depend on the following:

- The age of the patient
- Whether the cancer has spread to the brain or spinal cord
- Whether there are certain changes in the genes, including the Philadelphia chromosome
- Whether the cancer has been treated before or has recurred (come back)

Section 9.4

Childhood Acute Myeloid Leukemia

This section includes text excerpted from "Childhood Acute Myeloid Leukemia/Other Myeloid Malignancies Treatment (PDQ®)—Patient Version," National Cancer Institute (NCI), April 12, 2019.

What Is Childhood Acute Myeloid Leukemia?

Childhood acute myeloid leukemia (AML) is a cancer of the blood and bone marrow. AML is also called "acute myelogenous leukemia," "acute myeloblastic leukemia," "acute granulocytic leukemia," and "acute nonlymphocytic leukemia." Cancers that are acute usually get worse quickly if they are not treated. Cancers that are chronic usually get worse slowly.

Leukemia and Blood Stem Cells

Normally, the bone marrow makes blood stem cells (immature cells) that become mature blood cells over time. A blood stem cell may become a myeloid stem cell or a lymphoid stem cell. A lymphoid stem cell becomes a white blood cell (WBC).

A myeloid stem cell becomes one of three types of mature blood cells:

- Red blood cells (RBCs) that carry oxygen and other substances to all tissues of the body

- White blood cells that fight infection and disease

- Platelets that form blood clots to stop bleeding

In AML, the myeloid stem cells usually become a type of immature white blood cell called "myeloblasts" (or myeloid blasts). The myeloblasts, or leukemia cells, in AML are abnormal and do not become healthy white blood cells. The leukemia cells can build up in the blood and bone marrow, so there is less room for healthy white blood cells, red blood cells, and platelets. When this happens, infection, anemia, or easy bleeding may occur.

The leukemia cells can spread outside the blood to other parts of the body, including the central nervous system (brain and spinal cord), skin, and gums. Sometimes, leukemia cells form a solid tumor called a "granulocytic sarcoma" (GS) or "chloroma."

Recurring Acute Myeloid Leukemia or Myelodysplastic Syndromes

Cancer treatment with certain chemotherapy drugs and/or radiation therapy may cause therapy-related AML (t-AML) or therapy-related MDS (t-MDS). The risk of these therapy-related myeloid diseases depends on the total dose of the chemotherapy drugs used and the radiation dose and treatment field. Some patients also have an inherited risk for t-AML and t-MDS. These therapy-related diseases usually occur within seven years after treatment, but they are rare in children.

Risk Factors for Childhood Acute Myeloid Leukemia

Anything that increases your risk of getting a disease is called a "risk factor." Having a risk factor does not mean that you will get cancer; not having risk factors does not mean that you will not get cancer. Talk with your child's doctor if you think your child may be at risk. These and other factors may increase the risk of childhood AML, acute promyelocytic leukemia (APL), juvenile myelomonocytic leukemia (JMML), chronic myelogenous leukemia (CML), and myelodysplastic syndromes (MDS):

- Having a sister or brother, especially a twin, with leukemia
- Being Hispanic
- Being exposed to cigarette smoke or alcohol before birth
- Having a personal history of aplastic anemia
- Having a personal or family history of MDS
- Having a family history of AML
- Past treatment with chemotherapy or radiation therapy
- Being exposed to ionizing radiation or chemicals such as benzene
- Having certain syndromes or inherited disorders, such as:
  - Down syndrome
  - Aplastic anemia
  - Fanconi anemia
  - Neurofibromatosis type 1 (NF1)
  - Noonan syndrome
  - Shwachman-Diamond syndrome
  - Li-Fraumeni syndrome

Signs and Symptoms of Childhood Acute Myeloid Leukemia

These and other signs and symptoms may be caused by childhood AML, APL, JMML, CML, MDS, or by other conditions. Check with a doctor if your child has any of the following:

- Fever with or without an infection
- Night sweats
- Shortness of breath

- Weakness or feeling tired

- Easy bruising or bleeding

- Petechiae (flat, pinpoint spots under the skin that is caused by bleeding)

- Pain in the bones or joints

- Pain or feeling of fullness below the ribs

- Painless lumps in the neck, underarm, stomach, groin, or other parts of the body. In childhood AML, these lumps, called "leukemia cutis" (LC), may be blue or purple.

- Painless lumps that are sometimes around the eyes. These lumps, called "chloromas," are sometimes seen in childhood AML and may be blue-green.

- An eczema-like skin rash

The signs and symptoms of TAM may include the following:

- Swelling all over the body

- Shortness of breath

- Trouble breathing

- Weakness or feeling tired

- Bleeding a lot, even from a small cut

- Petechiae

- Pain below the ribs

- Skin rash

- Jaundice (yellowing of the skin and whites of the eyes)

- Headache, trouble seeing, and confusion

Sometimes, transient abnormal myelopoiesis does not cause any symptoms at all and is diagnosed after a routine blood test.

Diagnosis of Childhood Acute Myeloid Leukemia

The following tests and procedures may be used:

- **Physical exam and history:** An exam of the body to check general signs of health, including checking for signs of disease, such as lumps or anything else that seems unusual. A history of the patient's health habits and past illnesses and treatments will also be taken.

- **A complete blood count (CBC) with differential:** A procedure in which a sample of blood is drawn and checked for the following:

  - The number of red blood cells and platelets

  - The number and type of white blood cells

  - The amount of hemoglobin (the protein that carries oxygen) in the red blood cells

  - The portion of the blood sample made up of red blood cells

- **Blood chemistry studies:** A procedure in which a blood sample is checked to measure the amounts of certain substances released into the blood by organs and tissues in the body. An unusual (higher or lower than normal) amount of a substance can be a sign of disease.

- **Chest X-ray:** An X-ray of the organs and bones inside the chest. An X-ray is a type of energy beam that can go through the body and onto film, making a picture of areas inside the body.

- **Biopsy:** The removal of cells or tissues so they can be viewed under a microscope by a pathologist to check for signs of cancer. Biopsies that may be done include the following:

  - **Bone marrow aspiration and biopsy:** The removal of bone marrow, blood, and a small piece of bone by inserting a hollow needle into the hipbone or breastbone.

  - **Tumor biopsy:** A biopsy of a chloroma may be done.

  - **Lymph node biopsy:** The removal of all or part of a lymph node.

- **Immunophenotyping:** A process used to identify cells, based on the types of antigens or markers on the surface of the cell, that may include special staining of the blood and bone marrow cells. This process is used to diagnose the subtype of AML by comparing the cancer cells to normal cells of the immune system.

- **Cytogenetic analysis:** A laboratory test in which cells in a sample of blood or bone marrow are viewed under a microscope to look for certain changes in the chromosomes. Changes in the chromosomes include when part of one chromosome is switched with part of another chromosome, part of one chromosome is missing or repeated, or part of one chromosome is turned upside down.

The following test is a type of cytogenetic analysis:

- **Fluorescence in situ hybridization (FISH):** A laboratory technique used to look at genes or chromosomes in cells and tissues. Pieces of deoxyribonucleic acid (DNA) that contain a fluorescent dye are made in the laboratory and added to cells or tissues on a glass slide. When these pieces of DNA bind to specific genes or areas of chromosomes on the slide, they light up when viewed under a microscope with a special light.

- **Molecular testing:** A laboratory test to check for certain genes, proteins, or other molecules in a sample of blood or bone marrow. Molecular tests also check for certain changes in a gene or chromosome that may cause or affect the chance of developing AML. A molecular test may be used to help plan treatment, find out how well treatment is working, or make a prognosis.

- **Lumbar puncture (LP):** A procedure used to collect a sample of cerebrospinal fluid (CSF) from the spinal column. This is done by placing a needle between two bones in the spine and into the CSF around the spinal cord and removing a sample of the fluid. The sample of CSF is checked under a microscope for signs that leukemia cells have spread to the brain and spinal cord. This procedure is also called an "LP" or "spinal tap."

Factors Affecting Prognosis and Treatment Options

The prognosis (chance of recovery) and treatment options for childhood AML depend on the following:

- The age of the child when the cancer is diagnosed
- The race or ethnic group of the child
- Whether the child is greatly overweight
- Number of white blood cells in the blood at diagnosis
- Whether the AML occurred after previous cancer treatment
- The subtype of AML

- Whether there are certain chromosome or gene changes in the leukemia cells
- Whether the child has Down syndrome. Most children with AML and Down syndrome can be cured of their leukemia.
- Whether the leukemia is in the central nervous system (brain and spinal cord)
- How quickly the leukemia responds to treatment
- Whether the AML is newly diagnosed (untreated) or has recurred after treatment
- The length of time since treatment ended, for AML that has recurred

The prognosis for childhood APL depends on the following:

- Number of white blood cells in the blood at diagnosis
- Whether there are certain chromosome or gene changes in the leukemia cells
- Whether the APL is newly diagnosed or has recurred after treatment

The prognosis and treatment options for JMML depend on the following:

- The age of the child when the cancer is diagnosed
- The type of gene affected and the number of genes that have changed
- How many monocytes (a type of white blood cell) are in the blood
- How much hemoglobin is in the blood
- Whether the JMML is newly diagnosed or has recurred after treatment

The prognosis and treatment options for childhood CML depend on the following:

- How long it has been since the patient was diagnosed
- How many blast cells are in the blood
- Whether and how fully the blast cells disappear from the blood and bone marrow after therapy has started

- Whether the CML is newly diagnosed or has recurred after treatment

The prognosis and treatment options for MDS depend on the following:

- Whether the MDS was caused by previous cancer treatment

- How low the numbers of red blood cells, white blood cells, or platelets are

- Whether the MDS is newly diagnosed or has recurred after treatment

Section 9.5

Adult Acute Myeloid Leukemia

This section includes text excerpted from "Adult Acute Myeloid Leukemia Treatment (PDQ®)—Patient Version," National Cancer Institute (NCI), October 19, 2018.

What Is Adult Acute Myeloid Leukemia?

Adult acute myeloid leukemia (AML) is a cancer of the blood and bone marrow. This type of cancer usually gets worse quickly if it is not treated. It is the most common type of acute leukemia in adults. AML is also called "acute myelogenous leukemia," "acute myeloblastic leukemia," "acute granulocytic leukemia," and "acute nonlymphocytic leukemia."

Leukemia and Blood Stem Cells

Normally, the bone marrow makes blood stem cells (immature cells) that become mature blood cells over time. A blood stem cell may become a myeloid stem cell or a lymphoid stem cell. A lymphoid stem cell becomes a white blood cell (WBC).

A myeloid stem cell becomes one of three types of mature blood cells:

- Red blood cells (RBCs) that carry oxygen and other substances to all tissues of the body

- White blood cells that fight infection and disease

- Platelets that form blood clots to stop bleeding

In acute myeloid leukemia, the myeloid stem cells usually become a type of immature white blood cell called "myeloblasts" (or myeloid blasts). The myeloblasts in AML are abnormal and do not become healthy white blood cells. Sometimes in AML, too many stem cells become abnormal red blood cells or platelets. These abnormal white blood cells, red blood cells, or platelets are also called "leukemia cells" or "blasts." Leukemia cells can build up in the bone marrow and blood, so there is less room for healthy white blood cells, red blood cells, and platelets. When this happens, infection, anemia, or easy bleeding may occur. The leukemia cells can spread outside the blood to other parts of the body, including the central nervous system (brain and spinal cord), skin, and gums.

Subtypes of Acute Myeloid Leukemia

Most acute myeloid leukemia subtypes are based on how mature (developed) the cancer cells are at the time of diagnosis and how different they are from normal cells.

Acute promyelocytic leukemia (APL) is a subtype of AML that occurs when parts of two genes stick together. APL usually occurs in middle-aged adults. Signs of APL may include both bleeding and forming blood clots.

Risks of Adult Acute Myeloid Leukemia

Anything that increases your risk of getting a disease is called a "risk factor." Having a risk factor does not mean that you will get cancer; not having risk factors does not mean that you will not get cancer. Talk with your doctor if you think you may be at risk. Possible risk factors for AML include the following:

- Being male

- Smoking, especially after the age of 60

- Having had treatment with chemotherapy or radiation therapy in the past

- Having had treatment for childhood acute lymphoblastic leukemia (ALL) in the past

- Being exposed to radiation from an atomic bomb or to the chemical benzene

- Having a history of a blood disorder such as myelodysplastic syndrome

Signs and Symptoms of Adult Acute Myeloid Leukemia

The early signs and symptoms of AML may be similar to those caused by the flu or other common diseases. Check with your doctor if you have any of the following:

- Fever

- Shortness of breath

- Easy bruising or bleeding

- Petechiae (flat, pinpoint spots under the skin that are caused by bleeding)

- Weakness or feeling tired

- Weight loss or loss of appetite

Diagnosis of Adult Acute Myeloid Leukemia

The following tests and procedures may be used:

- **Physical exam and history:** An exam of the body to check general signs of health, including checking for signs of disease, such as lumps or anything else that seems unusual. A history of the patient's health habits and past illnesses and treatments will also be taken.

- **A complete blood count (CBC):** A procedure in which a sample of blood is drawn and checked for the following:

  - The number of red blood cells, white blood cells, and platelets

  - The amount of hemoglobin (the protein that carries oxygen) in the red blood cells

  - The portion of the sample made up of red blood cells

- **Peripheral blood smear:** A procedure in which a sample of blood is checked for blast cells, the number and kinds of white blood cells, the number of platelets, and changes in the shape of blood cells.

- **Bone marrow aspiration and biopsy:** The removal of bone marrow, blood, and a small piece of bone by inserting a hollow needle into the hipbone or breastbone. A pathologist views the bone marrow, blood, and bone under a microscope to look for signs of cancer.

- **Cytogenetic analysis:** A laboratory test in which the cells in a sample of blood or bone marrow are viewed under a microscope to look for certain changes in the chromosomes. Other tests, such as fluorescence in situ hybridization (FISH), may also be done to look for certain changes in the chromosomes.

- **Immunophenotyping:** A process used to identify cells, based on the types of antigens or markers on the surface of the cell. This process is used to diagnose the subtype of AML by comparing the cancer cells to normal cells of the immune system. For example, a cytochemistry study may test the cells in a sample of tissue using chemicals (dyes) to look for certain changes in the sample. A chemical may cause a color change in one type of leukemia cell but not in another type of leukemia cell.

- **Reverse transcription-polymerase chain reaction test (RT-PCR):** A laboratory test in which cells in a sample of tissue are studied using chemicals to look for certain changes in the structure or function of genes. This test is used to diagnose certain types of AML including acute promyelocytic leukemia (APL).

Factors Affecting Prognosis and Treatment Options

The prognosis (chance of recovery) and treatment options depend on:

- The age of the patient

- The subtype of AML

- Whether the patient received chemotherapy in the past to treat a different cancer

- Whether there is a history of a blood disorder such as myelodysplastic syndrome

- Whether the cancer has spread to the central nervous system

- Whether the cancer has been treated before or recurred (come back)

It is important that acute leukemia be treated right away.

Section 9.6

Chronic Lymphocytic Leukemia

This section includes text excerpted from "Chronic Lymphocytic Leukemia Treatment (PDQ®)—Patient Version," National Cancer Institute (NCI), January 22, 2019.

What Is Chronic Lymphocytic Leukemia?

Chronic lymphocytic leukemia (also called "CLL") is a blood and bone marrow disease that usually gets worse slowly. CLL is one of the most common types of leukemia in adults. It often occurs during or after middle age; it rarely occurs in children.

Leukemia and Blood Stem Cells

Normally, the body makes blood stem cells (immature cells) that become mature blood cells over time. A blood stem cell may become a myeloid stem cell or a lymphoid stem cell.

A myeloid stem cell becomes one of three types of mature blood cells:

- Red blood cells (RBCs) that carry oxygen and other substances to all tissues of the body

- White blood cells (WBCs) that fight infection and disease

- Platelets that form blood clots to stop bleeding

A lymphoid stem cell becomes a lymphoblast cell and then one of three types of lymphocytes (white blood cells):

- B lymphocytes that make antibodies to help fight infection

- T lymphocytes that help B lymphocytes make antibodies to fight infection

- Natural killer cells that attack cancer cells and viruses

In chronic lymphocytic leukemia, too many blood stem cells become abnormal lymphocytes and do not become healthy white blood cells. The abnormal lymphocytes may also be called "leukemia cells." The lymphocytes are not able to fight infection very well. Also, as the number of lymphocytes increases in the blood and bone marrow, there is less room for healthy white blood cells, red blood cells, and platelets. This may cause infection, anemia, and easy bleeding.

Risks of Chronic Lymphocytic Leukemia

Anything that increases your risk of getting a disease is called a "risk factor." Having a risk factor does not mean that you will get cancer; not having risk factors does not mean that you will not get cancer. Talk with your doctor if you think you may be at risk. Risk factors for CLL include the following:

- Being middle-aged or older, male, or White

- A family history of CLL or cancer of the lymph system

- Having relatives who are Russian Jews or Eastern European Jews

Signs and Symptoms of Chronic Lymphocytic Leukemia

Usually, chronic lymphocytic leukemia does not cause any signs or symptoms and is found during a routine blood test. Signs and symptoms may be caused by CLL or by other conditions. Check with your doctor if you have any of the following:

- Painless swelling of the lymph nodes in the neck, underarm, stomach, or groin

- Feeling very tired

- Pain or fullness below the ribs

- Fever and infection

- Weight loss for no known reason

Diagnosis of Chronic Lymphocytic Leukemia

The following tests and procedures may be used:

- **Physical exam and history:** An exam of the body to check general signs of health, including checking for signs of disease, such as lumps or anything else that seems unusual. A history of the patient's health habits and past illnesses and treatments will also be taken.

- **A complete blood count (CBC) with differential:** A procedure in which a sample of blood is drawn and checked for the following:

  - The number of red blood cells and platelets

  - The number and type of white blood cell

  - The amount of hemoglobin (the protein that carries oxygen) in the red blood cells

  - The portion of the blood sample made up of red blood cells

- **Immunophenotyping:** A laboratory test in which the antigens or markers on the surface of a blood or bone marrow cell are checked to see if they are lymphocytes or myeloid cells. If the cells are malignant lymphocytes (cancer), they are checked to see if they are B lymphocytes or T lymphocytes.

- **Fluorescence in situ hybridization (FISH):** A laboratory technique used to look at genes or chromosomes in cells and tissues. Pieces of deoxyribonucleic acid (DNA) that contain a fluorescent dye are made in the laboratory and added to cells or tissues on a glass slide. When these pieces of DNA bind to specific genes or areas of chromosomes on the slide, they light up when viewed under a microscope with a special light.

- **Flow cytometry:** A laboratory test that measures the number of cells in a sample, the percentage of live cells in a sample, and certain characteristics of cells, such as size, shape, and the presence of tumor markers on the cell surface. The cells are stained with a light-sensitive dye, placed in a fluid, and passed in a stream before a laser or other type of light.

The measurements are based on how the light-sensitive dye reacts to the light.

- *IgVH* **gene mutation test:** A laboratory test done on a bone marrow or blood sample to check for an *IgVH* gene mutation. Patients with an *IgVH* gene mutation have a better prognosis.

- **Bone marrow aspiration and biopsy:** The removal of bone marrow, blood, and a small piece of bone by inserting a hollow needle into the hipbone or breastbone. A pathologist views the bone marrow, blood, and bone under a microscope to look for abnormal cells.

Factors Affecting Treatment Options and Prognosis

Treatment options depend on:

- The stage of the disease
- Red blood cell, white blood cell, and platelet blood counts
- Whether there are signs or symptoms, such as fever, chills, or weight loss
- Whether the liver, spleen, or lymph nodes are larger than normal
- The response to initial treatment
- Whether the CLL has recurred (come back)

The prognosis (chance of recovery) depends on:

- Whether there is a change in the DNA and the type of change, if there is one
- Whether lymphocytes are spread throughout the bone marrow
- The stage of the disease
- Whether the CLL gets better with treatment or has recurred
- Whether the CLL progresses to lymphoma or prolymphocytic leukemia
- The patient's age and general health

Section 9.7

Chronic Myelogenous Leukemia

This section includes text excerpted from "Chronic Myelogenous Leukemia Treatment (PDQ®)—Patient Version," National Cancer Institute (NCI), January 30, 2019.

What Is Chronic Myelogenous Leukemia?

Chronic myelogenous leukemia (also called "CML" or "chronic granulocytic leukemia") is a slowly progressing blood and bone marrow disease that usually occurs during or after middle age, and rarely occurs in children.

Leukemia and Blood Stem Cells

Normally, the bone marrow makes blood stem cells (immature cells) that become mature blood cells over time. A blood stem cell may become a myeloid stem cell or a lymphoid stem cell. A lymphoid stem cell becomes a white blood cell.

A myeloid stem cell becomes one of three types of mature blood cells:

- Red blood cells (RBCs) that carry oxygen and other substances to all tissues of the body

- Platelets that form blood clots to stop bleeding

- Granulocytes (white blood cells) that fight infection and disease

In chronic myelogenous leukemia, too many blood stem cells become a type of white blood cell (WBC) called "granulocytes." These granulocytes are abnormal and do not become healthy white blood cells. They are also called "leukemia cells." The leukemia cells can build up in the blood and bone marrow, so there is less room for healthy white blood cells, red blood cells, and platelets. When this happens, infection, anemia, or easy bleeding may occur.

Signs and Symptoms of Chronic Myelogenous Leukemia

These and other signs and symptoms may be caused by CML or by other conditions. Check with your doctor if you have any of the following:

- Feeling very tired

- Weight loss for no known reason

- Night sweats

- Fever

- Pain or a feeling of fullness below the ribs on the left side

Sometimes, chronic myelogenous leukemia does not cause any symptoms at all.

Chronic Myelogenous Leukemia and Gene Mutation

Every cell in the body contains deoxyribonucleic acid (DNA) (genetic material) that determines how the cell looks and acts. DNA is contained inside chromosomes. In CML, part of the DNA from one chromosome moves to another chromosome. This change is called the "Philadelphia chromosome" (Ph). It results in the bone marrow making a protein, called "tyrosine kinase," that causes too many stem cells to become white blood cells (granulocytes or blasts).

The Philadelphia chromosome is not passed from parent to child.

Diagnosis of Chronic Myelogenous Leukemia

The following tests and procedures may be used:

- **Physical exam and history:** An exam of the body to check general signs of health, including checking for signs of disease such as an enlarged spleen. A history of the patient's health habits and past illnesses and treatments will also be taken.

- **A complete blood count (CBC) with differential:** A procedure in which a sample of blood is drawn and checked for the following:

  - The number of red blood cells and platelets

  - The number and type of white blood cells

  - The amount of hemoglobin (the protein that carries oxygen) in the red blood cells

  - The portion of the blood sample made up of red blood cells

- **Blood chemistry studies:** A procedure in which a blood sample is checked to measure the amounts of certain substances released into the blood by organs and tissues in the body. An unusual (higher or lower than normal) amount of a substance can be a sign of disease.

- **Bone marrow aspiration and biopsy:** The removal of bone marrow, blood, and a small piece of bone by inserting a needle into the hipbone or breastbone. A pathologist views the bone marrow, blood, and bone under a microscope to look for abnormal cells.

One of the following tests may be done on the samples of blood or bone marrow tissue that are removed:

- **Cytogenetic analysis:** A test in which cells in a sample of blood or bone marrow are viewed under a microscope to look for certain changes in the chromosomes, such as the Philadelphia chromosome.

- **Fluorescence in situ hybridization (FISH):** A laboratory technique used to look at genes or chromosomes in cells and tissues. Pieces of DNA that contain a fluorescent dye are made in the laboratory and added to cells or tissues on a glass slide. When these pieces of DNA bind to specific genes or areas of chromosomes on the slide, they light up when viewed under a microscope with a special light.

- **Reverse transcription-polymerase chain reaction (RT-PCR):** A laboratory test in which cells in a sample of tissue are studied using chemicals to look for certain changes in the structure or function of genes.

Factors Affecting Prognosis and Treatment Options

The prognosis (chance of recovery) and treatment options depend on the following:

- The patient's age
- The phase of CML
- The amount of blasts in the blood or bone marrow
- The size of the spleen at diagnosis
- The patient's general health

Section 9.8

Hairy Cell Leukemia

This section includes text excerpted from "Hairy Cell Leukemia
Treatment (PDQ®)—Patient Version," National Cancer
Institute (NCI), May 18, 2018.

What Is Hairy Cell Leukemia?

Hairy cell leukemia is a cancer of the blood and bone marrow. This
rare type of leukemia gets worse slowly or does not get worse at all.
The disease is called "hairy cell leukemia" because the leukemia cells
look "hairy" when viewed under a microscope.

Leukemia and Blood Stem Cells

Normally, the bone marrow makes blood stem cells (immature
cells) that become mature blood cells over time. A blood stem cell may
become a myeloid stem cell or a lymphoid stem cell.

A myeloid stem cell becomes one of three types of mature blood cells:

- Red blood cells (RBCs) that carry oxygen and other substances
  to all tissues of the body

- White blood cells (WBCs) that fight infection and disease

- Platelets that form blood clots to stop bleeding

A lymphoid stem cell becomes a lymphoblast cell and then turns
into one of three types of lymphocytes (white blood cells):

- B lymphocytes that make antibodies to help fight infection

- T lymphocytes that help B lymphocytes make antibodies to help
  fight infection

- Natural killer cells that attack cancer cells and viruses

In hairy cell leukemia, too many blood stem cells become lymphocytes. These lymphocytes are abnormal and do not become healthy
white blood cells. They are also called "leukemia cells." The leukemia
cells can build up in the blood and bone marrow, so there is less room
for healthy white blood cells, red blood cells, and platelets. This may
cause infection, anemia, and easy bleeding. Some of the leukemia cells
may collect in the spleen and cause it to swell.

Risks of Hairy Cell Leukemia

Anything that increases your chance of getting a disease is called a "risk factor." Having a risk factor does not mean that you will get cancer; not having risk factors does not mean that you will not get cancer. Talk with your doctor if you think you may be at risk. The cause of hairy cell leukemia is unknown. It occurs more often in older men.

Signs and Symptoms of Hairy Cell Leukemia

These and other signs and symptoms may be caused by hairy cell leukemia or by other conditions. Check with your doctor if you have any of the following:

- Weakness or feeling tired

- Fever or frequent infections

- Easy bruising or bleeding

- Shortness of breath

- Weight loss for no known reason

- Pain or a feeling of fullness below the ribs

- Painless lumps in the neck, underarm, stomach, or groin

Diagnosis of Hairy Cell Leukemia

The following tests and procedures may be used:

- **Physical exam and history:** An exam of the body to check general signs of health, including checking for signs of disease, such as a swollen spleen, lumps, or anything else that seems unusual. A history of the patient's health habits and past illnesses and treatments will also be taken.

- **A complete blood count (CBC):** A procedure in which a sample of blood is drawn and checked for the following:

  - The number of red blood cells, white blood cells, and platelets

  - The amount of hemoglobin (the protein that carries oxygen) in the red blood cells

  - The portion of the sample made up of red blood cells

- **Peripheral blood smear:** A procedure in which a sample of blood is checked for cells that look "hairy," the number and kinds of white blood cells, the number of platelets, and changes in the shape of blood cells.

- **Blood chemistry studies:** A procedure in which a blood sample is checked to measure the amounts of certain substances released into the blood by organs and tissues in the body. An unusual (higher or lower than normal) amount of a substance can be a sign of disease.

- **Bone marrow aspiration and biopsy:** The removal of bone marrow, blood, and a small piece of bone by inserting a hollow needle into the hipbone or breastbone. A pathologist views the bone marrow, blood, and bone under a microscope to look for signs of cancer.

- **Immunophenotyping:** A laboratory test in which the antigens or markers on the surface of a blood or bone marrow cell are checked to see what type of cell it is. This test is done to diagnose the specific type of leukemia by comparing the cancer cells to normal cells of the immune system.

- **Flow cytometry:** A laboratory test that measures the number of cells in a sample, the percentage of live cells in a sample, and certain characteristics of cells, such as size, shape, and the presence of tumor markers on the cell surface. The cells are stained with a light-sensitive dye, placed in a fluid, and passed in a stream before a laser or other type of light. The measurements are based on how the light-sensitive dye reacts to the light.

- **Cytogenetic analysis:** A laboratory test in which cells in a sample of tissue are viewed under a microscope to look for certain changes in the chromosomes.

- **Gene mutation test:** A laboratory test done on a bone marrow or blood sample to check for mutations in the *BRAF* gene. A *BRAF* gene mutation is often found in patients with hairy cell leukemia.

- **Computed tomography (CT or CAT scan):** A procedure that makes a series of detailed pictures of areas inside the body, taken from different angles. The pictures are made by a computer linked to an X-ray machine. A dye may be injected into a vein or swallowed to help the organs or tissues show up more clearly. This procedure is also called "computed tomography," "computerized tomography," or "computerized axial tomography." A CT scan of the abdomen may be done to check for swollen lymph nodes or a swollen spleen.

Factors Affecting Treatment Options and Prognosis

The treatment options may depend on the following:
The number of hairy (leukemia) cells and healthy blood cells in the blood and bone marrow.

- Whether the spleen is swollen

- Whether there are signs or symptoms of leukemia, such as infection

- Whether the leukemia has recurred (come back) after previous treatment

The prognosis (chance of recovery) depends on the following:

- Whether the hairy cell leukemia does not grow or grows so slowly it does not need treatment

- Whether the hairy cell leukemia responds to treatment

Treatment often results in a long-lasting remission (a period during which some or all of the signs and symptoms of the leukemia are gone). If the leukemia returns after it has been in remission, retreatment often causes another remission.

Chapter 10

Lymphoma

Chapter Contents

Section 10.1

Lymphoma: An Overview

This section includes text excerpted from "Lymphoma," Centers for Disease Control and Prevention (CDC), May 29, 2018.

What Is Lymphoma?

"Lymphoma" is a general term for cancers that start in the lymph system (the tissues and organs that produce, store, and carry white blood cells (WBCs) that fight infections). The two main kinds of lymphoma are:

- Hodgkin lymphoma (HL), which spreads in an orderly manner from one group of lymph nodes to another

- Non-Hodgkin lymphoma (NHL), which spreads through the lymphatic system in a non-orderly manner

Hodgkin lymphoma and non-Hodgkin lymphoma can occur in children, teens, and adults.

What Causes Lymphoma

Non-Hodgkin lymphoma becomes more common as people get older. Unlike most cancers, rates of Hodgkin lymphoma are highest among teens and young adults (individuals between the ages of 15 and 39) and again among older adults (individuals 75 years of age or older). White people are more likely than Black people to develop non-Hodgkin lymphoma, and men are more likely than women to develop lymphoma.

Scientists do not fully understand all of the causes of lymphoma, but research has found many links. For example:

- Research has shown that people who are infected with human immunodeficiency virus (HIV) are at a much higher risk of developing lymphoma.

- Other viruses, such as human T-cell lymphotropic virus and Epstein Barr virus, also have been linked with certain kinds of lymphoma.

- People exposed to high levels of ionizing radiation have a higher risk of developing non-Hodgkin lymphoma.

- Family history has been linked with a higher risk of Hodgkin lymphoma.

- Some studies suggest that specific ingredients in herbicides and pesticides may be linked with lymphoma, but scientists do not know how much is needed to raise the risk of developing lymphoma.

Symptoms of Lymphoma

Symptoms of Hodgkin lymphoma and non-Hodgkin lymphoma include swollen lymph nodes, especially in the part of the body where the lymphoma starts to grow. Other symptoms include fever, night sweats, feeling tired, and weight loss.

These symptoms can also come from other conditions. If you have any of them, talk to your doctor.

Section 10.2

Childhood Hodgkin Lymphoma

This section includes text excerpted from "Childhood Hodgkin Lymphoma Treatment (PDQ®)—Patient Version," National Cancer Institute (NCI), January 15, 2019.

What Is Childhood Hodgkin Lymphoma?

Childhood Hodgkin lymphoma (HL) is a type of cancer that develops in the lymph system. The lymph system is part of the immune system. It helps protect the body from infection and disease.

The lymph system is made up of the following:

- **Lymph:** Colorless, watery fluid that travels through the lymph vessels and carries T and B lymphocytes. Lymphocytes are a type of white blood cell (WBC).

- **Lymph vessels:** A network of thin tubes that collect lymph from different parts of the body and return it to the bloodstream.

- **Lymph nodes:** Small, bean-shaped structures that filter lymph and store white blood cells that help fight infection and disease. Lymph nodes are found along a network of lymph vessels throughout the body. Groups of lymph nodes are found in the neck, underarm, mediastinum, abdomen, pelvis, and groin.

- **Spleen:** An organ that makes lymphocytes, stores red blood cells (RBCs) and lymphocytes, filters the blood, and destroys old blood cells. The spleen is on the left side of the abdomen near the stomach.

- **Thymus:** An organ in which T lymphocytes mature and multiply. The thymus is in the chest behind the breastbone.

- **Tonsils:** Two small masses of lymph tissue at the back of the throat. There is one tonsil on each side of the throat.

- **Bone marrow:** The soft, spongy tissue in the center of certain bones, such as the hip bone and breastbone. White blood cells, red blood cells, and platelets are made in the bone marrow.

Lymph tissue is also found in other parts of the body, such as the stomach, thyroid gland, brain, and skin.

There are two general types of lymphoma: Hodgkin lymphoma and non-Hodgkin lymphoma (NHL). Hodgkin lymphoma often occurs in adolescents between 15 and 19 years of age. The treatment for children and adolescents is different than treatment for adults.

Types of Childhood Hodgkin Lymphoma

The two types of childhood Hodgkin lymphoma are:

- Classical Hodgkin lymphoma

- Nodular lymphocyte-predominant Hodgkin lymphoma

Classical Hodgkin lymphoma is divided into four subtypes, based on how the cancer cells look under a microscope:

- Lymphocyte-rich classical Hodgkin lymphoma

- Nodular sclerosis Hodgkin lymphoma

- Mixed cellularity Hodgkin lymphoma

- Lymphocyte-depleted Hodgkin lymphoma

Risks of Childhood Hodgkin Lymphoma

Anything that increases your risk of getting a disease is called a "risk factor." Having a risk factor does not mean that you will get cancer; not having risk factors does not mean that you will not get cancer. Talk with your child's doctor if you think your child may be at risk.

Risk factors for childhood Hodgkin lymphoma include the following:

- Being infected with the Epstein-Barr virus (EBV)

- Being infected with the human immunodeficiency virus (HIV)

- Having certain diseases of the immune system

- Having a personal history of mononucleosis ("mono")

- Having a parent or sibling with a personal history of Hodgkin lymphoma

Being exposed to common infections in early childhood may decrease the risk of Hodgkin lymphoma in children because of the effect it has on the immune system.

Signs of Childhood Hodgkin Lymphoma

These and other signs and symptoms may be caused by childhood Hodgkin lymphoma or by other conditions. Check with your child's doctor if your child has any of the following:

- Painless, swollen lymph nodes near the collarbone or in the neck, chest, underarm, or groin

- Fever for no known reason

- Weight loss for no known reason

- Night Sweats

- Fatigue

- Anorexia

- Itchy skin

- Pain in the lymph nodes

Fever, weight loss, and night sweats are called "B symptoms."

Diagnosis of Childhood Hodgkin Lymphoma

The following tests and procedures may be used:

- **Physical exam and history:** An exam of the body to check general signs of health, including checking for signs of disease, such as lumps or anything else that seems unusual. A history of the patient's health habits and past illnesses and treatments will also be taken.

- **Computed tomography (CT or CAT) scan:** A procedure that makes a series of detailed pictures of areas inside the body, such as the neck, chest, abdomen, or pelvis, taken from different angles. The pictures are made by a computer linked to an X-ray machine. A dye may be injected into a vein or swallowed to help the organs or tissues show up more clearly. This procedure is also called "computed tomography," "computerized tomography," or "computerized axial tomography."

- **Positron emission tomography (PET) scan:** A procedure to find malignant tumor cells in the body. A small amount of radioactive glucose (sugar) is injected into a vein. The PET scanner rotates around the body and makes a picture of where glucose is being used in the body. Malignant tumor cells show up brighter in the picture because they are more active and take up more glucose than normal cells do. Sometimes, a PET scan and a CT scan are done at the same time. If there is any cancer, this increases the chance that it will be found.

- **Chest X-ray:** An X-ray of the organs and bones inside the chest. An X-ray is a type of energy beam that can go through the body and onto film, making a picture of areas inside the body.

- **A complete blood count (CBC):** A procedure in which a sample of blood is drawn and checked for the following:

  - The number of red blood cells, white blood cells, and platelets

  - The amount of hemoglobin (the protein that carries oxygen) in the red blood cells

  - The portion of the blood sample made up of red blood cells

- **Blood chemistry studies:** A procedure in which a blood sample is checked to measure the amounts of certain substances released into the blood by organs and tissues in the body. An unusual (higher or lower than normal) amount of a substance can be a sign of disease.

- **Sedimentation rate:** A procedure in which a sample of blood is drawn and checked for the rate at which the red blood cells settle to the bottom of the test tube. The sedimentation rate is a measure of how much inflammation is in the body. A higher than normal sedimentation rate may be a sign of lymphoma. Also called "erythrocyte" "sedimentation rate," "sed rate," or "ESR."

- **Lymph node biopsy:** The removal of all or part of a lymph node. The lymph node may be removed during an image-guided CT scan or a thoracoscopy, mediastinoscopy, or laparoscopy. One of the following types of biopsies may be done:

  - **Excisional biopsy:** The removal of an entire lymph node

  - **Incisional biopsy:** The removal of part of a lymph node

  - **Core biopsy:** The removal of tissue from a lymph node using a wide needle

  - **Fine-needle aspiration (FNA) biopsy:** The removal of tissue from a lymph node using a thin needle

A pathologist views the lymph node tissue under a microscope to check for cancer cells, especially Reed-Sternberg cells. Reed-Sternberg cells are common in classical Hodgkin lymphoma.

The following test may be done on tissue that was removed:

- **Immunophenotyping:** A laboratory test used to identify cells, based on the types of antigens or markers on the surface of the cell. This test is used to diagnose the specific type of lymphoma by comparing the cancer cells to normal cells of the immune system.

Factors Affecting Prognosis and Treatment Options

The prognosis (chance of recovery) and treatment options depend on the following:

- The stage of the cancer

- The size of the tumor

- Whether there are B symptoms at diagnosis

- The type of Hodgkin lymphoma

- Certain features of the cancer cells

- Whether there are too many white blood cells or too few red blood cells at the time of diagnosis

- How well the tumor responds to initial treatment with chemotherapy

- Whether the cancer is newly diagnosed or has recurred (come back)

The treatment options also depend on:

- The child's age and sex

- The risk of long-term side effects

Most children and adolescents with newly diagnosed Hodgkin lymphoma can be cured.

Section 10.3

Adult Hodgkin Lymphoma

This section includes text excerpted from "Adult Hodgkin Lymphoma Treatment (PDQ®)—Patient Version," National Cancer Institute (NCI), February 14, 2019.

What Is Adult Hodgkin Lymphoma?

Adult Hodgkin lymphoma (HL) is a type of cancer that develops in the lymph system. The lymph system is part of the immune system. It helps protect the body from infection and disease.

The lymph system is made up of the following:

- **Lymph:** Colorless, watery fluid that travels through the lymph vessels and carries T and B lymphocytes. Lymphocytes are a type of white blood cell (WBC).

- **Lymph vessels:** A network of thin tubes that collect lymph from different parts of the body and return it to the bloodstream.

- **Lymph nodes:** Small, bean-shaped structures that filter lymph and store white blood cells that help fight infection and disease.

Lymph nodes are found along a network of lymph vessels throughout the body. Groups of lymph nodes are found in the neck, underarm, mediastinum, abdomen, pelvis, and groin.

- **Spleen:** An organ that makes lymphocytes, stores red blood cells (RBCs) and lymphocytes, filters the blood, and destroys old blood cells. The spleen is on the left side of the abdomen near the stomach.

- **Thymus:** An organ in which T lymphocytes mature and multiply. The thymus is in the chest behind the breastbone.

- **Tonsils:** Two small masses of lymph tissue at the back of the throat. There is one tonsil on each side of the throat.

- **Bone marrow:** The soft, spongy tissue in the center of certain bones, such as the hip bone and breastbone. White blood cells, red blood cells, and platelets are made in the bone marrow.

Lymph tissue is also found in other parts of the body, such as the stomach, thyroid gland, brain, and skin. Cancer can spread to the liver and lungs.

Lymphomas are divided into two general types: Hodgkin lymphoma and non-Hodgkin lymphoma (NHL). This section is about the treatment of adult Hodgkin lymphoma.

Hodgkin lymphoma can occur in both adults and children. Treatment for adults is different than treatment for children. Hodgkin lymphoma may also occur in patients who have acquired immunodeficiency syndrome (AIDS); these patients require special treatment.

Hodgkin lymphoma in pregnant women is the same as the disease in nonpregnant women of childbearing age. However, treatment is different for pregnant women. This summary includes information about treating Hodgkin lymphoma during pregnancy.

Types of Adult Hodgkin Lymphoma

Most Hodgkin lymphomas are the classical type. The classical type is broken down into the following four subtypes:

- Nodular sclerosing Hodgkin lymphoma

- Mixed cellularity Hodgkin lymphoma

- Lymphocyte depletion Hodgkin lymphoma

- Lymphocyte-rich classical Hodgkin lymphoma

Risks of Adult Hodgkin Lymphoma

Anything that increases your risk of getting a disease is called a "risk factor." Having a risk factor does not mean that you will get cancer; not having risk factors does not mean that you will not get cancer. Talk with your doctor if you think you may be at risk. Risk factors for adult Hodgkin lymphoma include the following:

- Being in young or late adulthood
- Being male
- Being infected with the Epstein-Barr virus
- Having a first-degree relative (parent, brother, or sister) with Hodgkin lymphoma

Pregnancy is not a risk factor for Hodgkin lymphoma.

Signs of Adult Hodgkin Lymphoma

These and other signs and symptoms may be caused by adult Hodgkin lymphoma or by other conditions. Check with your doctor if any of the following do not go away:

- Painless, swollen lymph nodes in the neck, underarm, or groin
- Fever for no known reason
- Drenching night sweats
- Weight loss for no known reason
- Itchy skin
- Feeling very tired

Diagnosis of Adult Hodgkin Lymphoma

The following tests and procedures may be used:

- **Physical exam and history:** An exam of the body to check general signs of health, including checking for signs of disease, such as lumps or anything else that seems unusual. A history of the patient's health, including fever, night sweats, and weight loss, past illnesses and treatments will also be taken.

- **A complete blood count (CBC):** A procedure in which a sample of blood is drawn and checked for the following:

- The number of red blood cells, white blood cells, and platelets

- The amount of hemoglobin (the protein that carries oxygen) in the red blood cells

- The portion of the sample made up of red blood cells

- **Blood chemistry studies:** A procedure in which a blood sample is checked to measure the amounts of certain substances released into the blood by organs and tissues in the body. An unusual (higher or lower than normal) amount of a substance can be a sign of disease.

- **Lactate dehydrogenase test (LDH):** A procedure in which a blood sample is checked to measure the amount of lactic dehydrogenase. An increased amount of LDH in the blood may be a sign of tissue damage, lymphoma, or other diseases.

- **Hepatitis B and hepatitis C test:** A procedure in which a sample of blood is checked to measure the amounts of hepatitis B virus-specific antigens and/or antibodies and the amounts of hepatitis C virus-specific antibodies. These antigens or antibodies are called "markers." Different markers or combinations of markers are used to determine whether a patient has a hepatitis B or C infection, has had a prior infection or vaccination, or is susceptible to infection.

- **Human immunodeficiency virus test (HIV):** A test to measure the level of HIV antibodies in a sample of blood. Antibodies are made by the body when it is invaded by a foreign substance. A high level of HIV antibodies may mean the body has been infected with HIV.

- **Sedimentation rate:** A procedure in which a sample of blood is drawn and checked for the rate at which the red blood cells settle to the bottom of the test tube. The sedimentation rate is a measure of how much inflammation is in the body. A higher than normal sedimentation rate may be a sign of lymphoma or another condition. This procedure is also called "erythrocyte sedimentation rate," "sed rate," or "ESR."

- **Computed tomography (CT or CAT) scan:** A procedure that makes a series of detailed pictures of areas inside the body, such as the neck, chest, abdomen, pelvis, and lymph nodes, taken from different angles. The pictures are made by a computer linked to an X-ray machine. A dye may be injected into a vein or swallowed to help the organs or tissues show up more clearly. This procedure is also called "computed tomography," "computerized tomography," or "computerized axial tomography."

- **Positron emission tomography-computed tomography (PET-CT) scan:** A procedure that combines the pictures from a positron emission tomography (PET) scan and a computed tomography (CT) scan. The PET and CT scans are done at the same time on the same machine. The pictures from both scans are combined to make a more detailed picture than either test would make by itself. A PET scan is a procedure to find malignant tumor cells in the body. A small amount of radioactive glucose (sugar) is injected into a vein. The PET scanner rotates around the body and makes a picture of where glucose is being used in the body. Malignant tumor cells show up brighter in the picture because they are more active and take up more glucose than normal cells do.

- **Lymph node biopsy:** The removal of all or part of a lymph node. A pathologist views the tissue under a microscope to look for cancer cells, especially Reed-Sternberg cells. Reed-Sternberg (RS) cells are common in classical Hodgkin lymphoma.

One of the following types of biopsies may be done:

- **Excisional biopsy:** The removal of an entire lymph node

- **Incisional biopsy:** The removal of part of a lymph node

- **Core biopsy:** The removal of tissue from a lymph node using a wide needle

Other areas of the body, such as the liver, lung, bone, bone marrow, and brain, may also have a sample of tissue removed and checked by a pathologist for signs of cancer.

The following test may be done on tissue that was removed:

- **Immunophenotyping:** A laboratory test used to identify cells, based on the types of antigens or markers on the surface of the cell. This test is used to diagnose the specific type of lymphoma by comparing the cancer cells to normal cells of the immune system.

For pregnant women with Hodgkin lymphoma, staging tests that protect the fetus from the harmful radiation are used. These include:

- **Magnetic resonance imaging (MRI):** A procedure that uses a magnet, radio waves, and a computer to make a series of detailed pictures of areas inside the body. This procedure is also called "nuclear magnetic resonance imaging" (NMRI).

- **Ultrasound exam:** A procedure in which high-energy sound waves (ultrasound) are bounced off internal tissues or organs and make echoes. The echoes form a picture of body tissues called a "sonogram."

Factors Affecting Prognosis and Treatment Options

The prognosis (chance of recovery) and treatment options depend on the following:

- The patient's signs and symptoms
- The stage of the cancer
- The type of Hodgkin lymphoma
- Blood test results
- The patient's age, sex, and general health
- Whether the cancer is recurrent or progressive

For Hodgkin lymphoma during pregnancy, treatment options also depend on:

- The wishes of the patient
- The age of the fetus

Adult Hodgkin lymphoma can usually be cured if found and treated early.

Section 10.4

Childhood Non-Hodgkin Lymphoma

This section includes text excerpted from "Childhood Non-Hodgkin Lymphoma Treatment (PDQ®)—Patient Version," National Cancer Institute (NCI), January 30, 2019.

What Is Childhood Non-Hodgkin Lymphoma?

Childhood non-Hodgkin lymphoma (NHL) is a type of cancer that forms in the lymph system, which is part of the body's immune system. It helps protect the body from infection and disease.

The lymph system is made up of the following:

- **Lymph:** Colorless, watery fluid that travels through the lymph vessels and carries T and B lymphocytes. Lymphocytes are a type of white blood cell (WBC).

- **Lymph vessels:** A network of thin tubes that collect lymph from different parts of the body and return it to the bloodstream.

- **Lymph nodes:** Small, bean-shaped structures that filter lymph and store white blood cells that help fight infection and disease. Lymph nodes are found along a network of lymph vessels throughout the body. Groups of lymph nodes are found in the neck, underarm, mediastinum, abdomen, pelvis, and groin.

- **Spleen:** An organ that makes lymphocytes, stores red blood cells (RBCs) and lymphocytes, filters the blood, and destroys old blood cells. The spleen is on the left side of the abdomen near the stomach.

- **Thymus:** An organ in which T lymphocytes mature and multiply. The thymus is in the chest behind the breastbone.

- **Tonsils:** Two small masses of lymph tissue at the back of the throat. There is one tonsil on each side of the throat.

- **Bone marrow:** The soft, spongy tissue in the center of certain bones, such as the hip bone and breastbone. White blood cells, red blood cells, and platelets are made in the bone marrow.

Non-Hodgkin lymphoma can begin in B lymphocytes, T lymphocytes, or natural killer cells. Lymphocytes can also be found in the blood and collect in the lymph nodes, spleen, and thymus.

Lymph tissue is also found in other parts of the body, such as the stomach, thyroid gland, brain, and skin.

Non-Hodgkin lymphoma can occur in both adults and children. Treatment for children is different than treatment for adults.

Types of Lymphoma

Lymphomas are divided into two general types: Hodgkin lymphoma and non-Hodgkin lymphoma. This section is about the treatment of childhood non-Hodgkin lymphoma.

Types of Childhood Non-Hodgkin Lymphoma

The type of lymphoma is determined by how the cells look under a microscope. The three major types of childhood non-Hodgkin lymphoma are:

Mature B-Cell Non-Hodgkin Lymphoma

Mature B-cell non-Hodgkin lymphomas include:

- **Burkitt and Burkitt-like lymphoma/leukemia:** Burkitt lymphoma and Burkitt leukemia are different forms of the same disease. Burkitt lymphoma/leukemia is an aggressive (fast-growing) disorder of B lymphocytes that is most common in children and young adults. It may form in the abdomen, Waldeyer ring, testicles, bone, bone marrow, skin, or central nervous system (CNS). Burkitt leukemia may start in the lymph nodes as Burkitt lymphoma and then spread to the blood and bone marrow, or it may start in the blood and bone marrow without forming in the lymph nodes first. Both Burkitt leukemia and Burkitt lymphoma have been linked to infection with the Epstein-Barr virus (EBV), although EBV infection is more likely to occur in patients in Africa than in the United States. Burkitt and Burkitt-like lymphoma/leukemia are diagnosed when a sample of tissue is checked and a certain change to the *MYC* gene is found.

- **Diffuse large B-cell lymphoma (DLBCL):** Diffuse large B-cell lymphoma is the most common type of non-Hodgkin lymphoma. It is a type of B-cell non-Hodgkin lymphoma that grows quickly in the lymph nodes. The spleen, liver, bone marrow, or other organs are also often affected. Diffuse large B-cell lymphoma occurs more often in adolescents than in children.

- **Primary mediastinal B-cell lymphoma:** A type of lymphoma that develops from B cells in the mediastinum (the area behind the breastbone). It may spread to nearby organs, including the lungs and the sac around the heart. It may also spread to lymph nodes and distant organs, including the kidneys. In children and adolescents, primary mediastinal B-cell lymphoma occurs more often in older adolescents.

Lymphoblastic Lymphoma

Lymphoblastic lymphoma is a type of lymphoma that mainly affects T-cell lymphocytes. It usually forms in the mediastinum. This causes trouble with breathing and/or swallowing, wheezing, or swelling of the head and neck. It may spread to the lymph nodes, bone, bone marrow, skin, the CNS, abdominal organs, and other areas. Lymphoblastic lymphoma is very similar to acute lymphoblastic leukemia (ALL).

Anaplastic Large Cell Lymphoma

Anaplastic large cell lymphoma is a type of lymphoma that mainly affects T-cell lymphocytes. It usually forms in the lymph nodes, skin, or bone, and sometimes forms in the gastrointestinal tract, lung, tissue that covers the lungs, and muscle. Patients with anaplastic large cell lymphoma have a receptor, called "CD30," on the surface of their T cells. In many children, anaplastic large cell lymphoma is marked by changes in the *ALK* gene that makes a protein called "anaplastic lymphoma kinase" (ALK). A pathologist checks for these cells and gene changes to help diagnose anaplastic large cell lymphoma.

Types of Non-Hodgkin Lymphoma

Some types of childhood non-Hodgkin lymphoma are less common. These include:

- **Pediatric-type follicular lymphoma:** In children, follicular lymphoma occurs mainly in males. It is more likely to be found in one area and does not spread to other places in the body. It usually forms in the tonsils and lymph nodes in the neck, but it may also form in the testicles, kidney, gastrointestinal tract, and salivary gland.

- **Marginal zone lymphoma:** Marginal zone lymphoma is a type of lymphoma that tends to grow and spread slowly and is usually found at an early stage. It may be found in the lymph nodes or in areas outside the lymph nodes. Marginal zone lymphoma found outside the lymph nodes in children is called "mucosa-associated lymphoid tissue (MALT) lymphoma." MALT lymphoma may be linked to Helicobacter pylori infection of the gastrointestinal tract and Chlamydophila psittaci infection of the conjunctival membrane, which lines the eye.

- **Primary central nervous system (CNS) lymphoma:** Primary CNS lymphoma is extremely rare in children.

- **Peripheral T-cell lymphoma:** Peripheral T-cell lymphoma is an aggressive (fast-growing) non-Hodgkin lymphoma that begins in mature T lymphocytes. The T lymphocytes mature in the thymus gland and travel to other parts of the lymph system, such as the lymph nodes, bone marrow, and spleen.

- **Cutaneous T-cell lymphoma:** Cutaneous T-cell lymphoma begins in the skin and can cause the skin to thicken or form a tumor. It is very rare in children, but it is more common in adolescents and young adults. There are different types of cutaneous T-cell lymphoma, such as cutaneous anaplastic large cell lymphoma, subcutaneous panniculitis-like T-cell lymphoma, gamma-delta T-cell lymphoma, and mycosis fungoides. Mycosis fungoides rarely occurs in children and adolescents.

Risks of Childhood Non-Hodgkin Lymphoma

Anything that increases your risk of getting a disease is called a "risk factor." Having a risk factor does not mean that you will get cancer; not having risk factors does not mean that you will not get cancer. Talk with your child's doctor if you think your child may be at risk.

Possible risk factors for childhood non-Hodgkin lymphoma include the following:

- Past treatment for cancer
- Being infected with the Epstein-Barr virus or human immunodeficiency virus (HIV)
- Having a weakened immune system after a transplant or from medicines given after a transplant
- Having certain inherited diseases (such as deoxyribonucleic acid (DNA) repair defect syndromes, which include ataxia-telangiectasia, Nijmegen breakage syndrome, and constitutional mismatch repair deficiency)

If lymphoma or lymphoproliferative disease is linked to a weakened immune system from certain inherited diseases, HIV infection, a transplant or medicines given after a transplant, the condition is called "lymphoproliferative disease associated with immunodeficiency." The different types of lymphoproliferative disease associated with immunodeficiency include:

- Lymphoproliferative disease associated with primary immunodeficiency

- HIV-associated non-Hodgkin lymphoma

- Posttransplant lymphoproliferative disease

Signs of Childhood Non-Hodgkin Lymphoma

These and other signs may be caused by childhood non-Hodgkin lymphoma or by other conditions. Check with a doctor if your child has any of the following:

- Trouble breathing

- Wheezing

- Coughing

- High-pitched breathing sounds

- Swelling of the head, neck, upper body, or arms

- Trouble swallowing

- Painless swelling of the lymph nodes in the neck, underarm, stomach, or groin

- Painless lump or swelling in a testicle

- Fever for no known reason

- Weight loss for no known reason

- Night sweats

Diagnosis of Childhood Non-Hodgkin Lymphoma

The following tests and procedures may be used:

- **Physical exam and history:** An exam of the body to check general signs of health, including checking for signs of disease, such as lumps or anything else that seems unusual. A history of the patient's health habits and past illnesses and treatments will also be taken.

- **Blood chemistry studies:** A procedure in which a blood sample is checked to measure the amounts of certain substances released into the blood by organs and tissues in the body, including electrolytes, lactate dehydrogenase (LDH), uric acid, blood urea nitrogen (BUN), creatinine, and liver function values. An unusual (higher or lower than normal) amount of a substance can be a sign of disease.

- **Liver function tests:** A procedure in which a blood sample is checked to measure the amounts of certain substances released into the blood by the liver. A higher than normal amount of a substance can be a sign of cancer.

- **Computed tomography (CT or CAT) scan:** A procedure that makes a series of detailed pictures of areas inside the body, taken from different angles. The pictures are made by a computer linked to an X-ray machine. A dye may be injected into a vein or swallowed to help the organs or tissues show up more clearly. This procedure is also called "computed tomography," "computerized tomography," or "computerized axial tomography."

- **Positron emission tomography (PET) scan:** A procedure to find malignant tumor cells in the body. A small amount of radioactive glucose (sugar) is injected into a vein. The PET scanner rotates around the body and makes a picture of where glucose is being used in the body. Malignant tumor cells show up brighter in the picture because they are more active and take up more glucose than normal cells do. Sometimes, a PET scan and a CT scan are done at the same time. If there is any cancer, this increases the chance that it will be found.

- **Magnetic resonance imaging (MRI):** A procedure that uses a magnet, radio waves, and a computer to make a series of detailed pictures of areas inside the body. This procedure is also called "nuclear magnetic resonance imaging" (NMRI).

- **Lumbar puncture:** A procedure used to collect cerebrospinal fluid (CSF) from the spinal column. This is done by placing a needle between two bones in the spine and into the CSF around the spinal cord and removing a sample of the fluid. The sample of CSF is checked under a microscope for signs that the cancer has spread to the brain and spinal cord. This procedure is also called an "LP" or "spinal tap."

- **Chest X-ray:** An X-ray of the organs and bones inside the chest. An X-ray is a type of energy beam that can go through the body and onto film, making a picture of areas inside the body.

- **Ultrasound exam:** A procedure in which high-energy sound waves (ultrasound) are bounced off internal tissues or organs and make echoes. The echoes form a picture of body tissues called a "sonogram." The picture can be printed to be looked at later.

Biopsy to Diagnose Childhood Non-Hodgkin Lymphoma

Cells and tissues are removed during a biopsy so they can be viewed under a microscope by a pathologist to check for signs of cancer. Because treatment depends on the type of non-Hodgkin lymphoma, biopsy samples should be checked by a pathologist who has experience in diagnosing childhood non-Hodgkin lymphoma.

One of the following types of biopsies may be done:

- **Excisional biopsy:** The removal of an entire lymph node or lump of tissue

- **Incisional biopsy:** The removal of part of a lump, lymph node, or sample of tissue

- **Core biopsy:** The removal of tissue or part of a lymph node using a wide needle

- **Fine-needle aspiration (FNA) biopsy:** The removal of tissue or part of a lymph node using a thin needle

The procedure used to remove the sample of tissue depends on where the tumor is in the body:

- **Bone marrow aspiration and biopsy:** The removal of bone marrow and a small piece of bone by inserting a hollow needle into the hipbone or breastbone

- **Mediastinoscopy:** A surgical procedure to look at the organs, tissues, and lymph nodes between the lungs for abnormal areas. An incision (cut) is made at the top of the breastbone, and a mediastinoscope is inserted into the chest. A mediastinoscope is a thin, tube-like instrument with a light and a lens for viewing.

It also has a tool to remove tissue or lymph node samples, which are checked under a microscope for signs of cancer.

- **Anterior mediastinotomy:** A surgical procedure to look at the organs and tissues between the lungs and between the breastbone and heart for abnormal areas. An incision is made next to the breastbone, and a mediastinoscope is inserted into the chest. It also has a tool to remove tissue or lymph node samples, which are checked under a microscope for signs of cancer. This is also called the "Chamberlain procedure."

- **Thoracentesis:** The removal of fluid from the space between the lining of the chest and the lung, using a needle. A pathologist views the fluid under a microscope to look for cancer cells.

If cancer is found, the following tests may be done to study the cancer cells:

- **Immunohistochemistry:** A laboratory test that uses antibodies to check for certain antigens in a sample of tissue. The antibody is usually linked to a radioactive substance or a dye that causes the tissue to light up under a microscope. This type of test may be used to tell the difference between different types of cancer.

- **Flow cytometry:** A laboratory test that measures the number of cells in a sample; the percentage of live cells in a sample; and certain characteristics of cells, such as size, shape, and the presence of tumor markers on the cell surface. The cells are stained with a light-sensitive dye, placed in a fluid, and passed in a stream before a laser or other type of light. The measurements are based on how the light-sensitive dye reacts to the light.

- **Cytogenetic analysis:** A laboratory test in which cells in a sample of tissue are viewed under a microscope to look for certain changes in the chromosomes.

- **Fluorescence in situ hybridization (FISH):** A laboratory test used to look at genes or chromosomes in cells and tissues. Pieces of DNA that contain a fluorescent dye are made in the laboratory and added to cells or tissues on a glass slide. When these pieces of DNA attach to certain genes or areas of chromosomes on the slide, they light up when viewed under a microscope with

161

a special light. This type of test is used to find certain gene changes.

- **Immunophenotyping:** A laboratory test used to identify cells, based on the types of antigens or markers on the surface of the cell. This test is used to diagnose specific types of lymphoma by comparing the cancer cells to normal cells of the immune system.

Factors Affecting Prognosis and Treatment Options

The prognosis (chance of recovery) and treatment options depend on:

- The type of lymphoma
- Where the tumor is in the body when the tumor is diagnosed
- The stage of the cancer
- Whether there are certain changes in the chromosomes
- The type of initial treatment
- Whether the lymphoma responded to initial treatment
- The patient's age and general health

Section 10.5

Adult Non-Hodgkin Lymphoma

This section includes text excerpted from "Adult Non-Hodgkin Lymphoma Treatment (PDQ®)—Patient Version," National Cancer Institute (NCI), January 25, 2019.

What Is Adult Non-Hodgkin Lymphoma?

Non-Hodgkin lymphoma (NHL) is a type of cancer that forms in the lymph system. The lymph system is part of the immune system. It helps protect the body from infection and disease.

The lymph system is made up of the following:

- **Lymph:** Colorless, watery fluid that travels through the lymph vessels and carries lymphocytes (white blood cells (WBCs)). There are three types of lymphocytes:

  - B lymphocytes that make antibodies to help fight infection. B lymphocytes are also called "B cells." Most types of non-Hodgkin lymphoma begin in B lymphocytes.

  - T lymphocytes that help B lymphocytes make the antibodies that help fight infection. T lymphocytes are also called "T cells."

  - Natural killer cells that attack cancer cells and viruses. Natural killer cells are also called "NK cells."

- **Lymph vessels:** A network of thin tubes that collect lymph from different parts of the body and return it to the bloodstream.

- **Lymph nodes:** Small, bean-shaped structures that filter lymph and store white blood cells that help fight infection and disease. Lymph nodes are found along a network of lymph vessels throughout the body. Groups of lymph nodes are found in the neck, underarm, mediastinum, abdomen, pelvis, and groin.

- **Spleen:** An organ that makes lymphocytes, stores red blood cells (RBCs) and lymphocytes, filters the blood, and destroys old blood cells. The spleen is on the left side of the abdomen near the stomach.

- **Thymus:** An organ in which T lymphocytes mature and multiply. The thymus is in the chest behind the breastbone.

- **Tonsils:** Two small masses of lymph tissue at the back of the throat. There is one tonsil on each side of the throat.

- **Bone marrow:** The soft, spongy tissue in the center of certain bones, such as the hip bone and breastbone. White blood cells, red blood cells, and platelets are made in the bone marrow.

Lymph tissue is also found in other parts of the body, such as the stomach, thyroid gland, brain, and skin. Cancer can spread to the liver and lungs.

Non-Hodgkin lymphoma during pregnancy is rare. Non-Hodgkin lymphoma in pregnant women is the same as the disease in nonpregnant women of childbearing age. However, treatment is different for pregnant women. This summary includes information on the treatment of non-Hodgkin lymphoma during pregnancy.

Non-Hodgkin lymphoma can occur in both adults and children. Treatment for adults is different than treatment for children.

Types of Lymphoma

Lymphomas are divided into two general types: Hodgkin lymphoma and non-Hodgkin lymphoma. This section is about the treatment of adult non-Hodgkin lymphoma.

Risks of Adult Non-Hodgkin Lymphoma

Anything that increases your risk of getting a disease is called a "risk factor." Having a risk factor does not mean that you will get cancer; not having risk factors does not mean that you will not get cancer. Talk with your doctor if you think you may be at risk.

These and other risk factors may increase the risk of certain types of adult non-Hodgkin lymphoma:

- Being older, male, or White
- Having one of the following medical conditions:
  - An inherited immune disorder (such as hypogammaglobulinemia or Wiskott-Aldrich syndrome)
  - An autoimmune disease (such as rheumatoid arthritis, psoriasis, or Sjögren syndrome)
  - Human immunodeficiency virus (HIV)/acquired immunodeficiency syndrome (AIDS)
  - Human T-lymphotropic virus type I or Epstein-Barr virus infection
  - *Helicobacter pylori* infection
- Taking immunosuppressant drugs after an organ transplant

Signs and Symptoms of Adult Non-Hodgkin Lymphoma

These signs and symptoms may be caused by adult non-Hodgkin lymphoma or by other conditions. Check with your doctor if you have any of the following:

- Swelling in the lymph nodes in the neck, underarm, groin, or stomach

- Fever for no known reason

- Recurring night sweats

- Feeling very tired

- Weight loss for no known reason

- Skin rash or itchy skin

- Pain in the chest, abdomen, or bones for no known reason

When fever, night sweats, and weight loss occur together, this group of symptoms is called "B symptoms."

Other signs and symptoms of adult non-Hodgkin lymphoma may occur and depend on the following:

- Where the cancer forms in the body

- The size of the tumor

- How fast the tumor grows

Diagnosis of Adult Non-Hodgkin Lymphoma

The following tests and procedures may be used:

- **Physical exam and history:** An exam of the body to check general signs of health, including checking for signs of disease, such as lumps or anything else that seems unusual. A history of the patient's health, including fever, night sweats, and weight loss, health habits, and past illnesses and treatments will also be taken.

- **A complete blood count (CBC):** A procedure in which a sample of blood is drawn and checked for the following:

  - The number of red blood cells, white blood cells, and platelets

  - The amount of hemoglobin (the protein that carries oxygen) in the red blood cells

  - The portion of the sample made up of red blood cells

- **Blood chemistry studies:** A procedure in which a blood sample is checked to measure the amounts of certain substances released into the blood by organs and tissues in the body.

An unusual (higher or lower than normal) amount of a substance can be a sign of disease.

- **Lactate dehydrogenase (LDH) test:** A procedure in which a blood sample is checked to measure the amount of lactic dehydrogenase. An increased amount of LDH in the blood may be a sign of tissue damage, lymphoma, or other diseases.

- **Hepatitis B and hepatitis C test:** A procedure in which a sample of blood is checked to measure the amounts of hepatitis B virus-specific antigens and/or antibodies and the amounts of hepatitis C virus-specific antibodies. These antigens or antibodies are called "markers." Different markers or combinations of markers are used to determine whether a patient has a hepatitis B or C infection, has had a prior infection or vaccination, or is susceptible to infection.

- **Human immunodeficiency test:** A test to measure the level of HIV antibodies in a sample of blood. Antibodies are made by the body when it is invaded by a foreign substance. A high level of HIV antibodies may mean that the body has been infected with HIV.

- **Computed tomography (CT or CAT) scan:** A procedure that makes a series of detailed pictures of areas inside the body, such as the neck, chest, abdomen, pelvis, and lymph nodes, taken from different angles. The pictures are made by a computer linked to an X-ray machine. A dye may be injected into a vein or swallowed to help the organs or tissues show up more clearly. This procedure is also called "computed tomography," "computerized tomography," or "computerized axial tomography."

- **Positron emission tomography (PET) scan:** A procedure to find malignant tumor cells in the body. A small amount of radioactive glucose (sugar) is injected into a vein. The PET scanner rotates around the body and makes a picture of where glucose is being used in the body. Malignant tumor cells show up brighter in the picture because they are more active and take up more glucose than normal cells do.

- **Bone marrow aspiration and biopsy:** The removal of bone marrow and a small piece of bone by inserting a needle into the hipbone or breastbone. A pathologist views the bone marrow and bone under a microscope to look for signs of cancer.

- **Lymph node biopsy:** The removal of all or part of a lymph node. A pathologist views the tissue under a microscope to check for cancer cells. One of the following types of biopsies may be done:

- **Excisional biopsy:** The removal of an entire lymph node
- **Incisional biopsy:** The removal of part of a lymph node
- **Core biopsy:** The removal of part of a lymph node using a wide needle

If cancer is found, the following tests may be done to study the cancer cells:

- **Immunohistochemistry:** A test that uses antibodies to check for certain antigens in a sample of tissue. The antibody is usually linked to a radioactive substance or a dye that causes the tissue to light up under a microscope. This type of test may be used to tell the difference between different types of cancer.

- **Cytogenetic analysis:** A laboratory test in which cells in a sample of tissue are viewed under a microscope to look for certain changes in the chromosomes

- **Fluorescence in situ hybridization (FISH):** A laboratory test used to look at genes or chromosomes in cells and tissues. Pieces of deoxyribonucleic acid (DNA) that contain a fluorescent dye are made in the laboratory and added to cells or tissues on a glass slide. When these pieces of DNA attach to certain genes or areas of chromosomes on the slide, they light up when viewed under a microscope with a special light. This type of test is used to look for certain genetic markers.

- **Immunophenotyping:** A process used to identify cells, based on the types of antigens or markers on the surface of the cell. This process is used to diagnose specific types of leukemia and lymphoma by comparing the cancer cells to normal cells of the immune system.

Other tests and procedures may be done depending on the signs and symptoms seen and where the cancer forms in the body.

Factors Affecting Prognosis and Treatment Options

The prognosis (chance of recovery) and treatment options depend on the following:

- The stage of the cancer

- The type of non-Hodgkin lymphoma

- The amount of lactate dehydrogenase (LDH) in the blood

- Whether there are certain changes in the genes

- The patient's age and general health

- Whether the lymphoma has just been diagnosed or has recurred (come back)

For non-Hodgkin lymphoma during pregnancy, the treatment options also depend on:

- The wishes of the patient

- Which trimester of pregnancy the patient is in

- Whether the baby can be delivered early

Some types of non-Hodgkin lymphoma spread more quickly than others do. Most non-Hodgkin lymphomas that occur during pregnancy are aggressive. Delaying treatment of aggressive lymphoma until after the baby is born may lessen the mother's chance of survival. Immediate treatment is often recommended, even during pregnancy.

Section 10.6

AIDS-Related Lymphoma

This section includes text excerpted from "Aids-Related Lymphoma Treatment (PDQ®)—Patient Version," National Cancer Institute (NCI), January 25, 2019.

What Is AIDS-Related Lymphoma?

Acquired immunodeficiency syndrome (AIDS) is caused by the human immunodeficiency virus (HIV), which attacks and weakens the body's immune system. A weakened immune system is unable to fight infection and disease. People with HIV have an increased risk of infection and lymphoma or other types of cancer. A person with HIV and certain types of infection or cancer, such as lymphoma, is diagnosed as having AIDS. Sometimes, people are diagnosed with AIDS and AIDS-related lymphoma at the same time.

Acquired immunodeficiency syndrome-related lymphoma is a type of cancer that affects the lymph system. The lymph system is part of the immune system. It helps protect the body from infection and disease.

The lymph system is made up of the following:

- **Lymph:** Colorless, watery fluid that travels through the lymph vessels and carries T and B lymphocytes. Lymphocytes are a type of white blood cell (WBC).

- **Lymph vessels:** A network of thin tubes that collect lymph from different parts of the body and return it to the bloodstream

- **Lymph nodes:** Small, bean-shaped structures that filter lymph and store white blood cells that help fight infection and disease. Lymph nodes are found along a network of lymph vessels throughout the body. Groups of lymph nodes are found in the neck, underarm, mediastinum, abdomen, pelvis, and groin.

- **Spleen:** An organ that makes lymphocytes, stores red blood cells (RBCs) and lymphocytes, filters the blood, and destroys old blood cells. The spleen is on the left side of the abdomen near the stomach.

- **Thymus:** An organ in which T lymphocytes mature and multiply. The thymus is in the chest behind the breastbone.

- **Tonsils:** Two small masses of lymph tissue at the back of the throat. There is one tonsil on each side of the throat.

- **Bone marrow:** The soft, spongy tissue in the center of certain bones, such as the hip bone and breastbone. White blood cells, red blood cells, and platelets are made in the bone marrow.

Lymph tissue is also found in other parts of the body, such as the brain, stomach, thyroid gland, and skin.

Sometimes, acquired immunodeficiency syndrome-related lymphoma occurs outside the lymph nodes in the bone marrow, liver, meninges (thin membranes that cover the brain), and gastrointestinal tract. Less often, it may occur in the anus, heart, bile duct, gingiva, and muscles.

Types of AIDS-Related Lymphoma

Lymphomas are divided into two general types:

- Hodgkin lymphoma

- Non-Hodgkin lymphoma (NHL)

Both non-Hodgkin lymphoma and Hodgkin lymphoma may occur in patients with AIDS, but non-Hodgkin lymphoma is more common. When a person with AIDS has non-Hodgkin lymphoma, it is called "AIDS-related lymphoma." When AIDS-related lymphoma occurs in the central nervous system (CNS), it is called "AIDS-related primary CNS lymphoma."

Non-Hodgkin lymphomas are grouped by the way their cells look under a microscope. They may be indolent (slow-growing) or aggressive (fast-growing). AIDS-related lymphomas are aggressive. There are two main types of AIDS-related non-Hodgkin lymphoma:

- Diffuse large B-cell lymphoma (including B-cell immunoblastic lymphoma)

- Burkitt or Burkitt-like lymphoma

Signs of AIDS-Related Lymphoma

These and other signs and symptoms may be caused by AIDS-related lymphoma or by other conditions. Check with your doctor if you have any of the following:

- Weight loss or fever for no known reason

- Night sweats

- Painless, swollen lymph nodes in the neck, chest, underarm, or groin

- A feeling of fullness below the ribs

Diagnosis of AIDS-Related Lymphoma

The following tests and procedures may be used:

- **Physical exam and history:** An exam of the body to check general signs of health, including checking for signs of disease, such as lumps or anything else that seems unusual. A history of the patient's health, including fever, night sweats, and weight loss, health habits, and past illnesses and treatments will also be taken.

- **A complete blood count (CBC):** A procedure in which a sample of blood is drawn and checked for the following:

  - The number of red blood cells, white blood cells, and platelets

  - The amount of hemoglobin (the protein that carries oxygen) in the red blood cells

  - The portion of the sample made up of red blood cells

- **Blood chemistry studies:** A procedure in which a blood sample is checked to measure the amounts of certain substances released into the blood by organs and tissues in the body. An unusual (higher or lower than normal) amount of a substance can be a sign of disease.

- **Lactic dehydrogenase (LDH) test:** A procedure in which a blood sample is checked to measure the amount of lactic dehydrogenase. An increased amount of LDH in the blood may be a sign of tissue damage, lymphoma, or other diseases.

- **Hepatitis B and hepatitis C test:** A procedure in which a sample of blood is checked to measure the amounts of hepatitis B virus-specific antigens and/or antibodies and the amounts of hepatitis C virus-specific antibodies. These antigens or antibodies are called "markers." Different markers or combinations of markers are used to determine whether a patient has a hepatitis B or C infection, has had a prior infection or vaccination, or is susceptible to infection.

- **Human immunodeficiency test:** A test to measure the level of HIV antibodies in a sample of blood. Antibodies are made by the body when it is invaded by a foreign substance. A high level of HIV antibodies may mean the body has been infected with HIV.

- **Computed tomography (CT or CAT) scan:** A procedure that makes a series of detailed pictures of areas inside the body, such as the neck, chest, abdomen, pelvis, and lymph nodes, taken from different angles. The pictures are made by a computer linked to an X-ray machine. A dye may be injected into a vein or swallowed to help the organs or tissues show up more clearly. This procedure is also called "computed tomography," "computerized tomography," or "computerized axial tomography."

- **Positron emission tomography (PET) scan:** A procedure to find malignant tumor cells in the body. A small amount of radioactive glucose (sugar) is injected into a vein. The PET scanner rotates around the body and makes a picture of where glucose is being used in the body. Malignant tumor cells show up brighter in the picture because they are more active and take up more glucose than normal cells do.

- **Bone marrow aspiration and biopsy:** The removal of bone marrow and a small piece of bone by inserting a hollow needle into the hipbone or breastbone. A pathologist views the bone marrow and bone under a microscope to look for signs of cancer.

- **Lymph node biopsy:** The removal of all or part of a lymph node. A pathologist views the tissue under a microscope to look for cancer cells. One of the following types of biopsies may be done:

  - **Excisional biopsy:** The removal of an entire lymph node

  - **Incisional biopsy:** The removal of part of a lymph node

  - **Core biopsy:** The removal of tissue from a lymph node using a wide needle

Other areas of the body, such as the liver, lung, bone, bone marrow, and brain, may also have a sample of tissue removed and checked by a pathologist for signs of cancer.

If cancer is found, the following tests may be done to study the cancer cells:

- **Immunohistochemistry:** A test that uses antibodies to check for certain antigens in a sample of tissue. The antibody is usually linked to a radioactive substance or a dye that causes the tissue to light up under a microscope. This type of test may be used to tell the difference between different types of cancer.

- **Cytogenetic analysis:** A laboratory test in which cells in a sample of tissue are viewed under a microscope to look for certain changes in the chromosomes.

- **Fluorescence in situ hybridization (FISH):** A laboratory test used to look at genes or chromosomes in cells and tissues. Pieces of deoxyribonucleic acid (DNA) that contain a fluorescent dye are made in the laboratory and added to cells or tissues on a glass slide. When these pieces of DNA attach to certain genes or areas of chromosomes on the slide, they light up when viewed under a microscope with a special light. This type of test is used to look for certain genetic markers.

- **Immunophenotyping:** A process used to identify cells, based on the types of antigens or markers on the surface of the cell. This process is used to diagnose specific types of leukemia and lymphoma by comparing the cancer cells to normal cells of the immune system.

Factors Affecting Prognosis and Treatment Options

The prognosis (chance of recovery) and treatment options depend on the following:

- The stage of the cancer

- The age of the patient

- The number of CD4 lymphocytes (a type of white blood cell) in the blood

- The number of places in the body lymphoma is found outside the lymph system

- Whether the patient has a history of intravenous (IV) drug use

- The patient's ability to carry out regular daily activities

Section 10.7

Mycosis Fungoides and Sézary Syndrome

This section includes text excerpted from "Mycosis Fungoides (Including Sezary Syndrome) Treatment (PDQ®)—Patient Version," National Cancer Institute (NCI), March 29, 2019.

What Are Mycosis Fungoides and Sézary Syndrome?

Normally, the bone marrow makes blood stem cells (immature cells) that become mature blood stem cells over time. A blood stem cell may become a myeloid stem cell or a lymphoid stem cell. A myeloid stem cell becomes a red blood cell (RBC), white blood cell (WBC), or platelet.

A lymphoid stem cell becomes a lymphoblast and then one of three types of lymphocytes (white blood cells):

- B-cell lymphocytes that make antibodies to help fight infection

- T-cell lymphocytes that help B-lymphocytes make the antibodies that help fight infection

- Natural killer cells that attack cancer cells and viruses

In mycosis fungoides, T-cell lymphocytes become cancerous and affect the skin. In Sézary syndrome, cancerous T-cell lymphocytes affect the skin and are in the blood.

Signs of Mycosis Fungoides

Mycosis fungoides may go through the following phases:

- **Premycotic phase:** A scaly, red rash in areas of the body that usually are not exposed to the sun. This rash does not cause symptoms and may last for months or years. It is hard to diagnose the rash as mycosis fungoides during this phase.

- **Patch phase:** Thin, reddened, eczema-like rash

- **Plaque phase:** Small raised bumps (papules) or hardened lesions on the skin, which may be reddened

- **Tumor phase:** Tumors form on the skin. These tumors may develop ulcers and the skin may get infected.

Check with your doctor if you have any of these signs.

Sézary Syndrome and Cancerous T-Cells

Skin all over the body is reddened, itchy, peeling, and painful. There may also be patches, plaques, or tumors on the skin. It is not known if Sézary syndrome is an advanced form of mycosis fungoides or a separate disease.

Diagnosis of Mycosis Fungoides and Sézary Syndrome

The following tests and procedures may be used:

- **Physical exam and history:** An exam of the body to check general signs of health, including checking for signs of disease, such as lumps, the number and type of skin lesions, or anything else that seems unusual. Pictures of the skin and a history of the patient's health habits and past illnesses and treatments will also be taken.

- **A complete blood count (CBC) with differential:** A procedure in which a sample of blood is drawn and checked for the following:

  - The number of red blood cells and platelets

  - The number and type of white blood cells

  - The amount of hemoglobin (the protein that carries oxygen) in the red blood cells

  - The portion of the blood sample made up of red blood cells

- **Peripheral blood smear:** A procedure in which a sample of blood is viewed under a microscope to count different circulating blood cells (red blood cells, white blood cells, platelets, etc.) and see whether the cells look normal

- **Skin biopsy:** The removal of cells or tissues so they can be viewed under a microscope to check for signs of cancer. The doctor may remove a growth from the skin, which will be examined by a pathologist. More than one skin biopsy may be needed to diagnose mycosis fungoides.

- **Immunophenotyping:** A process used to identify cells, based on the types of antigens or markers on the surface of the cell. This process may include special staining of the blood cells. It is used to diagnose specific types of leukemia and lymphoma by comparing the cancer cells to normal cells of the immune system.

- *T-cell receptor (TCR)* **gene rearrangement test:** A laboratory test in which cells in a sample of tissue are checked to see if there is a certain change in the genes. This gene change can lead to too many of one kind of T-cells (white blood cells that fight infection) to be made.

- **Flow cytometry:** A laboratory test that measures the number of cells in a sample of blood, the percentage of live cells in a sample, and certain characteristics of cells, such as size, shape, and the presence of tumor markers on the cell surface. The cells are stained with a light-sensitive dye, placed in a fluid, and passed in a stream before a laser or other type of light. The measurements are based on how the light-sensitive dye reacts to the light.

Factors Affecting Prognosis and Treatment Options

The prognosis (chance of recovery) and treatment options depend on the following:

- The stage of the cancer
- The type of lesion (patches, plaques, or tumors)
- The patient's age and sex

Mycosis fungoides and Sézary syndrome are hard to cure. Treatment is usually palliative, to relieve symptoms and improve the quality of life. Patients with early stage disease may live many years.

Section 10.8

Primary Central Nervous System Lymphoma

This section includes text excerpted from "Primary CNS Lymphoma Treatment (PDQ®)—Patient Version," National Cancer Institute (NCI), April 9, 2019.

What Is Primary Central Nervous System Lymphoma?

Lymphoma is a disease in which malignant (cancer) cells form in the lymph system. The lymph system is part of the immune system and is made up of the lymph, lymph vessels, lymph nodes, spleen, thymus, tonsils, and bone marrow. Lymphocytes (carried in the lymph) travel in and out of the central nervous system (CNS). It is thought that some of these lymphocytes become malignant and cause lymphoma to form in the CNS. Primary CNS lymphoma can start in the brain, spinal cord, or meninges (the layers that form the outer covering of the brain). Because the eye is so close to the brain, primary CNS lymphoma can also start in the eye (called "ocular lymphoma").

Risks of Primary Central Nervous System Lymphoma

Anything that increases your chance of getting a disease is called a "risk factor." Having a risk factor does not mean that you will get cancer; not having risk factors does not mean that you will not get cancer. Talk with your doctor if you think you may be at risk.

Primary central nervous system lymphoma may occur in patients who have acquired immunodeficiency syndrome (AIDS) or other disorders of the immune system or who have had a kidney transplant.

Diagnosis of Primary Central Nervous System Lymphoma

The following tests and procedures may be used:

- **Physical exam and history:** An exam of the body to check general signs of health, including checking for signs of disease, such as lumps or anything else that seems unusual. A history of the patient's health habits and past illnesses and treatments will also be taken.

- **Neurological exam:** A series of questions and tests to check the brain, spinal cord, and nerve function. The exam checks a person's mental status, coordination, ability to walk normally, and how well the muscles, senses, and reflexes work. This may also be called a "neuro exam" or a "neurologic exam."

- **Slit-lamp eye exam:** An exam that uses a special microscope with a bright, narrow slit of light to check the outside and inside of the eye

- **Magnetic resonance imaging (MRI):** A procedure that uses a magnet, radio waves, and a computer to make a series of detailed pictures of areas inside the brain and spinal cord. A substance called "gadolinium" is injected into the patient through a vein. The gadolinium collects around the cancer cells, so they show up brighter in the picture. This procedure is also called "nuclear magnetic resonance imaging" (NMRI).

- **Positron emission tomography (PET) scan:** A procedure to find malignant tumor cells in the body. A small amount of radioactive glucose (sugar) is injected into a vein. The PET scanner rotates around the body and makes a picture of where glucose is being used in the body. Malignant tumor cells show up brighter in the picture because they are more active and take up more glucose than normal cells do.

- **Lumbar puncture:** A procedure used to collect cerebrospinal fluid (CSF) from the spinal column. This is done by placing a needle between two bones in the spine and into the CSF around the spinal cord and removing a sample of the fluid. The sample of CSF is checked under a microscope for signs of tumor cells. The sample may also be checked for the amounts of protein and glucose. A higher than normal amount of protein or lower than normal amount of glucose may be a sign of a tumor. This procedure is also called an "LP" or "spinal tap."

- **Stereotactic biopsy:** A biopsy procedure that uses a computer and a three-dimensional (3-D) scanning device to find a tumor site and guide the removal of tissue so it can be viewed under a microscope to check for signs of cancer.

The following tests may be done on the samples of tissue that are removed:

- **Flow cytometry:** A laboratory test that measures the number of cells in a sample; the percentage of live cells in a sample; and certain characteristics of cells, such as size, shape, and the presence of tumor markers on the cell surface. The cells are stained with a light-sensitive dye, placed in a fluid, and passed in a stream before a laser or other type of light. The measurements are based on how the light-sensitive dye reacts to the light.

- **Immunohistochemistry:** A test that uses antibodies to check for certain antigens in a sample of tissue. The antibody is usually linked to a radioactive substance or a dye that causes the tissue to light up under a microscope. This type of test may be used to tell the difference between different types of cancer.

- **Cytogenetic analysis:** A laboratory test in which cells in a sample of tissue are viewed under a microscope to look for certain changes in the chromosomes. Other tests, such as fluorescence in situ hybridization (FISH), may also be done to look for certain changes in the chromosomes.

- **A complete blood count (CBC) with differential:** A procedure in which a sample of blood is drawn and checked for the following:

  - The number of red blood cells (RBCs) and platelets

- The number and type of white blood cells (WBCs)

- The amount of hemoglobin (the protein that carries oxygen) in the red blood cells

- The portion of the blood sample made up of red blood cells

- **Blood chemistry studies:** A procedure in which a blood sample is checked to measure the amounts of certain substances released into the blood by organs and tissues in the body. An unusual (higher or lower than normal) amount of a substance can be a sign of disease.

Factors Affecting Prognosis and Treatment Options

The prognosis (chance of recovery) depends on the following:

- The patient's age and general health

- The level of certain substances in the blood and cerebrospinal fluid

- Where the tumor is in the central nervous system, eye, or both

- Whether the patient has AIDS

Treatment options depend on the following:

- The stage of the cancer

- Where the tumor is in the central nervous system

- The patient's age and general health

- Whether the cancer has just been diagnosed or has recurred (come back)

Treatment of primary CNS lymphoma works best when the tumor has not spread outside the cerebrum (the largest part of the brain) and the patient is younger than 60 years of age, able to carry out most daily activities, and does not have AIDS or other diseases that weaken the immune system.

Section 10.9

Waldenström Macroglobulinemia

This section contains text excerpted from the following sources:
Text beginning with the heading "What Is Waldenström
Macroglobulinemia?" is excerpted from "Waldenström
Macroglobulinemia," Genetics Home Reference (GHR), National
Institutes of Health (NIH), April 16, 2019; Text under the heading
"Treatment of Waldenström Macroglobulinemia" is excerpted from
"Waldenström Macroglobulinemia," Genetic and Rare Diseases
Information Center (GARD), National Center for Advancing
Translational Sciences (NCATS), October 1, 2013.
Reviewed June 2019.

What Is Waldenström Macroglobulinemia?

Waldenström macroglobulinemia is a rare blood cell cancer characterized by an excess of abnormal white blood cells (WBCs) called "lymphoplasmacytic cells" in the bone marrow. This condition is classified as a lymphoplasmacytic lymphoma. The abnormal cells have characteristics of both white blood cells (lymphocytes), called "B cells," and of more mature cells derived from B cells, known as "plasma cells." These abnormal cells produce excess amounts of immunoglobulin, a type of protein known as "IgM;" the overproduction of this large protein is how the condition got its name ("macroglobulinemia").

Waldenström macroglobulinemia usually begins in a person's sixties and is a slow-growing (indolent) cancer. Some affected individuals have elevated levels of IgM and lymphoplasmacytic cells but no symptoms of the condition; in these cases, the disease is usually found incidentally by a blood test taken for another reason. These individuals are diagnosed with smoldering (or asymptomatic) Waldenström macroglobulinemia. It can be several years before this form of the condition progresses to the symptomatic form.

Individuals with symptomatic Waldenström macroglobulinemia can experience general symptoms, such as fever, night sweats, and weight loss. Several other signs and symptoms of the condition are related to the excess IgM, which can thicken blood and impair circulation, causing a condition known as "hyperviscosity syndrome." Features related to hyperviscosity syndrome include bleeding in the nose or mouth, blurring or loss of vision, headache, dizziness, and difficulty coordinating movements (ataxia). In some affected individuals, the

IgM proteins clump together in the hands and feet, where the body temperature is cooler than at the center of the body. These proteins are then referred to as "cryoglobulins," and their clumping causes a condition known as "cryoglobulinemia." Cryoglobulinemia can lead to pain in the hands and feet or episodes of Raynaud phenomenon, in which the fingers and toes turn white or blue in response to cold temperatures. The IgM protein can also build up in organs, such as the heart and kidneys, causing a condition called "amyloidosis," which can lead to heart and kidney problems. Some people with Waldenström macroglobulinemia develop a loss of sensation and weakness in the limbs (peripheral neuropathy). Doctors are unsure why this feature occurs, although they speculate that the IgM protein attaches to the protective covering of nerve cells (myelin) and breaks it down. The damaged nerves cannot carry signals normally, leading to neuropathy.

Other features of Waldenström macroglobulinemia are due to the accumulation of lymphoplasmacytic cells in different tissues. For example, accumulation of these cells can lead to an enlarged liver (hepatomegaly), spleen (splenomegaly), or lymph nodes (lymph-adenopathy). In the bone marrow, the lymphoplasmacytic cells interfere with normal blood cell development, causing a shortage of normal blood cells (pancytopenia). Excessive tiredness (fatigue) due to a reduction in red blood cells (anemia) is common in affected individuals.

People with Waldenström macroglobulinemia have an increased risk of developing other cancers of the blood or other tissues.

Frequency of Waldenström Macroglobulinemia

Waldenström macroglobulinemia affects an estimated 3 per million people each year in the United States. Approximately 1,500 new cases of the condition are diagnosed each year in the United States, and White individuals are more commonly affected than African Americans. For unknown reasons, the condition occurs twice as often in men than women.

Causes of Waldenström Macroglobulinemia

Waldenström macroglobulinemia is thought to result from a combination of genetic changes. The most common known genetic change associated with this condition is a mutation in the *MYD88* gene, which is found in more than 90 percent of affected individuals. Another gene commonly associated with Waldenström macroglobulinemia, *CXCR4*, is mutated in approximately 30 percent of affected individuals (most of whom also have the *MYD88* gene mutation). Other genetic changes believed to be involved in Waldenström macroglobulinemia have not yet been identified. Studies have found that certain regions of deoxyribonucleic acid (DNA) are deleted or added in some people with the condition; however, researchers are unsure which genes in these regions are important for development of the condition. The mutations that cause Waldenström macroglobulinemia are acquired during a person's lifetime and are present only in the abnormal blood cells.

The proteins produced from the *MYD88* and *CXCR4* genes are both involved in signaling within cells. The MYD88 protein relays signals that help prevent the self-destruction (apoptosis) of cells, thus aiding in cell survival. The CXCR4 protein stimulates signaling pathways inside the cell that help regulate cell growth and division (proliferation) and cell survival. Mutations in these genes lead to production of proteins that are constantly functioning (overactive). Excessive signaling through these overactive proteins allows survival and proliferation of abnormal cells that should undergo apoptosis, which likely contributes to the accumulation of lymphoplasmacytic cells in Waldenström macroglobulinemia.

Treatment of Waldenström Macroglobulinemia

For individuals who do not have any symptoms, doctors may decide to "watch and wait" and not treat the disease right away. This can last for many years for some individuals. For individuals requiring treatment, the type and severity of symptoms present, aggressiveness of the disease, and age all play a role in the type of therapy chosen.

Some affected individuals have a procedure called "plasmapheresis" to reverse or prevent the symptoms associated with the thickening of the blood (hyperviscosity). This involves removing the blood, passing it through a machine that removes the part of the blood with the IgM antibody, and returning the blood to the body. This may be combined with other treatments, such as various types of chemotherapy. Many different drugs can be used to manage this condition, both alone and/or in various combinations.

For many individuals, there is a delayed response to treatment, and the best response sometimes occurs several months after the treatment ends. Although the condition is not curable, many individuals do have a long-term response to treatment. Those who relapse after treatment or do not respond to initial treatment may consider secondary therapies. There are also several new drugs and drug combinations that are being studied in clinical trials.

Chapter 11

Myeloproliferative Disorders

Chapter Contents

Section 11.1

Myelodysplastic Syndromes

This section includes text excerpted from "Myelodysplastic Syndromes Treatment (PDQ®)—Patient Version," National Cancer Institute (NCI), March 28, 2019.

What Are Myelodysplastic Syndromes?

In a healthy person, the bone marrow makes blood stem cells (immature cells) that become mature blood cells over time.

A blood stem cell may become a lymphoid stem cell or a myeloid stem cell. A lymphoid stem cell becomes a white blood cell (WBC). A myeloid stem cell becomes one of three types of mature blood cells:

- Red blood cells (RBCs) that carry oxygen and other substances to all tissues of the body

- Platelets that form blood clots to stop bleeding

- White blood cells that fight infection and disease

In a patient with a myelodysplastic syndrome, the blood stem cells (immature cells) do not become mature red blood cells, white blood cells, or platelets in the bone marrow. These immature blood cells, called "blasts," do not work the way they should and either die in the bone marrow or soon after they go into the blood. This leaves less room for healthy white blood cells, red blood cells, and platelets to form in the bone marrow. When there are fewer healthy blood cells, infection, anemia, or easy bleeding may occur.

Types of Myelodysplastic Syndromes

- **Refractory anemia:** There are too few red blood cells in the blood, and the patient has anemia. The number of white blood cells and platelets is normal.

- **Refractory anemia with ring sideroblasts:** There are too few red blood cells in the blood, and the patient has anemia. The red blood cells have too much iron inside the cell. The number of white blood cells and platelets is normal.

- **Refractory anemia with excess blasts:** There are too few red blood cells in the blood, and the patient has anemia. 5 percent to

19 percent of the cells in the bone marrow are blasts. There also may be changes to the white blood cells and platelets. Refractory anemia with excess blasts may progress to acute myeloid leukemia (AML).

- **Refractory cytopenia with multilineage dysplasia:** There are too few of at least two types of blood cells (red blood cells, platelets, or white blood cells). Less than 5 percent of the cells in the bone marrow are blasts, and less than 1 percent of the cells in the blood are blasts. If red blood cells are affected, they may have extra iron. Refractory cytopenia may progress to acute myeloid leukemia.

- **Refractory cytopenia with unilineage dysplasia:** There are too few of one type of blood cell (red blood cells, platelets, or white blood cells). There are changes in 10 percent or more of 2 other types of blood cells. Less than 5 percent of the cells in the bone marrow are blasts, and less than 1 percent of the cells in the blood are blasts.

- **Unclassifiable myelodysplastic syndrome:** The numbers of blasts in the bone marrow and blood are normal, and the disease is not one of the other myelodysplastic syndromes.

- **Myelodysplastic syndrome associated with an isolated del(5q) chromosome abnormality:** There are too few red blood cells in the blood, and the patient has anemia. Less than 5 percent of the cells in the bone marrow and blood are blasts. There is a specific change in the chromosome.

- **Chronic myelomonocytic leukemia (CMML)**

Risks of Myelodysplastic Syndrome

Anything that increases your risk of getting a disease is called a "risk factor." Having a risk factor does not mean that you will get a disease; not having risk factors does not mean that you will not get a disease. Talk with your doctor if you think you may be at risk. Risk factors for myelodysplastic syndromes include the following:

- Past treatment with chemotherapy or radiation therapy for cancer

- Being exposed to certain chemicals, including tobacco smoke; pesticides; fertilizers; and solvents, such as benzene

- Being exposed to heavy metals, such as mercury or lead

187

The cause of myelodysplastic syndromes in most patients is not known.

Signs and Symptoms of a Myelodysplastic Syndrome

Myelodysplastic syndromes often do not cause early signs or symptoms. They may be found during a routine blood test. Signs and symptoms may be caused by myelodysplastic syndromes or by other conditions. Check with your doctor if you have any of the following:

- Shortness of breath
- Weakness or feeling tired
- Having skin that is paler than usual
- Easy bruising or bleeding
- Petechiae (flat, pinpoint spots under the skin caused by bleeding)

Diagnosis of Myelodysplastic Syndromes

The following tests and procedures may be used:

- **Physical exam and history:** An exam of the body to check general signs of health, including checking for signs of disease, such as lumps or anything else that seems unusual. A history of the patient's health habits and past illnesses and treatments will also be taken.

- **A complete blood count (CBC) with differential:** A procedure in which a sample of blood is drawn and checked for the following:
  - The number of red blood cells and platelets
  - The number and type of white blood cells
  - The amount of hemoglobin (the protein that carries oxygen) in the red blood cells
  - The portion of the blood sample made up of red blood cells

- **Peripheral blood smear:** A procedure in which a sample of blood is checked for changes in the number, type, shape, and size of blood cells and for too much iron in the red blood cells.

- **Cytogenetic analysis:** A test in which cells in a sample of blood or bone marrow are viewed under a microscope to look for certain changes in the chromosomes.

- **Blood chemistry studies:** A procedure in which a blood sample is checked to measure the amounts of certain substances, such as vitamin B_{12} and folate, released into the blood by organs and tissues in the body. An unusual (higher or lower than normal) amount of a substance can be a sign of disease.

- **Bone marrow aspiration and biopsy:** The removal of bone marrow, blood, and a small piece of bone by inserting a hollow needle into the hipbone or breastbone. A pathologist views the bone marrow, blood, and bone under a microscope to look for abnormal cells.

The following tests may be done on the sample of tissue that is removed:

- **Immunocytochemistry:** A test that uses antibodies to check for certain antigens in a sample of bone marrow. This type of test is used to tell the difference between myelodysplastic syndromes, leukemia, and other conditions.

- **Immunophenotyping:** A process used to identify cells, based on the types of antigens or markers on the surface of the cell. This process is used to diagnose specific types of leukemia and other blood disorders by comparing the cancer cells to normal cells of the immune system.

- **Flow cytometry:** A laboratory test that measures the number of cells in a sample; the percentage of live cells in a sample; and certain characteristics of cells, such as size, shape, and the presence of tumor markers on the cell surface. The cells are stained with a light-sensitive dye, placed in a fluid, and passed in a stream before a laser or other type of light. The measurements are based on how the light-sensitive dye reacts to the light.

- **Fluorescence in situ hybridization (FISH):** A laboratory technique used to look at genes or chromosomes in cells and tissues. Pieces of deoxyribonucleic acid (DNA) that contain a fluorescent dye are made in the laboratory and added to cells or tissues on a glass slide. When these pieces of DNA bind to specific genes or areas of chromosomes on the slide, they light up when viewed under a microscope with a special light.

Factors Affecting Prognosis and Treatment Options

The prognosis (chance of recovery) and treatment options depend on the following:

- The number of blast cells in the bone marrow

- Whether one or more types of blood cells are affected

- Whether the patient has signs or symptoms of anemia, bleeding, or infection

- Whether the patient has a low or high risk of leukemia

- Certain changes in the chromosomes

- Whether the myelodysplastic syndrome occurred after chemotherapy or radiation therapy for cancer

- The age and general health of the patient

Section 11.2

Myelodysplastic/Myeloproliferative Neoplasms

This section includes text excerpted from "Myelodysplastic/ Myeloproliferative Neoplasms Treatment (PDQ®)—Patient Version," National Cancer Institute (NCI), March 28, 2019.

What Is Myelodysplastic/Myeloproliferative Neoplasms?

Myelodysplastic/myeloproliferative neoplasms are diseases of the blood and bone marrow.

Normally, the bone marrow makes blood stem cells (immature cells) that become mature blood cells over time. A blood stem cell may become a myeloid stem cell or a lymphoid stem cell. A lymphoid stem cell becomes a white blood cell (WBC). A myeloid stem cell becomes one of three types of mature blood cells:

- Red blood cells (RBCs) that carry oxygen and other substances to all tissues of the body

- White blood cells that fight infection and disease

- Platelets that form blood clots to stop bleeding

Different Types of Myelodysplastic/Myeloproliferative Neoplasms

The three main types of myelodysplastic/myeloproliferative neoplasms include the following:

- Chronic myelomonocytic leukemia (CMML)

- Juvenile myelomonocytic leukemia (JMML)

- Atypical chronic myelogenous leukemia (CML)

When a myelodysplastic/myeloproliferative neoplasm does not match any of these types, it is called "myelodysplastic/myeloproliferative neoplasm, unclassifiable" (MDS/MPN-UC).

Myelodysplastic/myeloproliferative neoplasms may progress to acute leukemia.

Diagnosis of Myelodysplastic/Myeloproliferative Neoplasms

The following tests and procedures may be used:

- **Physical exam and history:** An exam of the body to check general signs of health, including checking for signs of disease such as an enlarged spleen and liver. A history of the patient's health habits and past illnesses and treatments will also be taken.

- **A complete blood count (CBC) with differential:** A procedure in which a sample of blood is drawn and checked for the following:

  - The number of red blood cells and platelets

  - The number and type of white blood cells

  - The amount of hemoglobin (the protein that carries oxygen) in the red blood cells

  - The portion of the sample made up of red blood cells

- **Peripheral blood smear:** A procedure in which a sample of blood is checked for blast cells, the number and kinds of white blood cells, the number of platelets, and changes in the shape of blood cells.

- **Blood chemistry studies:** A procedure in which a blood sample is checked to measure the amounts of certain substances released into the blood by organs and tissues in the body. An unusual (higher or lower than normal) amount of a substance can be a sign of disease.

- **Bone marrow aspiration and biopsy:** The removal of a small piece of bone and bone marrow by inserting a needle into the hipbone or breastbone. A pathologist views both the bone and bone marrow samples under a microscope to look for abnormal cells.

The following tests may be done on the sample of tissue that is removed:

- **Cytogenetic analysis:** A test in which cells in a sample of blood or bone marrow are viewed under a microscope to look for certain changes in the chromosomes. The cancer cells in myelodysplastic/myeloproliferative neoplasms do not contain the Philadelphia chromosome (Ph) that is present in chronic myelogenous leukemia.

- **Immunocytochemistry:** A test that uses antibodies to check for certain antigens in a sample of bone marrow. The antibody is usually linked to a radioactive substance or a dye that causes the cells in the sample to light up under a microscope. This type of test is used to tell the difference between myelodysplastic/myeloproliferative neoplasms, leukemia, and other conditions.

Section 11.3

Chronic Myeloproliferative Neoplasms

This section includes text excerpted from "Chronic Myeloproliferative Neoplasms Treatment (PDQ®)—Patient Version," National Cancer Institute (NCI), January 31, 2019.

What Are Myeloproliferative Neoplasms?

Normally, the bone marrow makes blood stem cells (immature cells) that become mature blood cells over time.

A blood stem cell may become a myeloid stem cell or a lymphoid stem cell. A lymphoid stem cell becomes a white blood cell (WBC). A myeloid stem cell becomes one of three types of mature blood cells:

- Red blood cells (RBCs) that carry oxygen and other substances to all tissues of the body

- White blood cells that fight infection and disease

- Platelets that form blood clots to stop bleeding

In myeloproliferative neoplasms, too many blood stem cells become one or more types of blood cells. The neoplasms usually get worse slowly as the number of extra blood cells increases.

Types of Chronic Myeloproliferative Neoplasms

The type of myeloproliferative neoplasm is based on whether too many red blood cells, white blood cells, or platelets are being made. Sometimes, the body will make too many of more than one type of blood cell, but usually, one type of blood cell is affected more than the others are. Chronic myeloproliferative neoplasms include the following six types:

- Chronic myelogenous leukemia (CML)

- Polycythemia vera (PV)

- Primary myelofibrosis (also called "chronic idiopathic myelofibrosis")

- Essential thrombocythemia (ET)

- Chronic neutrophilic leukemia

- Chronic eosinophilic leukemia

These types are described below. Chronic myeloproliferative neoplasms sometimes become acute leukemia, in which too many abnormal white blood cells are made.

Diagnosis of Chronic Myeloproliferative Neoplasms

The following tests and procedures may be used:

- **Physical exam and history:** An exam of the body to check general signs of health, including checking for signs of disease, such as lumps or anything else that seems unusual. A history of the patient's health habits and past illnesses and treatments will also be taken.

- **A complete blood count (CBC) with differential:** A procedure in which a sample of blood is drawn and checked for the following:

  - The number of red blood cells and platelets

  - The number and type of white blood cells

  - The amount of hemoglobin (the protein that carries oxygen) in the red blood cells

  - The portion of the blood sample made up of red blood cells

- **Peripheral blood smear:** A procedure in which a sample of blood is checked for the following:

  - Whether there are red blood cells shaped like teardrops.

  - The number and kinds of white blood cells

  - The number of platelets

  - Whether there are blast cells

- **Blood chemistry studies:** A procedure in which a blood sample is checked to measure the amounts of certain substances released into the blood by organs and tissues in the body. An unusual (higher or lower than normal) amount of a substance can be a sign of disease.

- **Bone marrow aspiration and biopsy:** The removal of bone marrow, blood, and a small piece of bone by inserting a hollow needle into the hipbone or breastbone. A pathologist views the bone marrow, blood, and bone under a microscope to look for abnormal cells.

- **Cytogenetic analysis:** A test in which cells in a sample of blood or bone marrow are viewed under a microscope to look for certain changes in the chromosomes. Certain diseases or disorders may be diagnosed or ruled out based on the chromosomal changes.

- **Gene mutation test:** A laboratory test done on a bone marrow or blood sample to check for mutations in *JAK2*, *MPL*, or *CALR* genes. A *JAK2* gene mutation is often found in patients with polycythemia vera, essential thrombocythemia, or primary myelofibrosis. *MPL* or *CALR* gene mutations are found in patients with essential thrombocythemia or primary myelofibrosis.

Section 11.4

Polycythemia Vera

This section includes text excerpted from "Polycythemia Vera," Genetic and Rare Diseases Information Center (GARD), National Center for Advancing Translational Sciences (NCATS), November 2, 2017.

What Is Polycythemia Vera?

Polycythemia vera (PV) is a condition characterized by an increased number of red blood cells (RBCs) in the bloodstream (erythrocytosis). Affected people may also have excess white blood cells (WBCs) and platelets. Conditions, where the body makes too many of these cells, are known as "myeloproliferative neoplasms" (MPN). These extra cells cause the blood to be thicker than normal, increasing the risk for blood clots that can block blood flow in arteries and veins. If a blood clot occurs in the veins deep in the arms and the legs, it is known as "deep vein thrombosis" (DVT). A DVT can sometimes travel through the bloodstream to the lungs, which can cause a pulmonary embolism (PE) and is very dangerous. A blood clot could also travel to the heart or brain, which leads to an increased risk for heart attack or stroke.

Most cases of PV are not inherited and are acquired during a person's lifetime. PV is more common as a person ages, and it typically presents for the first time around 60 years of age. PV occurs more frequently in men than it does in women. The condition has been associated with mutations in the *JAK2* and *TET2* genes. In rare cases, the risk for PV runs in families and may be inherited in an autosomal dominant manner.

Symptoms of Polycythemia Vera

Polycythemia vera is characterized by having too many red blood cells in the bloodstream. This can cause problems because the blood is thicker than it would normally be, which causes an increased risk for blood clots that can cause serious health problems, such as heart attack or stroke. Other symptoms of PV include headaches, dizziness, ringing in the ears (tinnitus), and impaired vision. The skin may also become itchy (pruritus) or reddened (erythema). Affected individuals may also have an enlarged spleen (splenomegaly) and an increased risk for heart disease, and there is a small chance that PV may progress to cause leukemia (cancer of the blood).

Causes of Polycythemia Vera

Polycythemia vera is frequently caused by mutations (changes) affecting the *JAK2* gene and less frequently by mutations affecting the *TET2* gene. *JAK2* is known to provide the body with instructions to produce blood cells. When there is a mutation in this gene, the gene is constantly turned on, and the body, therefore, produces too many red blood cells. Having too many red blood cells cause the blood to be thicker than normal, so it cannot travel as efficiently through the bloodstream. This causes an increased risk for blood clots, and it can cause the skin to be reddened. It also can mean that the organs of the body are not getting enough oxygen due to reduced blood flow, so the organs such as the spleen may swell resulting in splenomegaly.

Inheritance of Polycythemia Vera

Even though most people with polycythemia vera have mutations in *JAK2* or *TET2*, that does not mean that the condition is inherited from their parents. Instead, most cases of polycythemia vera are associated with genetic changes (mutations) that are somatic. This means that the mutations occur in the cells that produce red blood cells (hematopoietic stem cell), but generally not in the egg and sperm cells which pass on genetic information to offspring.

In rare cases, the mutation to a gene that causes PV does occur in the egg or sperm cells, which increases the risk that a person with PV will pass the mutation on to their children. In these cases, the condition appears to have an autosomal dominant pattern of inheritance. This means that only one altered copy of a gene is enough to give a person an increased risk for PV. However, not every person who has a mutation in *JAK2* or *TET2* will necessarily develop PV. Rather, if a person has a mutation in one of these genes, she or he has an increased risk to develop PV during her or his lifetime.

Section 11.5

Thrombocythemia and Thrombocytosis

This section includes text excerpted from "Thrombocythemia and Thrombocytosis," National Heart, Lung, and Blood Institute (NHLBI), August 19, 2012. Reviewed June 2019.

What Are Thrombocythemia and Thrombocytosis?

Thrombocythemia and thrombocytosis are conditions in which your blood has a higher than normal number of platelets.

Platelets are blood cell fragments. They are made in your bone marrow along with other kinds of blood cells.

Platelets travel through your blood vessels and stick together (clot). Clotting helps stop any bleeding that may occur if a blood vessel is damaged. Platelets also are called "thrombocytes" because a blood clot also is called a "thrombus."

A normal platelet count ranges from 150,000 to 450,000 platelets per microliter of blood.

Causes of Thrombocythemia and Thrombocytosis
Primary Thrombocythemia

In this condition, faulty stem cells in the bone marrow make too many platelets. What causes this to happen usually is not known.

When this process occurs without other blood cell disorders, it is called "essential thrombocythemia."

A rare form of thrombocythemia is inherited. ("Inherited" means the condition is passed from parents to children through the genes.) In some cases, a genetic mutation may cause the condition.

In addition to the bone marrow making too many platelets, the platelets also are abnormal in primary thrombocythemia. They may form blood clots or, surprisingly, cause bleeding when they do not work well.

Bleeding also can occur because of a condition that develops called "von Willebrand disease" (VWD). This condition affects the blood clotting process.

After many years, scarring of the bone marrow can occur.

Secondary Thrombocytosis

This condition occurs if another disease, condition, or outside factor causes the platelet count to rise. For example, 35 percent of people who have high platelet counts also have cancer—most often of the lung, gastrointestinal (GI), breast, ovarian, and lymphoma varieties. Sometimes, a high platelet count is the first sign of cancer.

Other conditions or factors that can cause a high platelet count are:

- Iron-deficiency anemia

- Hemolytic anemia

- Absence of a spleen (after surgery to remove the organ)

- Inflammatory or infectious diseases, such as connective tissue disorders, inflammatory bowel disease (IBD), and tuberculosis (TB)

- Reactions to medicine

Some conditions can lead to a high platelet count that lasts for only a short time. Examples of such conditions include:

- Recovery from serious blood loss

- Recovery from a very low platelet count caused by excessive alcohol use and lack of vitamin B_{12} or folate

- Acute (short-term) infection or inflammation

- Response to physical activity

Although the platelet count is high in secondary thrombocytosis, the platelets are normal (unlike in primary thrombocythemia). Thus, people who have secondary thrombocytosis have a lower risk of blood clots and bleeding.

Risk Factors for Thrombocythemia and Thrombocytosis

Primary Thrombocythemia

Thrombocythemia is not common. The exact number of people who have the condition is not known. Some estimates suggest that 24 out of every 100,000 people have primary thrombocythemia.

Primary thrombocythemia is more common in people between the ages of 50 and 70, but it can occur at any age. For unknown reasons, more women around the age of 30 have primary thrombocythemia than men of the same age.

Secondary Thrombocytosis

You might be at risk for secondary thrombocytosis if you have a disease, condition, or factor that can cause it.

Secondary thrombocytosis is more common than primary thrombocythemia. Studies have shown that most people who have platelet counts over 500,000 have secondary thrombocytosis.

Screening and Prevention of Thrombocythemia and Thrombocytosis

You cannot prevent primary thrombocythemia. However, you can take steps to reduce your risk for complications. For example, you can control many of the risk factors for blood clots, such as high blood cholesterol, high blood pressure, diabetes, and smoking.

To reduce your risk, quit smoking, adopt healthy lifestyle habits, and work with your doctor to manage your risk factors.

It is not always possible to prevent conditions that lead to secondary thrombocytosis. But, if you have routine medical care, your doctor may detect these conditions before you develop a high platelet count.

Signs, Symptoms, and Complications of Thrombocythemia and Thrombocytosis

People who have thrombocythemia or thrombocytosis may not have signs or symptoms. These conditions might be discovered only after routine blood tests.

However, people who have primary thrombocythemia are more likely than those who have secondary thrombocytosis to have serious signs and symptoms.

The signs and symptoms of a high platelet count are linked to blood clots and bleeding. They include weakness, bleeding, headache, dizziness, chest pain, and tingling in the hands and feet.

Blood Clots

In primary thrombocythemia, blood clots most often develop in the brain, hands, and feet. But, they can develop anywhere in the body, including in the heart and intestines.

Blood clots in the brain may cause symptoms such as chronic (ongoing) headache and dizziness. In extreme cases, stroke may occur.

Blood clots in the tiny blood vessels of the hands and feet leave them numb and red. This may lead to an intense burning and throbbing pain felt mainly on the palms of the hands and the soles of the feet.

Other signs and symptoms of blood clots may include:

- Changes in speech or awareness, ranging from confusion to passing out

- Seizures

- Upper body discomfort in one or both arms, the back, neck, jaw, or abdomen

- Shortness of breath and nausea (feeling sick to your stomach)

In pregnant women, blood clots in the placenta can cause miscarriage or problems with fetal growth and development.

Women who have primary thrombocythemia or secondary thrombocytosis and take birth control pills (BCPs) are at an increased risk for blood clots.

Blood clots are related to other conditions and factors as well. Older age, prior blood clots, diabetes, high blood pressure, and smoking also increase your risk for blood clots.

Bleeding

If bleeding occurs, it most often affects people who have platelet counts higher than 1 million platelets per microliter of blood. Signs of bleeding include nosebleeds, bruising, bleeding from the mouth or gums, or blood in the stools.

Although bleeding usually is associated with a low platelet count, it also can occur in people who have high platelet counts. Blood clots that develop in thrombocythemia or thrombocytosis may use up your body's platelets. This means that not enough platelets are left in your bloodstream to seal off cuts or breaks on the blood vessel walls.

Another cause of bleeding in people who have very high platelets counts is von Willebrand disease. This condition affects the blood clotting process.

In rare cases of primary thrombocythemia, the faulty bone marrow cells will cause a form of leukemia. Leukemia is a cancer of the blood cells.

Living with Thrombocythemia and Thrombocytosis

If you have thrombocythemia or thrombocytosis:

- See your doctor for ongoing medical care.

- Control risk factors for blood clots—for example, quit smoking and work to manage risk factors, such as high blood cholesterol, high blood pressure, and diabetes.

- Watch for signs and symptoms of blood clots and bleeding, and report them to your doctor right away.

- Take all medicines as prescribed.

If you are taking medicines to lower your platelet count, tell your doctor or dentist about them before any surgical or dental procedures. These medicines thin your blood and may increase bleeding during these procedures.

Medicines that thin the blood also may cause internal bleeding. Signs of internal bleeding include bruises, bloody or tarry-looking stools, pink or bloody urine, increased menstrual bleeding, bleeding gums, and nosebleeds. Contact your doctor right away if you have any of these signs.

Avoid over-the-counter (OTC) pain medicines, such as ibuprofen (except Tylenol®). These medicines may raise your risk of bleeding in the stomach or intestines and may limit the effect of aspirin. Be aware that cold and pain medicines and other over-the-counter products may contain ibuprofen.

Chapter 12

Plasma Cell Disorders

Chapter Contents

Section 12.1

Amyloidosis

This section includes text excerpted from "Amyloidosis and Kidney Disease," National Institute of Diabetes and Digestive and Kidney Diseases (NIDDK), September 2014. Reviewed June 2019.

What Is Amyloidosis?

Amyloidosis is a rare disease that occurs when amyloid proteins are deposited in tissues and organs. Amyloid proteins are abnormal proteins that the body cannot break down and recycle, as it does with normal proteins. When amyloid proteins clump together, they form amyloid deposits. The buildup of these deposits damages a person's organs and tissues. Amyloidosis can affect different organs and tissues in different people and can affect more than one organ at the same time. Amyloidosis most frequently affects the kidneys, heart, nervous system, liver, and digestive tract. The symptoms and severity of amyloidosis depend on the organs and tissues affected.

What Types of Amyloidosis Affect the Kidneys?

Primary amyloidosis and dialysis-related amyloidosis are the types of amyloidosis that can affect the kidneys.

Primary Amyloidosis of the Kidneys

The kidneys are the organs most commonly affected by primary amyloidosis. Amyloid deposits damage the kidneys and make it harder for them to filter wastes and break down proteins. When the kidneys become too damaged, they may no longer be able to function well enough to maintain health, resulting in kidney failure. Kidney failure can lead to problems, such as high blood pressure, bone disease, and anemia—a condition in which the body has fewer red blood cells (RBCs) than normal.

Dialysis-Related Amyloidosis

People who suffer from kidney failure and have been on long-term dialysis may develop dialysis-related amyloidosis. This type of amyloidosis occurs when a certain protein, called "beta-2 microglobulin," builds up in the blood because dialysis does not remove it completely. The two types of dialysis are:

- **Hemodialysis.** Hemodialysis uses a special filter called a "dialyzer" to remove wastes and extra fluid from the blood.

- **Peritoneal dialysis.** Peritoneal dialysis uses the lining of the abdominal cavity—the space in the body that holds organs, such as the stomach, intestines, and liver—to filter the blood.

Dialysis-related amyloidosis is a complication of kidney failure because neither hemodialysis nor peritoneal dialysis effectively filters beta-2 microglobulin from the blood. As a result, elevated amounts of beta-2 microglobulin remain in the blood.

What Are the Signs and Symptoms of Primary Amyloidosis of the Kidneys?

The most common sign of primary amyloidosis of the kidneys is nephrotic syndrome—a collection of signs that indicate kidney damage. The signs of nephrotic syndrome include:

- **Albuminuria**—an increased amount of albumin, a protein, in the urine. A person with nephrotic syndrome excretes more than half a teaspoon of albumin per day.

- **Hyperlipidemia**—a condition in which a person's blood has more-than-normal amounts of fats and cholesterol.

- **Edema**—swelling, typically in a person's legs, feet, or ankles, and less often in the hands or face.

- **Hypoalbuminemia**—a condition in which a person's blood has less-than-normal amounts of albumin.

Other signs and symptoms of primary amyloidosis may include:

- Fatigue, or feeling tired

- Shortness of breath

- Low blood pressure

- Numbness, tingling, or a burning sensation in the hands or feet

- Weight loss

What Are the Symptoms of Dialysis-Related Amyloidosis?

The symptoms of dialysis-related amyloidosis may include:

- Pain, stiffness, and fluid in the joints
- Abnormal, fluid-containing sacs, called "cysts," in some bones
- Carpal tunnel syndrome, caused by unusual buildup of amyloid proteins in the wrists. The symptoms of carpal tunnel syndrome include numbness or tingling, sometimes associated with muscle weakness, in the fingers and hands.

Dialysis-related amyloidosis most often affects bones, joints, and the tissues that connect muscle to bone, called "tendons." The disease may also affect the digestive tract and organs, such as the heart and lungs. Bone cysts caused by dialysis-related amyloidosis can lead to bone fractures. Dialysis-related amyloidosis can also cause tears in tendons and ligaments. Ligaments are tissues that connect bones to other bones.

Eating, Diet, and Nutrition

Researchers have not found that eating, diet, and nutrition play a role in causing or preventing primary amyloidosis of the kidneys or dialysis-related amyloidosis. People with nephrotic syndrome may make dietary changes, such as:

- Limiting dietary sodium, often from salt, to help reduce edema and lower blood pressure
- Decreasing liquid intake to help reduce edema and lower blood pressure
- Eating a diet low in saturated fat and cholesterol to help control more-than-normal amounts of fats and cholesterol in the blood

Healthcare providers may recommend that people with kidney disease eat moderate or reduced amounts of protein. Proteins break down into waste products that the kidneys filter from the blood. Eating more protein than the body needs may burden the kidneys and cause kidney function to decline faster. However, protein intake that is too low may lead to malnutrition, a condition that occurs when the body does not get enough nutrients.

People with kidney disease on a restricted protein diet should receive blood tests that can show low nutrient levels. People with primary amyloidosis of the kidneys or dialysis-related amyloidosis should talk with a healthcare provider about dietary restrictions to best manage their individual needs.

Learning as much as you can about your treatment will help make you an important member of your healthcare team.

Section 12.2

Cryoglobulinemia

This section includes text excerpted from "Cryoglobulinemia," Genetic and Rare Diseases Information Center (GARD), National Center for Advancing Translational Sciences (NCATS), May 7, 2015. Reviewed June 2019.

What Is Cryoglobulinemia?

Cryoglobulinemia is a type of vasculitis that is caused by abnormal proteins (antibodies) in the blood called "cryoglobulins." At cold temperatures, these proteins become solid or gel-like, which can block blood vessels and cause a variety of health problems. Many people affected by this condition will not experience any unusual signs or symptoms. When present, symptoms vary but may include breathing problems, fatigue, glomerulonephritis, joint or muscle pain purpura, Raynaud phenomenon, skin death, and/or skin ulcers. In some cases, the exact underlying cause is unknown; however, cryoglobulinemia can be associated with a variety of conditions, including certain types of infection, chronic inflammatory diseases (such as an autoimmune disease), and/or cancers of the blood or immune system. Treatment varies based on the severity of the condition, the symptoms present in each person, and the underlying cause.

How Is Cryoglobulinemia Diagnosed?

Cryoglobulinemia can be diagnosed by certain blood tests, examining a sample of skin (skin biopsy), urine tests (urinalysis, particularly to look for blood in the urine), taking images of the arteries (angiogram), a chest X-ray, and/or testing the function of the nerves in the arms or legs.

Treatment of Cryoglobulinemia

The treatment for cryoglobulinemia depends on the cause and severity of this condition. Avoiding cold temperatures may be enough to treat mild cases. Severe cases may be treated by taking medication to reduce the body's immune response (corticosteroids), by removing some of the blood and replacing it with fluid or donated blood (a process called "plasmapheresis"), or by specifically treating diseases that may cause cryoglobulinemia (such as hepatitis C).

What Are the Expected Outcomes for Individuals with Cryoglobulinemia?

Cryoglobulinemia is usually not deadly. The outcome usually depends on the disease-causing cryoglobulinemia, as well as each person's response to treatments. The outcome is not as good when a person's kidneys are affected.

Section 12.3

Gamma Heavy Chain Disease

This section includes text excerpted from "Gamma Heavy Chain Disease," Genetic and Rare Diseases Information Center (GARD), National Center for Advancing Translational Sciences (NCATS), July 25, 2010. Reviewed June 2019.

What Is Gamma Heavy Chain Disease?

Gamma heavy chain disease is characterized by the abnormal production of antibodies. Antibodies are made up of light chains and heavy chains. In this disorder, the heavy chain of the gamma antibody (IgG) is overproduced by the body. Gamma heavy chain disease mainly affects older adults and is similar to aggressive malignant (cancerous) lymphoma. However, some people with this disorder have no symptoms. People with symptoms may respond to chemotherapy drugs, corticosteroids, and radiation therapy. Approximately one-third of individuals with gamma heavy chain disease are also diagnosed with an autoimmune disorder.

What Are the Symptoms of Gamma Heavy Chain Disease?

The severity of symptoms varies widely among people with gamma heavy chain disease. Symptoms include fever, mild anemia, difficulty swallowing (dysphagia), recurrent upper respiratory infections, and an enlarged liver and spleen (hepatosplenomegaly).

What Causes Gamma Heavy Chain Disease

The causes or risk factors for gamma heavy chain disease are not known.

Treatment of Gamma Heavy Chain Disease

People with symptoms may respond to chemotherapy drugs, corticosteroids, and radiation therapy. Commonly used chemotherapeutic agents include cyclophosphamide, prednisone, vincristine, chlorambucil, and doxorubicin. Patients are most commonly treated and followed by oncologists and/or hematologists.

Section 12.4

Plasma Cell Neoplasms

This section includes text excerpted from "Plasma Cell Neoplasms
(Including Multiple Myeloma) Treatment (PDQ®)—Patient Version,"
National Cancer Institute (NCI), April 9, 2019.

What Are Plasma Cell Neoplasms?

Plasma cells develop from B lymphocytes (B cells), a type of white
blood cell (WBC) that is made in the bone marrow. Normally, when
bacteria or viruses enter the body, some of the B cells will change into
plasma cells. The plasma cells make antibodies to fight bacteria and
viruses in order to stop infection and disease.

Plasma cell neoplasms are diseases in which abnormal plasma cells
or myeloma cells form tumors in the bones or soft tissues of the body.
The plasma cells also make an antibody protein, called "M protein,"
that is not needed by the body and does not help fight infection. These
antibody proteins build up in the bone marrow and can cause the blood
to thicken or can damage the kidneys.

Types of Plasma Cell Neoplasms

Plasma cell neoplasms include the following:

Monoclonal Gammopathy of Undetermined Significance

In this type of plasma cell neoplasm, less than 10 percent of the
bone marrow is made up of abnormal plasma cells and there is no
cancer. The abnormal plasma cells make M protein, which is sometimes found during a routine blood or urine test. In most patients, the
amount of M protein stays the same, and there are no signs, symptoms,
or health problems.

In some patients, MGUS may later become a more serious condition, such as amyloidosis, or cause problems with the kidneys, heart,
or nerves. MGUS can also become cancer, such as multiple myeloma,
lymphoplasmacytic lymphoma, or chronic lymphocytic leukemia.

Plasmacytoma

In this type of plasma cell neoplasm, the abnormal plasma
cells (myeloma cells) are in one place and form one tumor, called a

"plasmacytoma." Sometimes, plasmacytoma can be cured. There are two types of plasmacytoma.

- In **isolated plasmacytoma of the bone,** one plasma cell tumor is found in the bone, less than 10 percent of the bone marrow is made up of plasma cells, and there are no other signs of cancer. Plasmacytoma of the bone often becomes multiple myeloma.

- In **extramedullary plasmacytoma,** one plasma cell tumor is found in soft tissue but, not in the bone or the bone marrow. Extramedullary plasmacytomas commonly form in tissues of the throat, tonsil, and paranasal sinuses.

Signs and symptoms depend on where the tumor is.

- In bone, the plasmacytoma may cause pain or broken bones.

- In soft tissue, the tumor may press on nearby areas and cause pain or other problems. For example, a plasmacytoma in the throat can make it hard to swallow.

Multiple Myeloma

In multiple myeloma, abnormal plasma cells (myeloma cells) build up in the bone marrow and form tumors in many bones of the body. These tumors may keep the bone marrow from making enough healthy blood cells. Normally, the bone marrow makes stem cells (immature cells) that become three types of mature blood cells:

- Red blood cells (RBCs) that carry oxygen and other substances to all tissues of the body

- White blood cells that fight infection and disease

- Platelets that form blood clots to help prevent bleeding

As the number of myeloma cells increases, fewer red blood cells, white blood cells, and platelets are made. The myeloma cells also damage and weaken the bone.

Sometimes, multiple myeloma does not cause any signs or symptoms. This is called "smoldering multiple myeloma" (SMM). It may be found when a blood or urine test is done for another condition. Signs and symptoms may be caused by multiple myeloma or other conditions. Check with your doctor if you have any of the following:

- Bone pain, especially in the back or ribs

- Bones that break easily

- Fever for no known reason or frequent infections

- Easy bruising or bleeding

- Trouble breathing

- Weakness of the arms or legs

- Feeling very tired

A tumor can damage the bone and cause hypercalcemia (too much calcium in the blood). This can affect many organs in the body, including the kidneys, nerves, heart, muscles, and digestive tract, and cause serious health problems.

Hypercalcemia may cause the following signs and symptoms:

- Loss of appetite

- Nausea or vomiting

- Feeling thirsty

- Frequent urination

- Constipation

- Feeling very tired

- Muscle weakness

- Restlessness

- Confusion or trouble thinking

Multiple Myeloma and Amyloidosis

In rare cases, multiple myeloma can cause peripheral nerves (nerves that are not in the brain or spinal cord) and organs to fail. This may be caused by a condition called "amyloidosis." Antibody proteins build up and stick together in peripheral nerves and organs, such as the kidney and heart. This can cause the nerves and organs to become stiff and unable to work the way they should.

Amyloidosis may cause the following signs and symptoms:

- Feeling very tired

- Purple spots on the skin

- Enlarged tongue

- Diarrhea

- Swelling caused by fluid in your body's tissues
- Tingling or numbness in your legs and feet

Risks of Plasma Cell Neoplasms

Anything that increases your risk of getting a disease is called a "risk factor." Having a risk factor does not mean that you will get cancer; not having risk factors does not mean that you will not get cancer. Talk with your doctor if you think you may be at risk.

Plasma cell neoplasms are most common in people who are middle-aged or older. For multiple myeloma and plasmacytoma, other risk factors include the following:

- Being Black
- Being male
- Having a personal history of MGUS or plasmacytoma
- Being exposed to radiation or certain chemicals

Diagnosis of Multiple Myeloma and Other Plasma Cell Neoplasms

The following tests and procedures may be used:

- **Physical exam and history:** An exam of the body to check general signs of health, including checking for signs of disease, such as lumps, or anything else that seems unusual. A history of the patient's health habits and past illnesses and treatments will also be taken.

- **Blood and urine immunoglobulin studies:** A procedure in which a blood or urine sample is checked to measure the amounts of certain antibodies (immunoglobulins). For multiple myeloma, beta-2-microglobulin, M protein, free light chains, and other proteins made by the myeloma cells are measured. A higher-than-normal amount of these substances can be a sign of disease.

- **Bone marrow aspiration and biopsy:** The removal of bone marrow, blood, and a small piece of bone by inserting a hollow needle into the hipbone or breastbone. A pathologist views the bone marrow, blood, and bone under a microscope to look for abnormal cells.

The following test may be done on the sample of tissue removed during the bone marrow aspiration and biopsy:

- **Cytogenetic analysis:** A test in which cells in a sample of bone marrow are viewed under a microscope to look for certain changes in the chromosomes. Other tests, such as fluorescence in situ hybridization (FISH) and flow cytometry, may also be done to look for certain changes in the chromosomes.

- **Skeletal bone survey:** In a skeletal bone survey, X-rays of all the bones in the body are taken. The X-rays are used to find areas where the bone is damaged. An X-ray is a type of energy beam that can go through the body and onto film, making a picture of areas inside the body.

- **Complete blood count (CBC) with differential:** A procedure in which a sample of blood is drawn and checked for the following:

  - The number of red blood cells and platelets

  - The number and type of white blood cells

  - The amount of hemoglobin (the protein that carries oxygen) in the red blood cells

  - The portion of the blood sample made up of red blood cells

- **Blood chemistry studies:** A procedure in which a blood sample is checked to measure the amounts of certain substances, such as calcium or albumin, released into the blood by organs and tissues in the body. An unusual (higher or lower than normal) amount of a substance can be a sign of disease.

- **24-hour urine test:** A test in which urine is collected for 24 hours to measure the amounts of certain substances. An unusual (higher or lower than normal) amount of a substance can be a sign of disease in the organ or tissue that makes it. A higher than normal amount of protein may be a sign of multiple myeloma.

- **Magnetic resonance imaging (MRI):** A procedure that uses a magnet, radio waves, and a computer to make a series of detailed pictures of areas inside the body. This procedure is also called "nuclear magnetic resonance imaging" (NMRI). An MRI of the spine and pelvis may be used to find areas where the bone is damaged.

- **Positron emission tomography (PET) scan:** A procedure to find malignant tumor cells in the body. A small amount of radioactive glucose (sugar) is injected into a vein. The PET scanner rotates around the body and makes a picture of where glucose is being used in the body. Malignant tumor cells show up brighter in the picture because they are more active and take up more glucose than normal cells do.

- **Computed tomography (CT or CAT) scan:** A procedure that makes a series of detailed pictures of areas inside the body, such as the spine, taken from different angles. The pictures are made by a computer linked to an X-ray machine. A dye may be injected into a vein or swallowed to help the organs or tissues show up more clearly. This procedure is also called "computed tomography," "computerized tomography," or "computerized axial tomography."

- **Positron emission tomography-computed tomography (PET-CT) scan:** A procedure that combines the pictures from a positron emission tomography (PET) scan and a computed tomography (CT) scan. The PET and CT scans are done at the same time with the same machine. The combined scans give more detailed pictures of areas inside the body, such as the spine, than either scan gives by itself.

Factors Affecting Prognosis and Treatment Options

The prognosis (chance of recovery) depends on the following:

- The type of plasma cell neoplasm
- The stage of the disease
- Whether a certain immunoglobulin (antibody) is present
- Whether there are certain genetic changes
- Whether the kidney is damaged
- Whether the cancer responds to initial treatment or recurs (comes back)

Treatment options depend on the following:

- The type of plasma cell neoplasm
- The age and general health of the patient

- Whether there are signs, symptoms, or health problems, such as kidney failure or infection, related to the disease

- Whether the cancer responds to initial treatment or recurs

Chapter 13

Rh Incompatibility

What Is Rh Incompatibility?

Rh incompatibility is a condition that occurs during pregnancy if a woman has Rh-negative blood and the fetus has Rh-positive blood.

"Rh-negative" and "Rh-positive" refer to whether your blood has Rh factor. Rh factor is a protein on red blood cells (RBCs). If you have Rh factor, you are Rh-positive. If you do not have it, you are Rh-negative. Rh factor is inherited (passed from parents to children through the genes). Most people are Rh-positive.

Whether you have Rh factor does not affect your general health. However, it can cause problems during pregnancy.

Other Names for Rh Incompatibility

- Rh disease

- Rh-induced hemolytic disease of the newborn

What Causes Rh Incompatibility

A difference in blood type between a pregnant woman and the fetus causes Rh incompatibility. The condition occurs if a woman is Rh-negative and the fetus is Rh-positive.

This chapter includes text excerpted from "Rh Incompatibility," National Heart, Lung, and Blood Institute (NHLBI), November 8, 2008. Reviewed June 2019.

When you are pregnant, blood from the fetus can cross into your bloodstream, especially during delivery. If you are Rh-negative and the fetus is Rh-positive, your body will react to the fetus's blood as a foreign substance.

Your body will create antibodies (proteins) against the fetus's Rh-positive blood. These antibodies can cross the placenta and attack the fetus's red blood cells. This can lead to hemolytic anemia in the fetus.

Rh incompatibility usually does not cause problems during a first pregnancy. The baby often is born before many of the antibodies develop.

However, once you have formed Rh antibodies, they remain in your body. Thus, the condition is more likely to cause problems in second or later pregnancies (if the fetus is Rh-positive).

With each pregnancy, your body continues to make Rh antibodies. As a result, each Rh-positive child you conceive becomes more at risk for serious problems, such as severe hemolytic anemia.

Risk Factors for Rh Incompatibility

An Rh-negative woman who conceives a child with an Rh-positive man is at risk for Rh incompatibility. If you are Rh-negative and the father is Rh-positive, the child has a 50 percent or more chance of having Rh-positive blood.

Simple blood tests can show whether you and the father are Rh-positive or Rh-negative.

If you are Rh-negative, your risk of problems from Rh incompatibility is higher if you were exposed to Rh-positive blood before the pregnancy.

This may have happened during:

- An earlier pregnancy (usually during delivery). You also may have been exposed to Rh-positive blood if you had bleeding or abdominal trauma (for example, from a car accident) during the pregnancy.

- An ectopic pregnancy, a miscarriage, or an induced abortion. (An ectopic pregnancy is a pregnancy that starts outside of the uterus, or womb.)

- A mismatched blood transfusion or blood and marrow stem cell transplant

- An injection or puncture with a needle or other object containing Rh-positive blood

Certain tests also can expose you to Rh-positive blood. Examples include amniocentesis and chorionic villus sampling (CVS).

Amniocentesis is a test that you may have during pregnancy. Your doctor uses a needle to remove a small amount of fluid from the sac around the fetus. The fluid is then tested for various reasons.

Chorionic villus sampling also may be done during pregnancy. For this test, your doctor threads a thin tube through the vagina and cervix to the placenta. She or he removes a tissue sample from the placenta using gentle suction. The tissue sample is tested for various reasons.

Unless you were treated with the medicine that prevents Rh antibodies (Rh immune globulin) after each of these events, you are at risk for Rh incompatibility during current and future pregnancies.

Screening and Prevention of Rh Incompatibility

Rh incompatibility can be prevented with Rh immune globulin, as long as the medicine is given at the correct times. Once you have formed Rh antibodies, the medicine will no longer help.

Thus, a woman who has Rh-negative blood must be treated with Rh immune globulin during and after each pregnancy, or after any other event that allows her blood to mix with Rh-positive blood.

Early prenatal care also can help prevent some of the problems linked to Rh incompatibility. For example, your doctor can find out early whether you are at risk for the condition.

If you are at risk, your doctor can closely monitor your pregnancy. She or he will watch for signs of hemolytic anemia in the fetus and provided treatment as needed.

Signs, Symptoms, and Complications of Rh Incompatibility

Rh incompatibility does not cause signs or symptoms in a pregnant woman. In a fetus, the condition can lead to hemolytic anemia. Hemolytic anemia is a condition in which red blood cells are destroyed faster than the body can replace them.

Red blood cells contain hemoglobin, an iron-rich protein that carries oxygen to the body. Without enough red blood cells and hemoglobin, the fetus would not get enough oxygen.

Hemolytic anemia can cause mild to severe signs and symptoms in a newborn, such as jaundice and a buildup of fluid.

Jaundice is a yellowish color of the skin and whites of the eyes. When red blood cells die, they release hemoglobin into the blood. The hemoglobin is broken down into a compound called "bilirubin." This compound gives the skin and eyes a yellowish color. High levels of bilirubin can lead to brain damage in the fetus.

The buildup of fluid is a result of heart failure. Without enough hemoglobin-carrying red blood cells, the fetus's heart has to work harder to move oxygen-rich blood through the body. This stress can lead to heart failure.

Heart failure can cause fluid to build up in many parts of the body. When this occurs in a fetus or newborn, the condition is called "hydrops fetalis."

Severe hemolytic anemia can be fatal to a newborn at the time of birth or shortly after.

How Is Rh Incompatibility Diagnosed?

Rh incompatibility is diagnosed with blood tests. To find out if a fetus has developed hemolytic anemia and how serious it is, doctors may use more advanced tests, such as ultrasound.

Specialists Involved

An obstetrician will screen for Rh incompatibility. This is a doctor who specializes in treating pregnant women. The obstetrician also will monitor the pregnancy and the fetus for problems related to hemolytic anemia. She or he also will oversee treatment to prevent problems with future pregnancies.

A pediatrician or hematologist treats newborns who have hemolytic anemia and related problems. A pediatrician is a doctor who specializes in treating children. A hematologist is a doctor who specializes in treating people who have blood diseases and disorders.

Diagnostic Tests

If you are pregnant, your doctor will order a simple blood test at your first prenatal visit to learn whether you are Rh-positive or Rh-negative.

If you are Rh-negative, you also may have another blood test called an "antibody screen." This test shows whether you have Rh antibodies in your blood. If you do, it means that you were exposed to Rh-positive blood before and you are at risk for Rh incompatibility.

If you are Rh-negative and you do not have Rh antibodies, the father also will be tested to find out his Rh type. If he is Rh-negative too, the fetus has no chance of having Rh-positive blood. Thus, there is no risk of Rh incompatibility.

However, if the father is Rh-positive, the fetus has a 50 percent or more chance of having Rh-positive blood. As a result, you are at a high risk of developing Rh incompatibility.

If the father is Rh-positive, or if it is not possible to find out his Rh status, your doctor may do a test called "amniocentesis."

For this test, your doctor inserts a hollow needle through your abdominal wall into your uterus. She or he removes a small amount of fluid from the sac around the fetus. The fluid is tested to learn whether the fetus is Rh-positive. (Rarely, an amniocentesis can expose you to Rh-positive blood).

Your doctor also may use this test to measure the fetus's bilirubin levels. Bilirubin builds up as a result of red blood cells dying too quickly. The higher the level of bilirubin is, the greater the chance that the fetus has hemolytic anemia.

If Rh incompatibility is known or suspected, you will be tested for Rh antibodies one or more times during your pregnancy. This test often is done at least once at your sixth or seventh month of pregnancy.

The results from this test also can suggest how severe the fetus's hemolytic anemia has become. Higher levels of antibodies suggest more severe hemolytic anemia.

To check the fetus for hemolytic anemia, your doctor also may use a test called "Doppler ultrasound." She or he will use this test to measure how fast blood is flowing through an artery in the fetus's head.

Doppler ultrasound uses sound waves to measure how fast blood is moving. The faster the blood flow is, the greater the risk of hemolytic anemia. This is because the anemia will cause the fetus's heart to pump more blood.

How Is Rh Incompatibility Treated?

Rh incompatibility is treated with a medicine called "Rh immune globulin." Treatment for a fetus with hemolytic anemia will vary based on the severity of the condition.

Goals of Treatment

The goals of treating Rh incompatibility are to ensure that the fetus is healthy and to lower your risk for the condition in future pregnancies.

Treatment of Rh Incompatibility

If Rh incompatibility is diagnosed during your pregnancy, you will receive Rh immune globulin in your seventh month of pregnancy and again within 72 hours of delivery.

You also may receive Rh immune globulin if the risk of blood transfer between you and the fetus is high (for example, if you have had a miscarriage, ectopic pregnancy, or bleeding during pregnancy).

Rh immune globulin contains Rh antibodies that attach to the Rh-positive blood cells in your blood. When this happens, your body does not react to the fetus's Rh-positive cells as a foreign substance. As a result, your body does not make Rh antibodies. Rh immune globulin must be given at the correct times to work properly.

Once you have formed Rh antibodies, the medicine will no longer help. That is why a woman who has Rh-negative blood must be treated with the medicine with each pregnancy or any other event that allows her blood to mix with Rh-positive blood.

Rh immune globulin is injected into the muscle of your arm or buttock. Side effects may include soreness at the injection site and a slight fever. The medicine also may be injected into a vein.

Treatment of Hemolytic Anemia

Several options are available for treating hemolytic anemia in a fetus. In mild cases, no treatment may be needed. If treatment is needed, the fetus may be given a medicine called "erythropoietin" and "iron supplements." These treatments can prompt the body to make red blood cells.

If the hemolytic anemia is severe, the fetus may get a blood transfusion through the umbilical cord. If the hemolytic anemia is severe and the fetus is almost full-term, your doctor may induce labor early. This allows the fetus's doctor to begin treatment right away.

A newborn who has severe anemia may be treated with a blood exchange transfusion. The procedure involves slowly removing the newborn's blood and replacing it with fresh blood or plasma from a donor.

Newborns also may be treated with special lights to reduce the amount of bilirubin in their blood. These babies may have jaundice (a yellowish color of the skin and whites of the eyes). High levels of bilirubin cause jaundice.

Reducing the blood's bilirubin level is important because high levels of this compound can cause brain damage. High levels of bilirubin often are seen in babies who have hemolytic anemia. This is because the compound forms when red blood cells break down.

Living with Rh Incompatibility

If you have Rh-negative blood, injections of Rh immune globulin can reduce your risk of Rh incompatibility in future pregnancies. It is important to get this medicine every time you give birth to an Rh-positive baby or come in contact with Rh-positive blood.

You also can be exposed to Rh-positive blood during certain tests, such as amniocentesis and chorionic villus sampling.

Unless you were treated with Rh immune globulin after each of these events, you are at risk for Rh incompatibility during current and future pregnancies.

Let your doctor know about your risk early in your pregnancy. This allows her or him to carefully monitor your pregnancy and promptly treat any problems that arise.

Chapter 14

White Blood Cell Disorders

Chapter Contents

Section 14.1

Hypereosinophilic Syndrome

This section includes text excerpted from "Hypereosinophilic Syndrome," Genetic and Rare Diseases Information Center (GARD), National Center for Advancing Translational Sciences (NCATS), April 11, 2019.

What Is Hypereosinophilic Syndrome?

Hypereosinophilic syndrome (HES) refers to a rare group of conditions that are associated with persistent eosinophilia with evidence of organ involvement. Signs and symptoms vary significantly based on which parts of the body are affected. Although any organ system can be involved in HES, the heart, central nervous system, skin, and respiratory tract are the most commonly affected. The condition was originally thought to be idiopathic, or of unknown cause. However, recent advances in diagnostic testing have allowed a cause to be identified in approximately a quarter of cases. Management varies based on the severity of the condition and whether or not an underlying cause has been identified but generally includes imatinib or corticosteroids as an initial treatment.

Symptoms of Hypereosinophilic Syndrome

The signs and symptoms of the hypereosinophilic syndrome can vary significantly depending on which parts of the body are affected.

Some of the most frequent symptoms, listed by the body system affected, include:

- **Skin.** Rashes, itching, and edema

- **Lung.** Asthma, cough, difficulty breathing, recurrent upper respiratory infections, and pleural effusion

- **Gastrointestinal.** Abdominal pain, vomiting, and diarrhea

- **Musculoskeletal.** Arthritis, muscle inflammation, muscle aches, and joint pain

- **Nervous system.** Vertigo, paresthesia, speech impairment, and visual disturbances

- **Heart.** Congestive heart failure, cardiomyopathy, pericardial effusion, and myocarditis

- **Blood.** Deep venous thrombosis and anemia

Affected people can also experience a variety of nonspecific symptoms, such as fever, weight loss, night sweats, and fatigue.

Causes of Hypereosinophilic Syndrome

When the term "hypereosinophilic syndrome" was originally coined in 1975, the condition was thought to be idiopathic or of an unknown cause. At present, in approximately 75 percent of cases, the underlying cause still remains unknown. However, recent advances in diagnostic techniques have lead researchers to believe that some people affected by HES may have eosinophilia due to a variety of causes, including:

- Myeloproliferative neoplasms (MPNs) or other disorders that affect the bone marrow (myeloproliferative disorders). This form is called "myeloproliferative HES."

- Increased production of interleukin-5 (a protein produced by certain types of white blood cell (WBC)). This form is called "lymphocytic HES."

- A change (mutation) in an unknown gene passed down through a family. This form is called "familial HES."

Inheritance of Hypereosinophilic Syndrome

Although most cases of hypereosinophilic syndrome (HES) are not inherited, some cases do appear to be passed down through a family. In these families, the exact underlying genetic cause is unknown, but the genetic mutation is thought to be inherited in an autosomal dominant manner.

In autosomal dominant conditions, an affected person only needs a mutation in one copy of the responsible gene in each cell. In some cases, an affected person inherits the mutation from an affected parent. Other cases may result from new (de novo) mutations in the gene. These cases occur in people with no history of the disorder in their family. A person with an autosomal dominant condition has a 50 percent chance with each pregnancy of passing along the altered gene to her or his child.

Section 14.2

Langerhans Cell Histiocytosis

This section includes text excerpted from "Langerhans
Cell Histiocytosis," Genetic and Rare Diseases Information
Center (GARD), National Center for Advancing Translational
Sciences (NCATS), October 18, 2014. Reviewed June 2019.

What Is Langerhans Cell Histiocytosis?

Langerhans cell histiocytosis (LCH) is a disorder that primarily
affects children but is also found in adults of all ages. People with LCH
produce too many Langerhans cells or histiocytes, a form of white blood
cell found in healthy people that is supposed to protect the body from
infection. In people with LCH, these cells multiply excessively and
build up in certain areas of the body, causing tumors called "granulomas" to form. The symptoms vary among affected individuals, and
the cause of LCH is unknown. In most cases, this condition is not
life-threatening. Some people do experience lifelong problems associated with LCH.

What Are the Signs and Symptoms of Langerhans Cell Histiocytosis?

Symptoms of Langerhans cell histiocytosis (LCH) can vary greatly
from person to person depending on how much of the body is involved
and what part(s) are affected. The disease can affect virtually every
organ, including skin, bones, lymph nodes, bone marrow, liver, spleen,
lungs, gastrointestinal tract, thymus, central nervous system, and
hormone glands. The symptoms may range from localized bone lesions
or skin disease to multiple organ involvement and severe dysfunction.

Below are the organs that may be affected, as well as the symptoms
that might be observed:

- **Skin.** Red, scaly papules in areas where opposing skin surfaces
  touch or rub (e.g., skin folds) are commonly seen in LCH. Infants
  with the skin presentation on the scalp are often misdiagnosed
  with cradle cap. The skin symptoms usually improve without
  treatment.

- **Bone.** Lesions that cause bone destruction are common, with
  the skull, lower limbs, ribs, pelvis, and vertebrae usually being

affected. Symptoms may include pain, swelling, limited motion, and an inability to bear weight.

- **Lymph node.** Lymph node involvement may be limited or associated with a skin or bone lesion or disseminated disease. Although any of the lymph nodes may be affected, the cervical lymph nodes are where the disease commonly occurs. Individuals usually only experience pain of the lymph node affected. If only one lymph node is affected, prognosis is normally good and treatment is unnecessary.

- **Liver.** Liver involvement at the time of diagnosis is generally associated with more severe disease. Symptoms may include ascites, jaundice, low levels of protein, and prolonged clotting time.

- **Central nervous system (CNS) and hormone.** CNS involvement is rare and may be devastating. The most common result of CNS involvement is the altering of hormonal function, with some individuals developing diabetes insipidus.

What Causes Langerhans Cell Histiocytosis

The cause of Langerhans cell histiocytosis is unknown. It may be triggered by an unusual reaction of the immune system to something commonly found in the environment. It is not considered to be an infection or cancer. It is not known to be hereditary or communicable.

Is Langerhans Cell Histiocytosis Inherited?

Although Langerhans cell histiocytosis is generally considered a sporadic, nonhereditary condition, it has reportedly affected more than one individual in a family in a very limited number of cases (particularly identical twins).

How Is Langerhans Cell Histiocytosis Diagnosed?

Testing for Langerhans cell histiocytosis (LCH) may include bronchoscopy with biopsy, X-ray, skin biopsy, bone marrow biopsy, complete blood count, and pulmonary function tests. Because LCH is sometimes associated with cancer, CT scans and a biopsy may be done to rule out possible cancer.

Treatment of Langerhans Cell Histiocytosis

Treatment for LCH depends upon the individual patient; it may differ depending on the type and severity of the condition, as well as what part(s) of the body are affected. In some cases, the disease will regress without any treatment at all. In other cases, limited surgery and small doses of radiation therapy or chemotherapy will be needed, depending on the extent of the disease. Treatment is planned after complete evaluation of the patient, with the goal of using as little treatment as possible to keep the disease under control.

What Is the Typical Prognosis for People with Langerhans Cell Histiocytosis?

The prognosis (chance of recovery) for people with LCH can vary greatly from patient to patient, but in the majority of children, the disease resolves itself. Prognosis seems to be dependent mainly on the number of organ systems involved, the severity of organ involvement, and to a lesser rate, the age at which symptoms occur. In general, patients who are young and those with disseminated disease and organ dysfunction tend to have a poorer prognosis. Newborns who present only with skin lesions tend to do well. Therefore, the age at presentation is only important when multiple organs are affected. Additionally, individuals who have liver, spleen, lung, or bone marrow involvement usually have a worse prognosis. In a study looking at patients from several centers, it was shown that the best prognostic indicator was the patient's response to chemotherapy during the first six weeks of therapy. Therefore, it has been recommended by some that individuals who do not respond positively within the first six weeks of treatment should be treated more aggressively.

Other Names for Langerhans Cell Histiocytosis

- LCH
- Histiocytosis X
- Eosinophilic granuloma (formerly)
- Letterer-Siwe disease (formerly)
- Hand-Schüller-Christian syndrome (formerly)

Section 14.3

Lymphocytopenia

This section includes text excerpted from
"Lymphocytopenia," National Heart, Lung, and Blood
Institute (NHLBI), November 25, 2014. Reviewed June 2019.

What Is Lymphocytopenia?

Lymphocytopenia is a disorder in which your blood does not have enough white blood cells called "lymphocytes."

These cells are made in the bone marrow along with other kinds of blood cells. Lymphocytes help protect your body from infection. Low numbers of lymphocytes can raise your risk of infection. Lymphocytopenia also is called "lymphopenia."

Causes of Lymphocytopenia

In general, lymphocytopenia occurs because:

- The body does not make enough lymphocytes.

- The body makes enough lymphocytes, but they are destroyed.

- The lymphocytes get stuck in the spleen or lymph nodes.

A combination of these factors also may cause a low lymphocyte count.

Many diseases, conditions, and factors can lead to a low lymphocyte count. These conditions can be acquired or inherited. "Acquired" means you are not born with the condition, but you develop it. "Inherited" means your parents passed the gene for the condition on to you.

Exactly how each disease, condition, or factor affects your lymphocyte count is not known. Some people have low lymphocyte counts with no underlying cause.

Acquired Causes

Many acquired diseases, conditions, and factors can cause lymphocytopenia. Examples include:

- Infectious diseases, such as acquired immunodeficiency syndrome (AIDS) viral hepatitis, tuberculosis, and typhoid fever

- Autoimmune disorders, such as lupus. (Autoimmune disorders occur if the body's immune system mistakenly attacks the body's cells and tissues.)

- Steroid therapy

- Blood cancer and other blood diseases, such as Hodgkin disease and aplastic anemia

- Radiation and chemotherapy (treatments for cancer)

Inherited Causes

Certain inherited diseases and conditions can lead to lymphocytopenia. Examples include DiGeorge anomaly, Wiskott-Aldrich syndrome, severe combined immunodeficiency syndrome, and ataxia-telangiectasia. These inherited conditions are rare.

Risk Factors of Lymphocytopenia

People at the highest risk for lymphocytopenia have one of the diseases, conditions, or factors that can cause a low lymphocyte count. This includes people who have:

- AIDS or other infectious diseases

- Autoimmune disorders

- Blood cancers or other blood diseases

- Certain inherited diseases or conditions

People who have had steroid therapy or radiation or chemotherapy also are at increased risk.

Signs, Symptoms, and Complications of Lymphocytopenia

A low lymphocyte count alone may not cause any signs or symptoms. The condition usually is found when a person is tested for other diseases or conditions, such as AIDS.

If you have unusual infections, repeat infections, and/or infections that will not go away, your doctor may suspect that you have lymphocytopenia. Fever is the most common symptom of infection.

Screening and Prevention of Lymphocytopenia

You cannot prevent lymphocytopenia that is caused by an inherited condition. However, you can take steps to control lymphocytopenia. Follow your treatment plan and take all medicines as your doctor advises.

Early diagnosis also can help control lymphocytopenia. In the United States, newborns are routinely screened for an immune condition that can lead to lymphocytopenia. This allows doctors to diagnose the disorder before serious problems develop.

Living with Lymphocytopenia

If you have mild lymphocytopenia with no underlying cause, you may not need treatment. The disorder may improve on its own.

If an underlying condition is causing your lymphocytopenia, you will need treatment for that condition. You will also need treatment for infections if your body is unable to fight them because of lymphocytopenia.

Treating and Preventing Infections

The main risk of lymphocytopenia is getting unusual infections, repeat infections, and/or infections that will not go away. If you have the disorder, you may receive treatments to prevent infections or to treat infections you already have.

You also can take other steps to prevent infections. For example:

- Stay away from people who are sick, and avoid large crowds of people.

- Avoid foods that can expose you to bacteria, such as uncooked foods.

- Wash your hands often.

- Brush and floss your teeth, and get regular dental care to reduce the risk of infection in your mouth and throat.

- Ask your doctor whether you should get a yearly flu shot and the pneumonia vaccine.

Know the signs of an infection, such as a fever. Call your doctor right away if you think you have an infection.

Treating an Underlying Disease or Condition

If you have a disease or condition that is causing lymphocytopenia, you will need treatment for that condition.

You will likely have regular tests to show how the treatment is working. For example, you may have blood tests to check the number of lymphocytes in your blood.

If the treatments for the underlying condition are working, the number of lymphocytes in your blood may go up.

Physical Activity

Talk with your doctor about what types and amounts of physical activity are safe for you. You may want to avoid activities that could result in injuries or increase your risk of infections.

Section 14.4

Neutropenia

This section includes text excerpted from "What You Need to Know Neutropenia and Risk for Infection," Centers for Disease Control and Prevention (CDC), October 20, 2011. Reviewed June 2019.

What Is Neutropenia?

Neutropenia is a decrease in the number of white blood cells (WBCs). These cells are the body's main defense against infection. Neutropenia is common after receiving chemotherapy and increases your risk for infections.

Why Does Chemotherapy Cause Neutropenia?

These cancer-fighting drugs work by killing fast-growing cells in the body—both good and bad. These drugs kill cancer cells, as well as healthy white blood cells.

How Do I Know If I Have Neutropenia?

Your doctor or nurse will tell you. Because neutropenia is common after receiving chemotherapy, your doctor may draw some blood to look for neutropenia.

When Will I Be Most Likely to Have Neutropenia?

Neutropenia often occurs between 7 and 12 days after you receive chemotherapy. This period can be different depending upon the chemotherapy you get. Your doctor or nurse will let you know exactly when your white blood cell count is likely to be at its lowest. You should carefully watch for signs and symptoms of infection during this time.

How Can I Prevent Neutropenia?

There is not much you can do to prevent neutropenia from occurring, but you can decrease your risk for getting an infection while your white blood cell count is low.

How Can I Prevent an Infection?

In addition to receiving treatment from your doctor, the following suggestions can help prevent infections:

- Clean your hands frequently.
- Try to avoid crowded places and contact with people who are sick.
- Do not share food; drink cups; utensils; or other personal items, such as toothbrushes.
- Shower or bathe daily, and use an unscented lotion to prevent your skin from becoming dry and cracked.
- Cook meat and eggs all the way through to kill any germs.
- Carefully wash raw fruits and vegetables.
- Protect your skin from direct contact with pet bodily waste (urine or feces) by wearing vinyl or household cleaning gloves when cleaning up after your pet. Wash your hands immediately afterward.
- Use gloves for gardening.

- Clean your teeth and gums with a soft toothbrush, and if your doctor or nurse recommends one, use a mouthwash to prevent mouth sores.

- Try and keep all your household surfaces clean.

- Get the seasonal flu shot as soon as it is available.

What If I Have to Go to the Emergency Room

Cancer patients receiving chemotherapy should not sit in a waiting room for a long time. While you are receiving chemotherapy, fever may be a sign of infection. Infections can become serious very quickly. When you check in, tell them right away that you are getting chemotherapy and have a fever. This may be an indication of an infection.

Part Three

Bleeding and Clotting Disorders

Chapter 15

What Are Hereditary Bleeding and Clotting Disorders?

Bleeding Disorders

The blood clotting process, known as "coagulation," occurs when an injury causes a wound to bleed. When a healthy person is injured and begins to bleed, blood platelets immediately begin bonding together to form a blood clot, stopping further blood loss. Bleeding disorders interfere with the body's ability to form blood clots. This can result in excessive or abnormal bleeding internally or externally, depending upon the nature of the wound.

In most cases, bleeding disorders are inherited. Certain chronic health conditions can also result in a person developing an acquired bleeding disorder. Bleeding disorders can result from anemia, human immunodeficiency virus (HIV), low red blood cell count, liver disease, leukemia, vitamin K deficiency, and use of certain medications known as "anticoagulants."

Types of Bleeding Disorders

Bleeding disorders are primarily caused by insufficient levels or the absence of blood proteins known as "clotting factors." There are 13

"What Are Bleeding and Clotting Disorders?" © 2016 Omnigraphics. Reviewed June 2019.

blood clotting factors that help blood clots to form. Bleeding disorders are diagnosed and categorized according to the specific clotting factor that is deficient in a person's blood.

Hemophilia A (factor VIII deficiency) and hemophilia B (factor IX deficiency) are bleeding disorders that result in excessive bleeding after an injury to deep tissue (for example, in joints and muscles).

Von Willebrand disease is an inherited bleeding disorder affecting the body's ability to form blood clots due to lack of the von Willebrand factor. People who live with von Willebrand disease experience excessive bleeding after injuries to skin or mucous membranes (for example, inside the nose, mouth, and intestines).

Bleeding disorders due to deficiencies in the remaining clotting factors occur more rarely than hemophilia and von Willebrand disease.

Symptoms and Risks

Bleeding disorder symptoms tend to be different for each condition. Most bleeding disorders share primary symptoms such as frequent unexplained bruising, frequent nosebleeds, excessive bleeding after minor cuts, scrapes, or dental surgery, bleeding into joints or pooling blood in joints, and excessive or prolonged menstrual bleeding.

Bleeding disorders can expose a person to serious health risks if left undiagnosed and/or untreated. Some bleeding disorders result in unseen complications, such as internal bleeding in the intestines, the brain, or joints. Women with untreated bleeding disorders can be at a greater risk for developing anemia, a condition in which the body lacks sufficient levels of red blood cells. Anemia can result in dizziness, shortness of breath, and persistent general fatigue.

Diagnosis

Most bleeding disorders are diagnosed through blood tests. These tests measure the levels of certain blood components, such as red and white blood cells, platelet function, and bleeding time. Health professionals typically analyze blood test results while also considering a person's medical history. A medical history interview may be conducted, with a focus on the frequency of episodes of excessive bleeding, how long it usually takes to stop bleeding after a wound, and whether any family members have been diagnosed with bleeding disorders.

Clotting Disorders

Clotting disorders are similar to bleeding disorders in that both types of conditions affect the body's ability to form blood clots properly. However, where bleeding disorders indicate a lack of proper blood clot formation, clotting disorders result in unnecessary or excessive blood clot formation.

Clotting disorders can be inherited or acquired. Acquired clotting disorders can result from traumatic injury, surgery, certain chronic health conditions, and the use of certain medications.

Types of Clotting Disorder

Clotting disorders are typically caused by abnormal levels of the blood proteins that prevent blood clotting. Similar to bleeding disorders, clotting disorders are also categorized and diagnosed according to the specific blood protein that is affected. The most common form of inherited clotting disorder is factor V Leiden, a condition that results in excessive blood clots. Other inherited clotting disorders are indicated by abnormal levels of antithrombin; protein C; protein S; homocysteine; fibrinogen; or factors VIII, IX, and XI. A genetic disorder known as "*prothrombin* gene mutation" also produces excessive blood clotting.

Many health conditions and treatments can result in an acquired clotting disorder. These include cancer and cancer treatments, central venous catheter placements, deep vein thrombosis, heart attack, heart failure, HIV/acquired immunodeficiency virus (AIDS), hormone replacement therapy, inflammatory bowel syndrome (IBS), liver disease, nephrotic syndrome, obesity, oral contraceptives (birth control pills), pregnancy, prolonged immobility due to bed rest or other reason, traumatic injury, stroke, and surgery. Clotting disorders can also arise from frequent, lengthy airplane travel.

Symptoms and Risks

Clotting disorders, also known as "hypercoagulable state" or "thrombophilia," can be dangerous if left undiagnosed and/or untreated. Clotting disorders can cause blood clots to form within blood vessels as blood travels through the body. This type of blood clot is known as a "thrombus" or "embolus" and can result in a clotting disorder known as "disseminated intravascular coagulation." Blood clots that form in blood vessels can move throughout the body's bloodstream, resulting in serious complications if the clot lodges in the lungs, liver, intestines, kidneys, or veins in the legs and arms. Blood clots that move through or become lodged in arteries can cause stroke, heart attack, or loss of a limb due to the restricted blood supply.

Clotting disorder symptoms vary according to each specific condition. Some common symptoms include pain or swelling of the arms or legs, changes in skin color or temperature (redness, warmth), chest pain, shortness of breath, rapid heartbeat, heart attack or stroke at a young age, and multiple pregnancies that end in miscarriage or stillbirth.

Diagnosis

Clotting disorders are most often diagnosed through a medical history interview; various blood tests and diagnostic imaging, such as magnetic resonance imaging (MRI), ultrasound, or computed tomography (CT) scan. Some important medical history considerations in the diagnosis of clotting disorders are unexplained or recurring blood clots, history of frequent miscarriages, stroke or heart attack at a young age, and family members who have been diagnosed with a clotting disorder.

References

1. Kahn, April. "What is a Bleeding Disorder?" Health Line. December 3, 2015.

2. "Bleeding Disorders," National Hemophilia Foundation (NHF), n.d.

3. "Blood Clotting Disorders (Hypercoagulable States)," Cleveland Clinic, December 2015.

4. "Coagulation Disorders," Riley Children's Health, n.d.

Chapter 16

Vitamin K Deficiency Bleeding

What Is Vitamin K and Why Is It Important?

Vitamin K is a substance that our body needs to form clots and to stop bleeding. We get vitamin K from the food we eat. Some vitamin K is also made by the good bacteria that live in our intestines. Babies are born with very small amounts of vitamin K stored in their bodies, which can lead to serious bleeding problems if not supplemented.

What Is Vitamin K Deficiency Bleeding?

Vitamin K deficiency bleeding (VKDB) occurs when babies cannot stop bleeding because their blood does not have enough vitamin K to form a clot. The bleeding can occur anywhere on the inside or outside of the body. When the bleeding occurs inside the body, it can be difficult to notice. Commonly, a baby with VKDB will bleed into her or his intestines or into the brain, which can lead to brain damage and even death. Infants who do not receive the vitamin K shot at birth can develop VKDB at any time up to six months of age. There are three types of VKDB, based on the age of the baby when the bleeding problems start: early, classical, and late.

This chapter includes text excerpted from "What Is Vitamin K Deficiency Bleeding?" Centers for Disease Control and Prevention (CDC), December 26, 2018.

Why Are Babies More Likely to Have Vitamin K Deficiency and to Get Vitamin K Deficiency Bleeding?

All infants, regardless of sex, race, or ethnic background, are at higher risk for VKDB until they start eating regular foods, usually at the age of four to six months, and until the normal intestinal bacteria start making vitamin K. This is because:

- At birth, babies have very little vitamin K stored in their bodies because only small amounts pass to them through the placenta from their mothers.

- The good bacteria that produce vitamin K are not yet present in the newborn's intestines.

- Breast milk contains low amounts of vitamin K, so exclusively breastfed babies do not get enough vitamin K from the breast milk alone.

What Can I Do to Prevent My Baby from Getting Vitamin K Deficiency and Vitamin K Deficiency Bleeding?

The good news is that VKDB is easily prevented by giving babies a vitamin K shot into a muscle in the thigh. One shot given just after birth will protect your baby from VKDB. In order to ensure immediate bonding and contact between the newborn and mother, however, giving the vitamin K shot can be delayed up to six hours after birth.

Is the Vitamin K Shot Safe?

Yes. Many studies have shown that vitamin K is safe when given to newborns.

What Might Cause Babies to Be Deficient in Vitamin K and Have Bleeding Problems?

Some things can put infants at a higher risk of developing VKDB. Babies at greater risk include:

- Babies who do not receive a vitamin K shot at birth. The risk is even higher if they are exclusively breastfed.

- Babies whose mothers used certain medications, such as isoniazid or medicines to treat seizures. These drugs interfere with how the body uses vitamin K.

- Babies who have liver disease; often, they cannot use the vitamin K their body stores.

- Babies who have diarrhea, celiac disease, or cystic fibrosis often have trouble absorbing vitamins, including vitamin K, from the foods they eat.

How Often Are Babies Affected with Vitamin K Deficiency Bleeding?

Since babies can be affected until they are six months of age, health-care providers divide VKDB into three types; early, classical and late. The list below helps explain these three different types.

- Early and classical vitamin K deficiency bleeding is more common, occurring in 1 in 60 to 1 in 250 newborns, although the risk is much higher for early VKDB among those infants whose mothers used certain medications during the pregnancy.

- Late vitamin K deficiency bleeding is rarer, occurring in 1 in 14,000 to 1 in 25,000 infants (1 to 3).

- Infants who do not receive a vitamin K shot at birth are 81 times more likely to develop late VKDB than infants who do receive a vitamin K shot at birth.

What Things Should I Look for in My Baby If I Think She or He Might Have Vitamin K Deficiency Bleeding?

Babies with vitamin K deficiency bleeding might develop any of the following signs:

- Bruises, especially around the baby's head and face

- Bleeding from the nose or umbilical cord

- Skin color that is paler than before. For darker skinned babies, the gums may appear pale.

- After the first three weeks of life, the white parts of your baby's eyes may turn yellow.

- Stool that has blood in it, is black or dark and sticky (also called "tarry"), or if your baby is vomiting blood

- Irritability, seizures, excessive sleepiness, or a lot of vomiting may all be signs of bleeding in the brain.

Chapter 17

Hemophilia

What Is Hemophilia?

Hemophilia is a rare bleeding disorder in which the blood does not clot normally.

If you have hemophilia, you may bleed for a longer time than others after an injury. You also may bleed inside your body (internally), especially in your knees, ankles, and elbows. This bleeding can damage your organs and tissues, and it may be life-threatening.

Causes of Hemophilia

A defect in one of the genes that determines how the body makes blood clotting factor VIII or IX causes hemophilia. These genes are located on the X chromosomes.

Chromosomes come in pairs. Females have two X chromosomes, while males have one X and one Y chromosome. Only the X chromosome carries the genes related to clotting factors.

A male who has a hemophilia gene on his X chromosome will have hemophilia. When a female has a hemophilia gene on only one of her X chromosomes, she is a "hemophilia carrier" and can pass the gene to her children. Sometimes, carriers have low levels of clotting factor and have symptoms of hemophilia, including bleeding. Clotting factors

---

This chapter includes text excerpted from "Hemophilia," National Heart, Lung, and Blood Institute (NHLBI), February 28, 2018.

are proteins in the blood that work together with platelets to stop or control bleeding.

Very rarely, a girl may be born with a very low clotting factor level and have a greater risk for bleeding, similar to boys who have hemophilia and very low levels of clotting factor. There are several hereditary and genetic causes of this much rarer form of hemophilia in females.

Some males who have the disorder are born to mothers who are not carriers. In these cases, a mutation (random change) occurs in the gene as it is passed to the child.

Below are two examples of how the hemophilia gene is inherited.

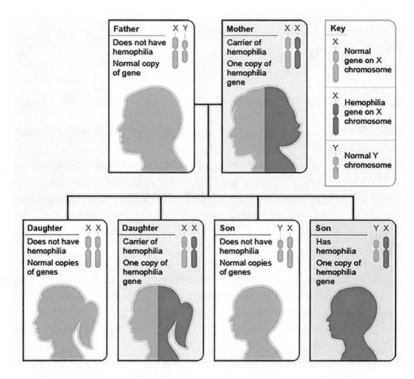

Figure 17.1. *Inheritance Pattern for Hemophilia—Example 1*

The image shows one example of how the hemophilia gene is inherited. In this example, the father does not have hemophilia (that is, he has two normal chromosomes—X and Y). The mother is a carrier of hemophilia (that is, she has one hemophilia gene on one X chromosome and one normal X chromosome).

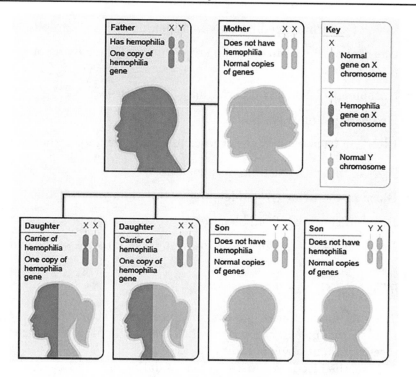

Figure 17.2. *Inheritance Pattern for Hemophilia—Example 2*

The image shows one example of how the hemophilia gene is inherited. In this example, the father has hemophilia (that is, he has the hemophilia gene on the X chromosome). The mother is not a hemophilia carrier (that is, she has two normal X chromosomes).

Signs, Symptoms, and Complications of Hemophilia

The major signs and symptoms of hemophilia are excessive bleeding and easy bruising.

Excessive Bleeding

The extent of bleeding depends on how severe the hemophilia is.

Children who have mild hemophilia may not have signs unless they have excessive bleeding from a dental procedure, an accident, or surgery. Males who have severe hemophilia may bleed heavily after circumcision.

Bleeding can occur on the body's surface (external bleeding) or internally.

Signs of external bleeding may include:

- Bleeding in the mouth from a cut or bite or from cutting or losing a tooth

- Nosebleeds for no obvious reason

- Heavy bleeding from a minor cut

- Bleeding from a cut that resumes after stopping for a short time

Signs of internal bleeding may include:

- Blood in the urine (from bleeding in the kidneys or bladder)

- Blood in the stool (from bleeding in the intestines or stomach)

- Large bruises (from bleeding into the large muscles of the body)

Bleeding in the Joints

Bleeding in the knees, elbows, or other joints is another common form of internal bleeding in people who have hemophilia. This bleeding can occur without obvious injury.

At first, the bleeding causes tightness in the joint with no real pain or any visible signs of bleeding. The joint then becomes swollen, hot to touch, and painful to bend.

Swelling continues as the bleeding continues. Eventually, movement in the joint is temporarily lost. Pain can be severe. Joint bleeding that is not treated quickly can damage the joint.

Bleeding in the Brain

Internal bleeding in the brain is a very serious complication of hemophilia. It can happen after a simple bump on the head or a more serious injury. The signs and symptoms of bleeding in the brain include:

- Long-lasting, painful headaches or neck pain or stiffness

- Repeated vomiting

- Sleepiness or changes in behavior

- Sudden weakness or clumsiness of the arms or legs or problems walking

- Double vision

- Convulsions or seizures

Living with Hemophilia

If you or your child has hemophilia, you can take steps to prevent bleeding problems. Thanks to improvements in treatment, a child who has hemophilia is likely to live a normal lifespan.

Hemophilia Treatment Centers

The federal government funds a nationwide network of hemophilia treatment centers (HTCs). These centers are an important resource for people who have hemophilia and their families.

The medical experts at HTCs provide treatment, education, and support. They can teach you or your family members how to do home treatments. Center staff also can provide your doctor with information.

People who get care at HTCs are less likely than those who get care elsewhere to have bleeding complications and hospitalizations. They are also more likely to have a better quality of life. This may be due to the centers' emphasis on bleeding prevention and the education and support provided to patients and their caregivers.

More than 100 federally funded HTCs are located throughout the United States. Many HTCs are located at major university medical and research centers. The hemophilia teams at these centers include:

- Nurse coordinators

- Pediatricians (doctors who treat children) and adult and pediatric hematologists (doctors who specialize in blood disorders)

- Social workers (who can help with financial issues, transportation, mental health, and other issues)

- Physical therapists and orthopedists (doctors who specialize in disorders of the bones and joints)

- Dentists

Many people who have hemophilia go to HTCs for annual checkups, even if it means traveling some distance to do so.

At a hemophilia treatment center, you or your child may be able to take part in clinical research and benefit from the latest hemophilia research findings. The HTC team also will work with your local healthcare providers to help meet your needs or your child's needs.

Ongoing Care

If you have hemophilia, you can take steps to avoid complications. For example:

- Follow your treatment plan exactly as your doctor prescribes.

- Have regular checkups and vaccinations as recommended.

- Tell all of your healthcare providers—such as your doctor, dentist, and pharmacist—that you have hemophilia. You also may want to tell people such as your employee health nurse, gym trainer, and sports coach about your condition.

- Have regular dental care. Dentists at the HTCs are experts in providing dental care for people who have hemophilia. If you see another dentist, tell her or him that you have hemophilia. The dentist can provide medicine that will reduce bleeding during dental work.

- Know the signs and symptoms of bleeding in joints and other parts of the body. Know when to call your doctor or when to go to the emergency room. For example, you will need care if you have:

  - Heavy bleeding that cannot be stopped or a wound that continues to ooze blood

  - Any signs or symptoms of bleeding in the brain. Such bleeding is life-threatening and requires emergency care.

  - Limited motion, pain, or swelling of any joint

It is a good idea to keep a record of all previous treatments. Be sure to take this information with you to medical appointments and to the hospital or emergency room.

If Your Child Is Diagnosed with Hemophilia

You may have emotional, financial, social, or other strains as you adjust to having a child who has hemophilia. Learn all you can about the disorder, and get the support you need.

Talk with doctors and other healthcare providers about treatment, prevention of bleeding, and what to do during an emergency.

The care teams at HTCs can provide your child with treatment and help educate and support you. The social worker on the team can help with emotional issues, financial and transportation problems, and other concerns.

Seek the many resources available through the Internet, books, and other materials, including those provided by national and local hemophilia organizations.

Look into support groups that offer a variety of activities for children who have hemophilia and for family members. Some groups offer summer camps for children who have hemophilia. Ask your doctor, nurse coordinator, or social worker about these groups and camps.

Challenges will occur as your child grows and becomes more active. In addition to treatment and regular health and dental care, your child needs information about hemophilia that she or he can understand.

Children who have hemophilia also need ongoing support, and they need to be reassured that the condition is not their fault.

Young children who have hemophilia need extra protection from things in the home and elsewhere that could cause injuries and bleeding:

- Protect toddlers with knee pads, elbow pads, and protective helmets. All children should wear safety helmets when riding tricycles or bicycles.

- Be sure to use the safety belts and straps in highchairs, car seats, and strollers to protect your child from falls.

- Remove furniture with sharp corners or pad them while your child is a toddler.

- Keep small, sharp objects and other items that could cause bleeding or harm out of reach or locked away.

- Check play equipment and outdoor play areas for possible hazards.

You also should learn how to examine your child for and recognize signs of bleeding. Learn to prepare for bleeding episodes when they occur. Keep a cold pack in the freezer ready to use as directed or to take along with you to treat bumps and bruises.

Popsicles work fine when there is minor bleeding in the mouth. You also might want to keep a bag ready to go with items you will need if you must take your child to the emergency room or elsewhere.

Be sure that anyone who is responsible for your child knows that she or he has hemophilia. Talk with your child's babysitters, day care providers, teachers, other school staff, and coaches or leaders of after-school activities about when to contact you or to call 911 for emergency care.

Your child should wear a medical identification (ID) bracelet or necklace. If your child is injured, the ID will alert anyone caring for your child about her or his hemophilia.

Physical Activity and Hemophilia

Physical activity helps keep muscles flexible, strengthens joints, and helps maintain a healthy weight. Children and adults who have hemophilia should be physically active, but they may have limits on what they can do safely.

People who have mild hemophilia can take part in many activities. Those who have severe hemophilia should avoid contact sports and other activities that are likely to lead to injuries that could cause bleeding. Examples of these activities include football, hockey, and wrestling.

Physical therapists at HTCs can develop exercise programs tailored to your needs and teach you how to exercise safely.

Talk with your doctor or physical therapist about recommended types of physical activity and sports. In general, some safe physical activities are swimming, biking (while wearing a helmet), walking, and golf.

To prevent bleeding, you also may be able to take clotting factors prior to exercise or a sporting event.

Medicine Precautions

Some medicines increase the risk of bleeding, such as:

• Aspirin and other medicines that contain salicylates

• Ibuprofen, naproxen, and some other nonsteroidal anti-inflammatory medicines

Talk with your doctor or pharmacist about which medicines are safe for you to take.

Treatment at Home and When Traveling

Home treatment with replacement therapy has many benefits. It lets you treat bleeding early, before complications are likely to develop. Home treatment also can prevent frequent trips to the doctor's office or hospital. This can give you more independence and control over your hemophilia.

However, if you are treating yourself or your child with clotting factors at home, you should take some steps for safety:

- Follow instructions for storage, preparation, and use of clotting factors and treatment materials.

- Keep a record of all medical treatment.

- Know the signs and symptoms of bleeding, infection, or an allergic reaction, and know the correct way to respond.

- Have someone with you when you treat yourself.

- Know when to call the doctor or 911.

When you are traveling, be sure to take enough treatment supplies along. You also should carry a letter from your doctor describing your hemophilia and treatment. It is a good idea to find out in advance where to go for care when you are out of town.

Cost Issues

Clotting factors are very costly. Many health insurance companies will only pay for clotting factors on a case-by-case basis. It is important to know:

- What your insurance covers

- Whether your insurance has a limit on the dollar amount it will cover and what that amount is

- Whether restrictions or waiting periods apply

As children grow, it is important to learn about available options for insurance. Look into what kinds of health insurance are offered when seeking a job.

Chapter 18

Von Willebrand Disease

Von Willebrand disease (VWD) is a blood disorder in which the blood does not clot properly. Blood contains many proteins that help the body stop bleeding. One of these proteins is called "von Willebrand factor" (VWF). People with VWD either have a low level of VWF in their blood or the VWF protein does not work the way it should.

Normally, when a person is injured and starts to bleed, the VWF in the blood attaches to small blood cells called "platelets." This helps the platelets stick together, similar to glue, to form a clot at the site of injury and stop the bleeding. When a person has VWD because the VWF does not work the way it should, the clot might take longer to form or not form the way it should, and bleeding might take longer to stop. This can lead to heavy, hard-to-stop bleeding. Although rare, the bleeding can be severe enough to damage joints or internal organs, or even be life-threatening.

Who Is Affected?

Von Willebrand disease is the most common bleeding disorder, found in up to one percent of the U.S. population. This means that 3.2 million (or about 1 in every 100) people in the United States have the disease. Although VWD occurs among men and women equally, women are more likely to notice the symptoms because of heavy or abnormal bleeding during their menstrual periods and after childbirth.

This chapter includes text excerpted from "What Is Von Willebrand Disease?" Centers for Disease Control and Prevention (CDC), October 23, 2018.

Types of Von Willebrand Disease
Type 1

This is the most common and mildest form of VWD, in which a person has lower than normal levels of VWF. A person with Type 1 VWD also might have low levels of factor VIII, another type of blood-clotting protein. This should not be confused with hemophilia, in which there are low levels or a complete lack of factor VIII but normal levels of VWF. About 85 percent of people treated for VWD have Type 1.

Type 2

With this type of VWD, although the body makes normal amounts of the VWF, the factor does not work the way it should. Type 2 is further broken down into four subtypes—2A, 2B, 2M, and 2N—depending on the specific problem with the person's VWF. Because the treatment is different for each type, it is important that a person knows which subtype she or he has.

Type 3

This is the most severe form of VWD, in which a person has very little or no VWF and low levels of factor VIII. This is the rarest type of VWD. Only three percent of people with VWD have Type 3.

Causes of Von Willebrand Disease

Most people who have VWD are born with it. It almost always is inherited, or passed down, from a parent to a child. VWD can be passed down from either the mother or the father, or both, to the child.

While rare, it is possible for a person to get VWD without a family history of the disease. This happens when a spontaneous mutation occurs. That means there has been a change in the person's gene. Whether the child received the affected gene from a parent or as a result of a mutation, once the child has it, the child can later pass it along to her or his children. Rarely, a person who is not born with VWD can acquire it or have it first occur later in life. This can happen when a person's own immune system destroys her or his VWF, often as a result of the use of a medication or as a result of another disease. If VWD is acquired, meaning it was not inherited from a parent, it cannot be passed along to any children.

How Von Willebrand Disease Is Inherited

Most people who have von Willebrand disease are born with it. It almost always is inherited, or passed down, from a parent to a child. VWD can be passed down from either the mother or the father, or both, to the child.

The child of a parent with VWD has a 50 percent chance of getting the gene for the condition and, therefore, of having VWD. In types 1 and 2, if even one parent has the gene for the disease and passes it to a child, the child will have the disease. In type 3, the child usually gets the gene for the disease from both parents. If both parents have VWD, the child could get either a mild (50 percent chance) or severe (25 percent chance) form of the disease. If neither parent shows the disease (recessive VWD), the child could get the severe form (25%). VWD Type 2N is also inherited as a recessive trait.

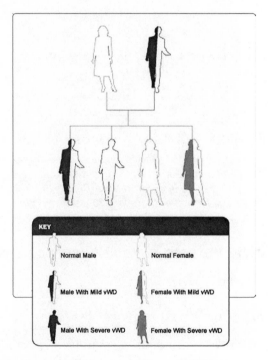

Figure 18.1. *Inheritance of Type 1 and Type 2 VWD*

The Inheritance of Type 1 and Type 2 VWD occurs in a pattern. They can have VWD because they inherited the gene from either parent who has the same changed gene or they could have a new change in the VWD gene which has occurred for the first time in the family. Someone with Type 1 or Type 2 VWD has a 50-50 chance to pass on the changed gene to each child.

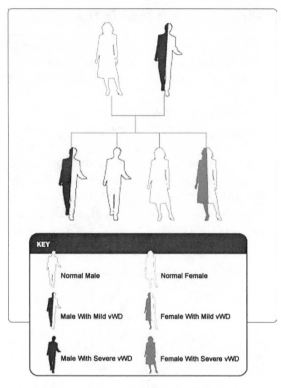

Figure 18.2. *Inheritance of Type 3 VWD and Type 2N VWD*

Type 3 is the common type of VWD and is caused by having both changed genes. This is a recessive inheritance pattern. Recessive means that a person must inherit two changed copies of the gene in order to have Type 3 VWD. If both parents have mild VWD and have a child together there is a 25 percent chance that the child will inherit both changed genes (one from each parent) and have Type 3 VWD.

Signs and Symptoms of Von Willebrand Disease

The major signs of VWD are:

Frequent or Hard-to-Stop Nosebleeds

People with von Willebrand disease might have nosebleeds that:

- Start without injury (spontaneous)
- Occur often, usually five times or more in a year
- Last more than 10 minutes
- Need packing or cautery to stop the bleeding

260

Easy Bruising

People with von Willebrand disease might experience easy bruising that:

- Occurs with very little or no trauma or injury
- Occurs often (one to four times per month)
- Is larger than the size of a quarter
- Is not flat and has a raised lump

Heavy Menstrual Bleeding

Women with von Willebrand disease might have heavy menstrual periods during which:

- Clots larger than the size of a quarter are passed
- More than one pad is soaked through every two hours
- A diagnosis of anemia (not having enough red blood cells) is made as a result of bleeding from heavy periods

Longer than Normal Bleeding after Injury, Surgery, Childbirth, or Dental Work

People with von Willebrand disease might have longer than normal bleeding after injury, surgery, or childbirth, for example:

- After a cut to the skin, the bleeding lasts more than five minutes.
- Heavy or longer bleeding occurs after surgery. Bleeding sometimes stops but starts up again hours or days later.
- Heavy bleeding occurs during or after childbirth

People with von Willebrand disease might have longer than normal bleeding during or after dental work, for example:

- Heavy bleeding occurs during or after dental surgery.
- The surgery site oozes blood longer than three hours after the surgery.
- The surgery site needs packing or cautery to stop the bleeding.

The amount of bleeding depends on the type and severity of VWD. Other common bleeding events include:

- Blood in the stool (feces) from bleeding into the stomach or intestines

- Blood in the urine from bleeding into the kidneys or bladder

- Bleeding into the joints or internal organs, in severe cases (Type 3)

Chapter 19

Factor V Leiden

Factor V Leiden thrombophilia is a genetic disorder that makes it more likely for you to develop a blood clot sometime during your life. Still, it is estimated that 95 percent of people with factor V Leiden never develop a clot. When a clot does form, the clot most often occurs in your leg (deep venous thrombosis or DVT) or lungs (pulmonary embolism or PE). "Factor V Leiden" is the name of a specific gene mutation in the *F5 gene*. This gene plays a role in how your body forms blood clots after an injury. People can inherit one or two copies of the factor V Leiden gene mutation.

Symptoms of Factor V Leiden

People with factor V Leiden thrombophilia have a higher risk for blood clots. However, the severity of factor V Leiden thrombophilia varies greatly from person to person. Only 5 percent of people with 1 factor V Leiden mutation develop a clot by 65 years of age.

The chance a person with a factor V Leiden gene mutation develops a blood clot is affected by a number of factors, such as having a family history of clots, a second factor V Leiden gene mutation, a second genetic or acquired blood clotting disorder, and other nongenetic risk factors. Nongenetic risk factors include surgery, long periods of not moving (such as sitting on a long airplane ride), birth control pills and

This chapter includes text excerpted from "Factor V Leiden Thrombophilia," Genetic and Rare Diseases Information Center (GARD), National Center for Advancing Translational Sciences (NCATS), January 24, 2017.

other female hormones, childbirth within the last six months, non-O blood group, cancer, and injuries (such as bone fractures).

The most common type of blood clots associated with factor V Leiden thrombophilia are deep venous thrombosis or DVT and pulmonary embolism or PE. Signs and symptoms of DVT include leg pain, tenderness, swelling, increased warmth, or redness in one leg. Signs and symptoms of pulmonary embolism usually include cough, chest pain, shortness of breath, or a rapid heartbeat or breathing.

While less common, other possible sites of blood clots include superficial veins of the leg, veins carrying blood from the digestive organs and spleen to the liver, veins carrying blood away from the liver, and veins supplying the brain. Factor V Leiden thrombophilia may contribute a small amount of risk toward a heart attack, stroke, or pregnancy complication.

Causes of Factor V Leiden

Factor V Leiden thrombophilia is caused by a specific mutation in the *F5* or *Factor V* gene. F5 plays a critical role in the formation of blood clots in response to injury. Genes are our body's instructions for making proteins. F5 instructs the body how to make a protein called "coagulation factor V." Coagulation factor V is involved in a series of chemical reactions that hold blood clots together. A molecule called "activated protein C" (APC) prevents blood clots from growing too large by inactivating factor V. Factor V Leiden gene mutations cause factor V to be inactivated more slowly than normal. This leaves more time for blood clots to form.

Inheritance of Factor V Leiden

We all inherit two copies of the *F5* or *Factor V* gene. We inherit one copy from our mother and the other from our father. As a result, our risk for having factor V Leiden thrombophilia depends on the genetic status of each of our parents.

Most people with factor V Leiden thrombophilia have one normal *F5* gene and one with the factor V Leiden gene mutation. People with one copy of the mutation are called "heterozygotes." Assuming this person and a person without the mutation have a child, this couple would have a 50 percent, or 1 in 2, chance of having a child with a single F5 mutation.

Factor V Leiden thrombophilia is a relatively common condition. In some families, both parents have the F5 mutation. In this scenario, each child of the couple would have a 25 percent, or 1 in 4, chance of having 2 mutations; a 25 percent chance of having no mutation, and a 50 percent chance of having a 1 mutation.

People with two copies of the F5 mutation are said to be "homozygotes." They will always pass one copy of the mutated gene to their children. A child's risk for a second mutation will depend on whether or not her or his other parent has the F5 mutation.

Diagnosis of Factor V Leiden

A diagnosis of factor V Leiden thrombophilia may be considered in people with a notable personal or family history of venous thromboembolism (VTE), such as having a VTE at an atypically young age, in an unusual location, or having multiple VTEs. A doctor may confirm the diagnosis by ordering a genetic or APC resistance test. Alternatively, it is becoming more common for people to learn they have a factor V Leiden gene mutation from an advertised genetic test they purchased directly.

The APC resistance assay, a coagulation screening test, measures the anticoagulant response to APC. This screening test has a sensitivity and specificity for factor V Leiden approaching 100 percent. The sensitivity of a test is a measure of the test's ability to detect a positive result when someone has the condition, while the specificity is a measure of the test's ability to identify negative results.

Targeted mutation analysis (a type of DNA test) of the *F5 gene* for the Leiden mutation is considered definitive and has a mutation detection frequency of approximately 100 percent. This means that approximately all individuals who have the factor V Leiden mutation will be detected by this genetic test. It is generally recommended that individuals who test positive by another means should then have the DNA test both for confirmation and to distinguish heterozygotes (individuals with a mutation in one copy of the gene) from homozygotes (individuals with mutations in both copies of the gene).

Treatment of Factor V Leiden

Treatment of factor V Leiden thrombophilia varies depending on the patient's medical history and current circumstances.

People with factor V Leiden thrombophilia who have had a deep venous thrombosis (DVT) or pulmonary embolism (PE) are usually treated with blood thinners, or anticoagulants (such as heparin and warfarin). Anticoagulants are given for varying amounts of time depending on the person's situation. It is not usually recommended that people with factor V Leiden be treated lifelong with anticoagulants if they have had only one DVT or PE, unless they have additional blood clot risk factors.

People who have factor V Leiden but have never had a blood clot are not routinely treated with an anticoagulant. Instead, they are counseled about reducing or eliminating other factors that add to their risk for clots. They may require temporary treatment with an anticoagulant during periods of particularly high risk, such as major surgery.

Women with factor V Leiden thrombophilia most often have normal pregnancies. Treatment with an anticoagulant during pregnancy and/or following delivery is often not needed, but it may be recommended depending on the woman's personal and family health history, method of delivery, and other risk factors.

Chapter 20

Prothrombin Thrombophilia

Prothrombin thrombophilia is an inherited disorder of blood clotting. Thrombophilia is an increased tendency to form abnormal blood clots in blood vessels. People who have prothrombin thrombophilia are at a somewhat higher-than-average risk for a type of clot called a "deep venous thrombosis," which typically occurs in the deep veins of the legs. Affected people also have an increased risk of developing a pulmonary embolism, which is a clot that travels through the bloodstream and lodges in the lungs. Most people with prothrombin thrombophilia never develop abnormal blood clots, however.

Some research suggests that prothrombin thrombophilia is associated with a somewhat increased risk of pregnancy loss (miscarriage) and may also increase the risk of other complications during pregnancy. These complications may include pregnancy-induced high blood pressure (preeclampsia), slow fetal growth, and early separation of the placenta from the uterine wall (placental abruption). It is important to note, however, that most women with prothrombin thrombophilia have normal pregnancies.

Frequency of Prothrombin Thrombophilia

Prothrombin thrombophilia is the second most common inherited form of thrombophilia after factor V Leiden thrombophilia.

This chapter includes text excerpted from "Prothrombin thrombophilia," Genetics Home Reference (GHR), National Institutes of Health (NIH), May 28, 2019.

Approximately 1 in 50 people in the White population in the United States and Europe has prothrombin thrombophilia. This condition is less common in other ethnic groups, occurring in less than 1 percent of African American, Native American, or Asian populations.

Causes of Prothrombin Thrombophilia

Prothrombin thrombophilia is caused by a particular mutation in the *F2 gene*. The *F2 gene* plays a critical role in the formation of blood clots in response to injury. The protein produced from the *F2 gene*, prothrombin (also called "coagulation factor II"), is the precursor to a protein called "thrombin" that initiates a series of chemical reactions in order to form a blood clot. The particular mutation that causes prothrombin thrombophilia results in an overactive *F2 gene* that causes too much prothrombin to be produced. An abundance of prothrombin leads to more thrombin, which promotes the formation of blood clots.

Other factors also increase the risk of blood clots in people with prothrombin thrombophilia. These factors include increasing age, obesity, trauma, surgery, smoking, the use of oral contraceptives (birth control pills) or hormone replacement therapy, and pregnancy. The combination of prothrombin thrombophilia and mutations in other genes involved in blood clotting can also influence the risk.

Inheritance Pattern

The risk of developing an abnormal clot in a blood vessel depends on whether a person inherits 1 or 2 copies of the *F2* gene mutation that causes prothrombin thrombophilia. In the general population, the risk of developing an abnormal blood clot is about 1 in 1,000 people per year. Inheriting one copy of the *F2* gene mutation increases that risk to 2 to 3 in 1,000. People who inherit 2 copies of the mutation, 1 from each parent, may have a risk as high as 20 in 1,000.

Chapter 21

Factor Deficiencies

Chapter Contents

Section 21.1

Factor V Deficiency

This section includes text excerpted from "Factor V Deficiency," Genetic and Rare Diseases Information Center (GARD), National Center for Advancing Translational Sciences (NCATS), April 17, 2017.

Factor V deficiency is an inherited bleeding disorder that prevents blood clots from forming properly. This disorder is caused by mutations in the *F5* gene, which leads to a deficiency of a protein called "coagulation factor V." The reduced amount of factor V may lead to nosebleeds, easy bruising, and excessive bleeding following surgery or trauma. This condition is inherited in an autosomal recessive manner. Treatment includes fresh blood plasma or fresh frozen plasma infusions during bleeding episodes.

Symptoms of Factor V Deficiency

The symptoms of factor V deficiency may include:

- Bleeding into the skin
- Excessive bruising
- Nosebleeds
- Bleeding of the gums
- Excessive menstrual bleeding
- Prolonged or excessive loss of blood with surgery, trauma, or following childbirth
- Umbilical stump bleeding
- In severe cases, bleeding into the skull, lungs, or gastrointestinal tract

Cause of Factor V Deficiency

Factor V deficiency is caused by mutations in the *F5* gene. These mutations prevent the production of a functional factor V protein, or they decrease the amount of the protein in the bloodstream. Mutations are present in both copies of the *F5* gene in each cell, which prevents blood from clotting normally.

Inheritance of Factor V Deficiency

Factor V deficiency is inherited in an autosomal recessive manner. This means that to be affected, a person must have a mutation in both copies of the responsible gene in each cell. Affected people inherit one mutated copy of the gene from each parent, who is referred to as a carrier. Carriers of an autosomal recessive condition typically do not have any signs or symptoms (they are unaffected). When two carriers of an autosomal recessive condition have children, each child has a:

- 25 percent chance to be affected

- 50 percent chance to be an unaffected carrier, such as each parent

- 25 percent chance to be unaffected and not a carrier

Section 21.2

Factor VIII Deficiency

This section includes text excerpted from "Hemophilia A," Genetic and Rare Diseases Information Center (GARD), National Center for Advancing Translational Sciences (NCATS), December 3, 2018.

Hemophilia A is an inherited bleeding disorder in which the blood does not clot normally. People with hemophilia A will bleed more than normal after an injury, surgery, or dental procedure. This disorder can be severe, moderate, or mild. In severe cases, heavy bleeding occurs after minor injury or even when there is no injury (spontaneous bleeding). Bleeding into the joints, muscles, brain, or organs can cause pain and other serious complications. In milder forms, there is no spontaneous bleeding, and the disorder might only be diagnosed after a surgery or serious injury. Hemophilia A is caused by having low levels of a protein called "factor VIII." Factor VIII is needed to form blood clots. The disorder is inherited in an X-linked recessive manner and is caused by changes (mutations) in the *F8* gene. The diagnosis of hemophilia A is made through clinical symptoms and specific laboratory tests to measure the amount of clotting factors in the blood. The main treatment is replacement therapy, during which clotting factor VIII is dripped or injected slowly into a vein. Hemophilia A mainly affects males. With treatment, most people with this disorder do well. Some people with severe hemophilia A may have a shortened lifespan due to the presence of other health conditions and rare complications of the disorder.

Symptoms of Hemophilia A

The symptoms of hemophilia A and the age symptoms appear vary depending on the amount of factor VIII a person's body makes. Infants with the severe form may bleed abnormally from their mouth and develop "goose eggs" on their heads (collections of blood under the scalp). Other symptoms of the severe form include bleeding without any known cause (spontaneous bleeding) into the muscles, joints, and organs. Children with the moderate form may bruise easily and bleed too much after minor injuries, dental work, or surgery. People with the mild form of hemophilia A may not be diagnosed until they bleed more than normal after a major injury or surgery. With the mild form, there are no episodes of spontaneous bleeds.

Cause of Hemophilia A

Hemophilia A is caused by genetic changes (mutations) in the *F8* gene. This gene is responsible for making the Factor VIII protein, an important protein that helps start the formation of blood clots. Mutations in the *F8* gene lead to reduced or absent levels of Factor VIII in the blood, making it hard for the body to form blood clots.

Inheritance Hemophilia A

The *F8* gene is located on the X-chromosome. Therefore, hemophilia A is inherited in an X-linked recessive pattern. In males (who have only one X chromosome), one mutated copy of the *F8* gene in each cell is enough to cause hemophilia A. In females (who have two X chromosomes), a mutation needs to occur in both copies of the *F8* gene to cause the disorder. Because it is unlikely that females will have two mutated copies of this gene, hemophilia A, as with other X-linked recessive disorders, affects males much more frequently than females. Females who have a mutation in one copy of the *F8* gene are called "carriers." Most carriers have no signs or symptoms; however, about 10 percent of female carriers of hemophilia A will experience some abnormal bleeding.

A female who carries one *F8* gene mutation has a 50 percent, or 1 in 2, the chance of having a son with hemophilia A. A male with hemophilia A cannot pass on the disorder to his sons, but all of his daughters will be carriers for hemophilia A.

When a male child is the first person in a family with hemophilia A, further testing may be needed to determine if the child inherited the disorder from his mother, or if the mutation occurred by chance for the first time in the child.

Section 21.3

Factor X Deficiency

This section includes text excerpted from "Factor X Deficiency," Genetic and Rare Diseases Information Center (GARD), National Center for Advancing Translational Sciences (NCATS), January 22, 2019.

Factor X deficiency is a rare disorder that affects the blood's ability to clot. The severity of the disorder and the associated signs and symptoms can vary significantly from person to person. Common features of factor X deficiency may include easy bruising, frequent nosebleeds, bleeding gums, blood in the urine, and prolonged bleeding after minor injuries. Women with factor X deficiency may also experience heavy menstrual bleeding and may have an increased risk for first trimester miscarriages. Acquired (noninherited) factor X deficiency, which is the most common form of the disorder, generally occurs in people with no family history of the disorder. Acquired factor X deficiency has a variety of causes, including liver disease, vitamin K deficiency, exposure to certain medications that affect clotting, and certain types of cancer. The inherited form of factor X deficiency (also called "congenital factor X deficiency") is caused by changes (mutations) in the *F10* gene and is inherited in an autosomal recessive manner. Factor X deficiency can be diagnosed based on the symptoms and through laboratory tests to measure clotting time. The goal of treatment is to control bleeding through intravenous (IV) infusions of plasma or concentrates of clotting factors.

Symptoms of Factor X Deficiency

The symptoms of factor X deficiency can be different for each person and can start at any age. Symptoms may include frequent nosebleeds, bruising easily, bleeding under the skin, and increased bleeding in the gums. Women with factor X deficiency may have extra heavy bleeding during their periods and during childbirth and are at increased risk for pregnancy complications. In more severe forms of Factor X deficiency, symptoms may include bleeding into joints and into the brain (intracranial hemorrhage).

Cause of Factor X Deficiency

There are two forms of factor X deficiency, an inherited form and a noninherited form. The inherited form is caused by a genetic change (mutation) in the *F10* gene that affects how the factor X protein is made. Factor X protein is important for helping blood clot properly. Mutations in the *F10* gene lead to lower amounts of factor X protein or a factor X protein that does not work correctly.

The noninherited form of factor X deficiency is caused by other health conditions, including liver disease, amyloidosis, vitamin K deficiency, and others.

Inheritance of Factor X Deficiency

The inherited form of factor X deficiency is passed down in families in an autosomal recessive pattern. Everyone inherits two copies of each gene. To inherit factor X deficiency, a person must have a genetic mutation in both copies of the *F10* gene in each cell. There is nothing either parent can do, before or during pregnancy, to cause a child to have this.

People with autosomal recessive disorders inherit one copy of the gene with a mutation from each of their parents. In most cases, each parent has a mutation in only one copy of the gene and is known as a "carrier." Carriers of an autosomal recessive disorder typically do not have any signs or symptoms (they are unaffected). When two carriers of factor X deficiency have children, each child has a:

- 25 percent (1 in 4) chance to have factor X deficiency

- 50 percent (1 in 2) chance to be a carrier, such as each parent

- 25 percent (1 in 4) chance to be unaffected and not be a carrier

Section 21.4

Factor XI Deficiency

This section includes text excerpted from "Factor XI Deficiency," Genetics Home Reference (GHR), National Institutes of Health (NIH), August 2018.

Factor XI deficiency is a disorder that can cause abnormal bleeding due to a shortage (deficiency) of the factor XI protein, which is involved in blood clotting. This condition is classified as either partial or severe based on the degree of deficiency of the factor XI protein. However, regardless of the severity of protein deficiency, most affected individuals have relatively mild bleeding problems, and some people with this disorder have few if any symptoms. The most common feature of factor XI deficiency is prolonged bleeding after trauma or surgery, especially involving the inside of the mouth and nose (oral and nasal cavities) or the urinary tract. If the bleeding is left untreated after surgery, solid swellings consisting of congealed blood (hematomas) can develop in the surgical area.

Other signs and symptoms of this disorder can include frequent nosebleeds, easy bruising, bleeding under the skin, and bleeding of the gums. Women with this disorder can have heavy or prolonged menstrual bleeding (menorrhagia) or prolonged bleeding after childbirth. In contrast to some other bleeding disorders, spontaneous bleeding into the urine (hematuria), gastrointestinal tract, or skull cavity are not common in factor XI deficiency, although they can occur in severely affected individuals. Bleeding into the muscles or joints, which can cause long-term disability in other bleeding disorders, generally does not occur in this condition.

Frequency of Factor XI Deficiency

Factor XI deficiency is estimated to affect approximately 1 in 1 million people worldwide. The severe deficiency disorder is much more common in people with central and eastern European (Ashkenazi) Jewish ancestry, occurring in about 1 in 450 individuals in that population. Researchers suggest that the actual prevalence of factor XI deficiency may be higher than reported because mild cases of the disorder often do not come to medical attention.

Causes of Factor XI Deficiency

Most cases of factor XI deficiency are caused by mutations in the *F11* gene, which provides instructions for making the factor XI protein.

This protein plays a role in the coagulation cascade, which is a series of chemical reactions that forms blood clots in response to injury. After an injury, clots seal off blood vessels to stop bleeding and trigger blood vessel repair.

Mutations in the *F11* gene result in a shortage (deficiency) of functional factor XI. This deficiency impairs the coagulation cascade, slowing the process of blood clotting and leading to the bleeding problems associated with this disorder. The amount of functional factor XI remaining varies depending on the particular mutation and whether one or both copies of the *F11* gene in each cell have mutations. However, the severity of the bleeding problems in affected individuals does not necessarily correspond to the amount of factor XI in the bloodstream and can vary even within the same family. Other genetic and environmental factors likely play a role in determining the severity of this condition.

Some cases of factor XI deficiency are not caused by *F11* gene mutations. In these cases, the condition is called "acquired factor XI deficiency." It can be caused by other disorders, such as conditions in which the immune system malfunctions and attacks the factor XI protein. Because factor XI is made primarily by cells in the liver, acquired factor XI deficiency can also occur as the result of severe liver disease or receiving a transplanted liver from an affected individual. In addition, approximately 25 percent of people with another disorder called "Noonan syndrome" have factor XI deficiency.

Chapter 22

Hereditary Hemorrhagic Telangiectasia

Hereditary hemorrhagic telangiectasia (HHT) is a disorder in which some blood vessels do not develop properly. A person with HHT may form blood vessels without the capillaries (tiny blood vessels that pass blood from arteries to veins) that are usually present between arteries and veins. The space between an artery and a vein is often fragile and can burst and bleed much more easily than other blood vessels. Men, women, and children from all racial and ethnic groups can be affected by HHT and experience the problems associated with this disorder, some of which are serious and potentially life-threatening. Fortunately, if HHT is discovered early, effective treatments are available. However, there is no cure for HHT.

Signs of Hereditary Hemorrhagic Telangiectasia

Nosebleeds are the most common sign of HHT, resulting from small abnormal blood vessels within the inside layer of the nose. Abnormal blood vessels in the skin can appear on the hands, fingertips, face, lips, lining of the mouth, and nose as delicate red or purplish spots that lighten briefly when touched. Bleeding within the stomach or

This chapter includes text excerpted from "Facts about Hereditary Hemorrhagic Telangiectasia," National Institute on Alcohol Abuse and Alcoholism (NIAAA), February 8, 2019.

intestines is another possible indicator of HHT that occurs because of abnormal blood vessels lining the digestive tract. Additional signs of HHT include abnormal artery-vein connections within the brain, lungs, and liver, which often do not display any warning signs before rupturing.

Causes of Hereditary Hemorrhagic Telangiectasia

Hereditary hemorrhagic telangiectasia is a genetic disorder. Each person with HHT has 1 gene that is altered (mutated), which causes HHT, as well as 1 normal gene. It takes only 1 mutant gene to cause HHT. When someone with HHT has children, each child has a 50 percent chance to receive the mutant gene from her or his parent and, therefore, to have HHT as well. Each child also has a 50 percent chance to receive the normal gene and not be affected with HHT. At least 5 different genes can cause HHT, 3 of which are known.

Diagnosis of Hereditary Hemorrhagic Telangiectasia

Hereditary hemorrhagic telangiectasia can be diagnosed by performing genetic testing. Genetic testing can detect a gene mutation in about three-fourths of families with signs of HHT, which, if found, can establish the diagnosis of HHT in individuals and families who are unsure about whether they have HHT. HHT can also be diagnosed by using clinical criteria (presence of signs and a history of signs in a parent, sibling, or child).

Complications and Treatments of Hereditary Hemorrhagic Telangiectasia

The complications of hereditary hemorrhagic telangiectasia can vary widely, even among people affected by HHT in the same family. Complications and treatment of HHT depend on the parts of the body that are affected by this disorder. Treatment may include controlling bleeding and anemia and preventing complications from abnormal artery-vein connections in the lungs and brain.

Chapter 23

Bruises

A bruise, also known as a "contusion" or "ecchymosis," happens when soft tissues of the body get hurt. When these body tissues are hurt, small veins and capillaries under the skin rupture, causing red blood cells to leak. The trapped blood then makes a red or purplish mark on the skin.

Bruises change color as the body begins to heal itself. The change of color indicates that the body is breaking down the blood cells in the skin.

Who Gets Bruises

Bruises typically are caused by an injury, such as falling or bumping into something. Bruises are more common in elderly people, as the blood vessels tend to become more fragile with aging. Causes of bruises depend upon the following:

- **The toughness of the skin.** Bruises occur more frequently for people who have thinner skin.

- **Sun damage.** Over-exposure to the sun may cause skin to lose its resilience. This means that any injury can lead to a bruise.

- **Underlying medical conditions.** Certain blood disorders, and other medical conditions tend to cause bruising easily and frequently.

"Bruises," © 2019 Omnigraphics. Reviewed June 2019.

- **Medications or drugs.** Medications that prevent blood clotting may be likely to cause quick bruising.

How Long Do Bruises Last?

A person may be able to estimate how old a bruise is from its color. The healing of a bruise undergoes a number of phases, and they are as follows:

- Initially, the bruise is a reddish color because of the blood's rich oxygen content. This phase happens immediately after the injury.

- After one or two days, the blood begins to lose oxygen. As a result, the color appears to be blue or purple.

- In about 5 to 10 days, the bruise changes to a yellow or greenish color. This color comes from two compounds called "biliverdin" and "bilirubin," which are produced by the body while breaking down hemoglobin.

- In 10 to 14 days, the bruise changes to light brown and begins to fade.

When to See a Doctor

Most often, bruises will heal within two weeks and without any treatment. However, it is recommended to consult a doctor if the bruise does not show any improvement over a long period of time. Also, check with a doctor if:

- Bruises occur often and seem to develop for no reason.

- It causes swelling and excess pain in the area.

- You cannot move a joint and feel as if you have a broken joint.

- The bruise is near the eye.

Exams and Tests

The doctor performs exams and tests if:

- There is severe pain or swelling. In this case, the doctor may recommend an X-ray of the area to make sure that there are no broken bones.

- Bruises occur often and for no specific reason. In this case, the doctor may recommend blood tests to check for the presence of a bleeding disorder.

How to Speed Up the Healing

There are many ways to speed up the healing process of a bruise, some of which are:

- Apply a cold compress for 15 to 20 minutes to reduce blood flow in the injured area. This helps keep inflammation and swelling down. In order to be effective, the cold compress must be used for a day or two, depending on the severity of pain.

- If the bruise takes up a large area on a leg or foot, the leg should be elevated while sleeping for one or two days. This prevents excess blood flow in the injured area.

- Over-the-counter (OTC) medicines, such as acetaminophen, can be taken to reduce the pain caused by a bruise.

- After 48 hours, apply pressure with a warm washcloth for 10 or 15 minutes to increase blood flow. This allows the skin to absorb blood more quickly.

- Use creams, such as vitamin B-3 or vitamin K, to speed up bruise healing.

How Can I Prevent Bruises?

Bruises are hard to avoid completely, but they can be prevented by using protective gear, such as pads and shin guards while playing soccer, riding bikes, etc. To prevent bruises, capillaries must be strong enough in order to avoid any leaking under the skin, and a well-balanced diet can help keep them strong. Foods rich in bioflavonoids, such as dark, leafy greens; onions; dark-colored berries; and garlic, can be included in any daily diet.

References

1. "Bruises," WebMD, November 18, 2017.

2. Fletcher, Jenna. "What Do the Colors of a Bruise Mean?" Medical News Today, August 10, 2018.

3. "What's a Bruise?" The Nemours Foundation/KidsHealth®, March 2018.

4. "Bruising Easily? Tips to Treat and Prevent Bruises," Elastoplast, September 8, 2016.

Chapter 24

Antiphospholipid Antibody Syndrome

What Is Antiphospholipid Antibody Syndrome?

Antiphospholipid antibody syndrome (APS) is an autoimmune disorder. Autoimmune disorders occur if the body's immune system makes antibodies that attack and damage tissues or cells.

Antibodies are a type of protein. They usually help defend the body against infections. In APS, however, the body makes antibodies that mistakenly attack phospholipids—a type of fat.

Phospholipids are found in all living cells and cell membranes, including blood cells and the lining of blood vessels.

When antibodies attack phospholipids, cells are damaged. This damage causes blood clots to form in the body's arteries and veins. (These are the vessels that carry blood to your heart and body.)

Usually, blood clotting is a normal bodily process. Blood clots help seal small cuts or breaks on blood vessel walls. This prevents you from losing too much blood. In APS, however, too much blood clotting can block blood flow and damage the body's organs.

This chapter includes text excerpted from "Antiphospholipid Antibody Syndrome," National Heart, Lung, and Blood Institute (NHLBI), September 30, 2008. Reviewed June 2019.

Causes of Antiphospholipid Antibody Syndrome

Antiphospholipid antibody syndrome occurs if the body's immune system makes antibodies (proteins) that attack phospholipids.

Phospholipids are a type of fat found in all living cells and cell membranes, including blood cells and the lining of blood vessels. What causes the immune system to make antibodies against phospholipids is not known.

Antiphospholipid antibody syndrome causes unwanted blood clots to form in the body's arteries and veins. Usually, blood clotting is a normal bodily process. It helps seal small cuts or breaks on blood vessel walls. This prevents you from losing too much blood. In APS, however, too much blood clotting can block blood flow and damage the body's organs.

Researchers do not know why APS antibodies cause blood clots to form. Some believe that the antibodies damage or affect the inner lining of the blood vessels, which causes blood clots to form. Others believe that the immune system makes antibodies in response to blood clots damaging the blood vessels.

Risk Factors of Antiphospholipid Antibody Syndrome

Antiphospholipid antibody syndrome can affect people of any age. The disorder is more common in women than men, but it affects both sexes.

Antiphospholipid antibody syndrome also is more common in people who have other autoimmune or rheumatic disorders, such as lupus. ("Rheumatic" refers to disorders that affect the joints, bones, or muscles.)

About 10 percent of all people who have lupus also have APS. About half of all people who have APS also have another autoimmune or rheumatic disorder.

Some people have APS antibodies but do not ever have signs or symptoms of the disorder. The mere presence of APS antibodies does not mean that you have APS. To be diagnosed with APS, you must have APS antibodies and a history of health problems related to the disorder.

However, people who have APS antibodies but no signs or symptoms are at risk of developing APS. Health problems, other than autoimmune disorders, that can trigger blood clots include:

- Smoking

- Prolonged bed rest

- Pregnancy and the postpartum period
- Birth control pills (BCPs) and hormone therapy
- Cancer and kidney disease

Signs, Symptoms, and Complications of Antiphospholipid Antibody Syndrome

The signs and symptoms of antiphospholipid antibody syndrome are related to abnormal blood clotting. The outcome of a blood clot depends on its size and location.

Blood clots can form in, or travel to, the arteries or veins in the brain, heart, kidneys, lungs, and limbs. Clots can reduce or block blood flow. This can damage the body's organs and may cause death.

Major Signs and Symptoms

Major signs and symptoms of blood clots include:

- Chest pain and shortness of breath
- Pain, redness, warmth, and swelling in the limbs
- Ongoing headaches
- Speech changes
- Upper body discomfort in the arms, back, neck, and jaw
- Nausea (feeling sick to your stomach)

Blood clots can lead to stroke, heart attack, kidney damage, deep vein thrombosis (DVT), and pulmonary embolism (PE).

Pregnant women who have APS can have successful pregnancies. However, they are at a higher risk for miscarriages; stillbirths; and other pregnancy-related problems, such as preeclampsia.

Preeclampsia is high blood pressure that occurs during pregnancy. This condition may progress to eclampsia. Eclampsia is a serious condition that causes seizures in pregnant women.

Some people who have APS may develop thrombocytopenia. This is a condition in which your blood has a lower than normal number of blood cell fragments called "platelets."

Mild to serious bleeding causes the main signs and symptoms of thrombocytopenia. Bleeding can occur inside the body (internal bleeding) or underneath or from the skin (external bleeding).

Other Signs and Symptoms

Other signs and symptoms of APS include chronic (ongoing) headaches, memory loss, and heart valve problems. Some people who have APS also get a lacy-looking red rash on their wrists and knees.

Living with Antiphospholipid Antibody Syndrome

Antiphospholipid antibody syndrome has no cure. However, you can take steps to control the disorder and prevent complications.

Take all medicines as your doctor prescribes and get ongoing medical care. Talk with your doctor about healthy lifestyle changes and any concerns you have.

Medicines

You may need to take anticoagulants, or "blood thinners, to prevent blood clots or to keep them from getting larger. You should take these medicines exactly as your doctor prescribes.

Tell your doctor about all other medicines you are taking, including over-the-counter (OTC) or herbal medicines. Some medicines, including over-the-counter ibuprofen or aspirin, can thin your blood. Your doctor may not want you to take two medicines that thin your blood because of the risk of bleeding.

Women who have APS should not use birth control or hormone therapy that contains estrogen. Estrogen increases the risk of blood clots. Talk with your doctor about other options.

Ongoing Medical Care

If you have antiphospholipid antibody syndrome, getting regular medical checkups is important. Have blood tests done as your doctor directs. These tests help track how well your blood is clotting.

The medicines used to treat APS increase the risk of bleeding. Bleeding might occur internally or externally. Know the warning signs of bleeding, so you can get help right away. They include:

- Unexplained bleeding from the gums and nose

- Increased menstrual flow

- Bright red vomit or vomit that looks like coffee grounds

- Bright red blood in your stools or black, tarry stools

- Pain in your abdomen or severe pain in your head

- Sudden changes in vision

- Sudden loss of movement in your limbs

- Memory loss or confusion

A lot of bleeding after a fall or injury or easy bruising or bleeding also might mean that your blood is too thin. Ask your doctor about these warning signs and when to seek emergency care.

Lifestyle Changes

Talk with your doctor about lifestyle changes that can help you stay healthy. Ask her or him whether your diet may affect your medicines. Some foods or drinks may increase or decrease the effects of warfarin.

Ask your doctor what amount of alcohol is safe for you to drink if you are taking medicine. If you smoke, talk with your doctor about programs and products that can help you quit. Smoking can damage your blood vessels and raise your risk for many health problems.

Antiphospholipid antibody syndrome medicines might increase your risk of bleeding. Thus, your doctor may advise you to avoid activities that have a high risk of injury, such as some contact sports.

Other Concerns
Pregnancy

Antiphospholipid antibody syndrome can raise the risk of pregnancy-related problems. Talk with your doctor about how to manage your APS if you are pregnant or planning a pregnancy.

With proper treatment, women who have APS are more likely to carry babies to term than women whose APS is not treated.

Surgery

If you need surgery, your doctor may adjust your medicines before, during, and after the surgery to prevent dangerous bleeding.

Chapter 25

Disseminated Intravascular Coagulation

What Is Disseminated Intravascular Coagulation?

Disseminated intravascular coagulation, or DIC, is a condition in which blood clots form throughout the body's small blood vessels. These blood clots can reduce or block blood flow through the blood vessels, which can damage the body's organs.

In disseminated intravascular coagulation, the increased clotting uses up platelets and clotting factors in the blood. Platelets are blood cell fragments that stick together to seal small cuts and breaks on blood vessel walls and stop bleeding. Clotting factors are proteins needed for normal blood clotting.

With fewer platelets and clotting factors in the blood, serious bleeding can occur. DIC can cause internal and external bleeding.

Internal bleeding occurs inside the body. External bleeding occurs underneath or from the skin or mucosa. (The mucosa is the tissue that lines some organs and body cavities, such as your nose and mouth.)

Disseminated intravascular coagulation can cause life-threatening bleeding.

This chapter includes text excerpted from "Disseminated Intravascular Coagulation," National Heart, Lung, and Blood Institute (NHLBI), February 19, 2010. Reviewed June 2019.

Causes of Disseminated Intravascular Coagulation

Some diseases and conditions can disrupt the body's normal blood clotting process and lead to disseminated intravascular coagulation. These diseases and conditions include:

- Sepsis (an infection in the bloodstream)

- Surgery and trauma

- Cancer

- Serious complications of pregnancy and childbirth

Examples of less common causes of DIC are bites from poisonous snakes (such as rattlesnakes and other vipers), frostbite, and burns.

The two types of DIC are acute and chronic. Acute DIC begins with clotting in the small blood vessels and quickly leads to serious bleeding. Chronic DIC causes blood clotting, but it usually does not lead to bleeding. Cancer is the most common cause of chronic DIC.

Similar Clotting Conditions

Two other conditions cause blood clotting in the small blood vessels. However, their causes and treatments differ from those of DIC.

These conditions are thrombotic thrombocytopenic purpura, or TTP, and hemolytic-uremic syndrome (HUS). HUS is more common in children than adults. It is also more likely to cause kidney damage than TTP.

Risk Factors of Disseminated Intravascular Coagulation

Disseminated intravascular coagulation is the result of an underlying disease or condition. People who have one or more of the following conditions are most likely to develop DIC:

- Sepsis (an infection in the bloodstream)

- Surgery and trauma

- Cancer

- Serious complications of pregnancy and childbirth

People who are bitten by poisonous snakes (such as rattlesnakes and other vipers), or those who have frostbite or burns, also are at risk for DIC.

Signs, Symptoms, and Complications of Disseminated Intravascular Coagulation

Signs and symptoms of disseminated intravascular coagulation depend on its cause and whether the condition is acute or chronic.

Acute disseminated intravascular coagulation develops quickly (over hours or days) and is very serious. Chronic DIC develops more slowly (over weeks or months). It lasts longer and usually is not recognized as quickly as acute DIC.

With acute disseminated intravascular coagulation, blood clotting in the blood vessels usually occurs first, followed by bleeding. However, bleeding may be the first obvious sign. Serious bleeding can occur very quickly after developing acute DIC. Thus, emergency treatment in a hospital is needed.

Blood clotting also occurs with chronic DIC, but it usually does not lead to bleeding. Sometimes, chronic DIC has no signs or symptoms.

Signs and Symptoms of Excessive Blood Clotting

In disseminated intravascular coagulation, blood clots form throughout the body's small blood vessels. These blood clots can reduce or block blood flow through the blood vessels. This can cause the following signs and symptoms:

- Chest pain and shortness of breath if blood clots form in the blood vessels in your lungs and heart

- Pain, redness, warmth, and swelling in the lower leg if blood clots form in the deep veins of your leg.

- Headaches, speech changes, paralysis (an inability to move), dizziness, and trouble speaking and understanding if blood clots form in the blood vessels in your brain. These signs and symptoms may indicate a stroke.

- Heart attack and lung and kidney problems if blood clots lodge in your heart, lungs, or kidneys. These organs may even begin to fail.

Signs and Symptoms of Bleeding

In disseminated intravascular coagulation, the increased clotting activity uses up the platelets and clotting factors in the blood. As a result, serious bleeding can occur. DIC can cause internal and external bleeding.

Internal Bleeding

Internal bleeding can occur in your body's organs, such as in the kidneys, intestines, and brain. This bleeding can be life-threatening. Signs and symptoms of internal bleeding include:

- Blood in your urine from bleeding in your kidneys or bladder

- Blood in your stools from bleeding in your intestines or stomach. Blood in your stools can appear red or as a dark, tarry color. (Taking iron supplements also can cause dark, tarry stools.)

- Headaches, double vision, seizures, and other symptoms from bleeding in your brain

External Bleeding

External bleeding can occur underneath or from the skin, such as at the site of cuts or an intravenous (IV) needle. External bleeding also can occur from the mucosa.

External bleeding may cause purpura or petechiae. Purpura are purple, brown, and red bruises. This bruising may happen easily and often. Petechiae are small red or purple dots on your skin.

Purpura and Petechiae

Other signs of external bleeding include:

- Prolonged bleeding, even from minor cuts

- Bleeding or oozing from your gums or nose, especially nosebleeds or bleeding from brushing your teeth

- Heavy or extended menstrual bleeding in women

Living with Disseminated Intravascular Coagulation

If you have disseminated intravascular coagulation, ask your doctor how often you should schedule follow-up care and blood tests. Blood tests help track how well your blood is clotting.

You may need to take blood-thinning medicines to help prevent blood clots or to keep existing clots from getting larger. If you take blood thinners, let everyone on your healthcare team know.

Blood thinners may thin your blood too much and cause bleeding. A lot of bleeding after a fall or injury or easy bruising or bleeding may mean that your blood is too thin.

Call your doctor right away if you have any signs of bleeding. If you have severe bleeding, call 911 right away.

Also, you should talk with your doctor before using any over-the-counter (OTC) medicines or products, such as vitamins, supplements, or herbal remedies. Some of these products also can affect blood clotting and bleeding. For example, aspirin and ibuprofen may thin your blood too much. This can increase your risk of bleeding.

If you need surgery, your doctor may adjust the amount of medicine you take before, during, and after the surgery to prevent bleeding. This also may happen for dental work, but it is less common.

Chapter 26

Hypercoagulation

Chapter Contents

Section 26.1

Excessive Blood Clotting

Excessive blood clotting is a medical disorder known as "hypercoagulation." In healthy people, a wound that causes bleeding triggers an immediate response in the body. Blood platelets begin to stick together in masses called "blood clots." This process is known as "coagulation" and is the body's primary means of stopping blood loss. Hypercoagulation means that the body has an abnormal blood clotting response. Hypercoagulation can manifest as an overactive blood clot response, in which blood clots form too easily or too often. It can also refer to persistent blood clots that are not dissolved by the body, or blood clots that form inside blood vessels or arteries.

Causes of Excessive Blood Clotting

Excessive blood clotting disorders can be inherited or acquired. Acquired clotting disorders can result from traumatic injury, surgery, long-term bed rest, pregnancy, obesity, smoking, severe dehydration, certain chronic health conditions, and the use of certain medications. Excessive blood clotting can also be caused by sitting for long periods of time during car or airplane trips. Certain medical history factors can also indicate a person's likelihood of having excessive blood clotting disorder. These include family members who have been diagnosed with an excessive blood clotting disorder, a history of excessive blood clots before 40 years of age, and history of pregnancies that ended in miscarriage.

Symptoms and Risks of Excessive Blood Clotting

Symptoms of excessive blood clotting disorders vary depending on where excessive blood clots form in the body.

Chest pain; shortness of breath; and pain in the upper arms, back, neck, or jaw can be symptoms of a blood clot in the heart or lungs. This type of blood clot can result in a heart attack, which restricts or blocks blood flow to part of the heart. An undiagnosed or untreated heart attack can result in serious long-term complications, including death.

Persistent headaches, changes in the ability to speak, difficulty understanding others talking, dizziness, or paralysis can indicate a blood clot in the brain. This type of blood clot can result in a stroke. A stroke causes restricted blood flow to the brain, which can result in serious complications including death if left undiagnosed or untreated.

Swelling, pain, redness, or warm skin on the arms or legs can indicate a type of blood clot known as a "deep vein thrombosis." These types of blood clots can travel through the bloodstream and cause serious complications if they reach the brain, heart, or lungs.

Excessive blood clots during pregnancy can cause complications such as high blood pressure (hypertension), miscarriage, or stillbirth.

Diagnosis of Excessive Blood Clotting

Excessive blood clotting disorders are diagnosed through a physical exam, a medical history interview, and diagnostic blood tests. Blood tests for excessive clotting measure the levels of various blood components, such as red and white blood cells, platelets, and blood clotting protein factors. Blood tests also analyze the clotting behavior of the blood samples to identify normal or abnormal clotting function. Medical history factors are evaluated to assess a person's risk for an excessive blood clotting disorder. Some factors that indicate a possible blood clotting disorder diagnosis include family members who have been diagnosed with a blood clotting disorder, a history of blood clots before 40 years of age, frequent unexplained bruising, or multiple pregnancies that ended in miscarriage.

References

1. "What Is Excessive Blood Clotting (Hypercoagulation)?" American Heart Association (AHA), November 30, 2015.

2. "Hypercoagulation," FamilyDoctor.org, March 2014.

Section 26.2

Deep Vein Thrombosis

This section includes text excerpted from "Deep Vein
Thrombosis (DVT)," Centers for Disease Control and
Prevention (CDC), September 15, 2017.

What Is the Problem?

Deep vein thrombosis (DVT) is a medical condition that occurs when
a blood clot forms in a deep vein. These clots usually develop in the
lower leg, thigh, or pelvis, but they can also occur in the arm. Some of
the most common symptoms and signs of DVT are a recent swelling
of the limb, unexplained pain or tenderness, skin that may be warm
to the touch, and redness of the skin.

Deep vein thrombosis can cause a life-threatening complication
called "pulmonary embolism" (PE). This is when part or all of a clot
breaks off and travels through the bloodstream and into the lungs. A
blood clot in the lungs can be life-threatening.

Who Is at Risk?

The precise number of people affected by DVT/PE is unknown,
but estimates range from 300,000 to 900,000 each year in the United
States. Among people who have had DVT, one-half will have long-term
complications, such as swelling, pain, discoloration, and scaling in the
affected limb. Some risk factors for developing DVT include injury
to a vein—often caused by fractures, severe muscle injury, or major
surgery; slow blood flow—often caused by confinement to bed, limited
movement, sitting for a long time, and recent paralysis; increased
estrogen—often caused by birth control pills (BPCs), hormone replacement therapy (HRT), and/or pregnancy (for up to 6 weeks after giving
birth); certain chronic medical illnesses, such as heart disease, lung
disease, cancer and its treatment, and inflammatory bowel disease
(IBD); previous or family history of DVT or PE; age; obesity; a catheter
located in a central vein; and inherited clotting disorders.

*Medical Conditions**

Certain medical conditions can increase your risk of developing
DVT. Some conditions are more closely linked to getting a DVT than
others and include the following:

- **Spinal cord injury.** In addition to damaging veins deep in your body, spinal cord injury may cause paralysis, which can reduce blood flow and raise your risk of venous thromboemlism (VTE). The risk is highest in the first weeks after the injury.

- **A broken hip or leg bone or other trauma**

- **Cancers,** such as advanced brain, breast, colon, and pancreatic cancer. Cancer chemotherapy, surgical treatment, and placement of a central venous catheter—a tube inserted into a vein to deliver chemotherapy treatment or other medicine—all increase the risk of VTE. Some cancers release substances that can make it easier for blood to clot. Some cancerous tumors may directly block blood flow by pressing on a vein. A central venous catheter increases the risk for VTE in arm veins, especially in children.

- **Heart conditions,** such as heart attack or congestive heart failure.

- **Stroke**

- **Obesity**

- **Varicose veins.** Most varicose veins do not cause problems, but large, untreated varicose veins can lead to VTE.

- **Infections**

- **Sickle cell disease.** This condition makes the blood clot more easily and can be a risk factor for VTE.*

* *Excerpted from "Venous Thromboembolism," National Heart, Lung, and Blood Institute (NHLBI), May 26, 2018.*

Can Deep Vein Thrombosis Be Prevented?

Yes, deep vein thrombosis may be prevented. If discovered early, it may also be treatable. Some measures can be taken to prevent DVT and PE, and they include maintaining a healthy weight, avoiding a sedentary lifestyle, and adhering to doctor recommendations. Medication may be used to prevent and treat DVT. Compression stockings are sometimes recommended to prevent DVT and to relieve pain and swelling. Medicines may be given in cases of severe, life-threatening PE to dissolve the clot and anticoagulants to prevent more clots from forming.

Section 26.3

Pulmonary Embolism

This section includes text excerpted from "Pulmonary Embolism,"
MedlinePlus, National Institutes of Health (NIH), August 10, 2018.

What Is a Pulmonary Embolism?

A pulmonary embolism (PE) is a sudden blockage in a lung artery.
It usually happens when a blood clot breaks loose and travels through
the bloodstream to the lungs. PE is a serious condition that can cause:

- Permanent damage to the lungs

- Low oxygen levels in your blood

- Damage to other organs in your body from not getting enough
  oxygen

A pulmonary embolism can be life-threatening, especially if a clot
is large, or if there are many clots.

What Causes a Pulmonary Embolism

The cause is usually a blood clot in the leg called a "deep vein thrombosis" (DVT) that breaks loose and travels through the bloodstream
to the lung.

Who Is at Risk for a Pulmonary Embolism?

Anyone can get a pulmonary embolism, but certain things can raise
your risk of PE:

- **Having surgery,** especially joint replacement surgery
- **Certain medical conditions,** including:
  - Cancers
  - Heart diseases
  - Lung diseases
  - A broken hip or leg bone or other trauma
- **Hormone-based medicines,** such as birth control pills (BCP)
  or hormone replacement therapy (HRT)

- **Pregnancy and childbirth.** The risk is at its highest around six weeks after childbirth.

- **Not moving for long periods,** such as being on bed rest, having a cast, or taking a long plane flight

- **Age.** Your risk increases as you get older, especially after the age of 40.

- **Family history and genetics.** Certain genetic changes can increase your risk of blood clots and PE.

- **Obesity**

What Are the Symptoms of a Pulmonary Embolism?

Half of the people who have pulmonary embolism have no symptoms. If you do have symptoms, they can include shortness of breath, chest pain, or coughing up blood. Symptoms of a blood clot include warmth, swelling, pain, tenderness, and redness of the leg.

Can Pulmonary Embolism Be Prevented?

Preventing new blood clots can prevent PE. Prevention may include:

- Continuing to take blood thinners. It is also important to get regular checkups with your provider to make sure that the dosage of your medicines is working to prevent blood clots and not causing any bleeding.

- Heart-healthy lifestyle changes, such as heart-healthy eating, exercise, and, if you smoke, quitting smoking

- Using compression stockings to prevent deep vein thrombosis

- Moving your legs when sitting for long periods of time (such as when on long trips)

- Moving around as soon as possible after surgery or being confined to a bed

Chapter 27

Thrombocytopenia

What Is Thrombocytopenia?

Thrombocytopenia is a condition in which your blood has a lower-than-normal number of blood cell fragments called "platelets."

Platelets are made in your bone marrow along with other kinds of blood cells. They travel through your blood vessels and stick together (clot) to stop any bleeding that may happen if a blood vessel is damaged. Platelets also are called "thrombocytes" because a clot also is called a "thrombus."

Causes of Thrombocytopenia

Many factors can cause thrombocytopenia. The condition can be inherited or acquired. "Inherited" means your parents pass the gene for the condition to you. "Acquired" means you are not born with the condition, but you develop it. Sometimes, the cause of thrombocytopenia is not known.

In general, a low platelet count occurs because:

- The body's bone marrow does not make enough platelets.

- The bone marrow makes enough platelets, but the body destroys them or uses them up.

- The spleen holds on to too many platelets.

This chapter includes text excerpted from "Thrombocytopenia," National Heart, Lung, and Blood Institute (NHLBI), January 31, 2008. Reviewed June 2019.

A combination of the above factors also may cause a low platelet count.

The Bone Marrow Does not Make Enough Platelets

Bone marrow is the sponge-like tissue inside the bones. It contains stem cells that develop into red blood cells (RBCs), white blood cells (WBCs), and platelets. When stem cells are damaged, they do not grow into healthy blood cells.

Many conditions and factors can damage stem cells.

Cancer

Cancer, such as leukemia or lymphoma, can damage the bone marrow and destroy blood stem cells. Cancer treatments, such as radiation and chemotherapy, also destroy the stem cells.

Aplastic Anemia

Aplastic anemia is a rare, serious blood disorder in which the bone marrow stops making enough new blood cells. This lowers the number of platelets in your blood.

Toxic Chemicals

Exposure to toxic chemicals—such as pesticides, arsenic, and benzene—can slow the production of platelets.

Medicines

Some medicines, such as diuretics and chloramphenicol (an antibiotic), can slow the production of platelets. Chloramphenicol rarely is used in the United States.

Common over-the-counter (OTC) medicines, such as aspirin or ibuprofen, also can affect platelets.

Alcohol

Alcohol also slows the production of platelets. A temporary drop in the platelet count is common among heavy drinkers, especially if they are eating foods that are low in iron, vitamin B_{12}, or folate.

Viruses

Chickenpox, mumps, rubella, Epstein-Barr virus (EBV), or parvovirus can decrease your platelet count for a while. People who have acquired immunodeficiency syndrome (AIDS) often develop thrombocytopenia.

Genetic Conditions

Some genetic conditions can cause low numbers of platelets in the blood. Examples include Wiskott-Aldrich and May-Hegglin syndromes.

The Body Destroys Its Own Platelets

A low platelet count can occur even if the bone marrow makes enough platelets. The body may destroy its own platelets due to auto-immune diseases, certain medicines, infections, surgery, pregnancy, and some conditions that cause too much blood clotting.

Autoimmune Diseases

Autoimmune diseases occur if the body's immune system mistakenly attacks healthy cells in the body. If an autoimmune disease destroys the body's platelets, thrombocytopenia can occur.

One example of this type of autoimmune disease is immune thrombocytopenia (ITP). ITP is a bleeding disorder in which the blood does not clot as it should. An autoimmune response is thought to cause most cases of ITP.

Normally, your immune system helps your body fight off infections and diseases. But if you have ITP, your immune system attacks and destroys its own platelets. Why this happens is not known. (ITP also may occur if the immune system attacks your bone marrow, which makes platelets.)

Other autoimmune diseases that destroy platelets include lupus and rheumatoid arthritis.

Medicines

A reaction to medicine can confuse your body and cause it to destroy its platelets. Examples of medicines that may cause this to happen include quinine; antibiotics that contain sulfa; and some medicines for seizures, such as Dilantin, vancomycin, and rifampin. (Quinine is a substance often found in tonic water and nutritional health products.)

Heparin is a medicine commonly used to prevent blood clots. But, an immune reaction may trigger the medicine to cause blood clots and thrombocytopenia. This condition is called "heparin-induced thrombocytopenia" (HIT). HIT rarely occurs outside of a hospital.

In heparin-induced thrombocytopenia, the body's immune system attacks a substance formed by heparin and a protein on the surface of the platelets. This attack activates the platelets, and they start to form blood clots.

Blood clots can form deep in the legs (deep vein thrombosis), or they can break loose and travel to the lungs (pulmonary embolism).

Infection

A low platelet count can occur after blood poisoning from a widespread bacterial infection. A virus, such as mononucleosis or cytomegalovirus, also can cause a low platelet count.

Surgery

Platelets can be destroyed when they pass through human-made heart valves, blood vessel grafts, or machines and tubing used for blood transfusions or bypass surgery.

Pregnancy

About five percent of pregnant women develop mild thrombocytopenia when they are close to delivery. The exact cause is not known for sure.

Rare and Serious Conditions That Cause Blood Clots

Some rare and serious conditions can cause a low platelet count. Two examples are thrombotic thrombocytopenic purpura (TTP) and disseminated intravascular coagulation (DIC).

Thrombotic thrombocytopenic purpura is a rare blood condition. It causes blood clots to form in the body's small blood vessels, including vessels in the brains, kidneys, and heart.

Disseminated intravascular coagulation is a rare complication of pregnancy, severe infections, or severe trauma. Tiny blood clots form suddenly throughout the body.

In both conditions, the blood clots use up many of the blood's platelets.

The Spleen Holds On to Too Many Platelets

Usually, one-third of the body's platelets are held in the spleen. If the spleen is enlarged, it will hold on to too many platelets. This means that not enough platelets will circulate in the blood.

An enlarged spleen often is due to cancer or severe liver disease, such as cirrhosis. Cirrhosis is a disease in which the liver is scarred. This prevents it from working well.

An enlarged spleen also might be due to a bone marrow condition, such as myelofibrosis. With this condition, the bone marrow is scarred and not able to make blood cells.

Risk Factors of Thrombocytopenia

People who are at the highest risk for thrombocytopenia includes people who:

- Have certain types of cancer, aplastic anemia, or autoimmune diseases

- Are exposed to certain toxic chemicals

- Have a reaction to certain medicines

- Have certain viruses

- Have certain genetic conditions

People at the highest risk also include heavy alcohol drinkers and pregnant women.

Screening and Prevention of Thrombocytopenia

Whether you can prevent thrombocytopenia depends on its specific cause. Usually, the condition cannot be prevented. However, you can take steps to prevent health problems associated with thrombocytopenia. For example:

- Avoid heavy drinking. Alcohol slows the production of platelets.

- Try to avoid contact with toxic chemicals. Chemicals, such as pesticides, arsenic, and benzene, can slow the production of platelets.

- Avoid medicines that you know have decreased your platelet count in the past.

- Be aware of medicines that may affect your platelets and raise your risk of bleeding. Two examples of such medicines are aspirin and ibuprofen. These medicines may thin your blood too much.

• Talk with your doctor about getting vaccinated for viruses that can affect your platelets. You may need vaccines for mumps, measles, rubella, and chickenpox. You may want to have your child vaccinated for these viruses as well. Talk with your child's doctor about these vaccines.

Signs, Symptoms, and Complications of Thrombocytopenia

Mild to serious bleeding causes the main signs and symptoms of thrombocytopenia. Bleeding can occur inside your body (internal bleeding) or underneath your skin or from the surface of your skin (external bleeding).

Signs and symptoms can appear suddenly or over time. Mild thrombocytopenia often has no signs or symptoms. Many times, it is found during a routine blood test.

Check with your doctor if you have any signs of bleeding. Severe thrombocytopenia can cause bleeding in almost any part of the body. Bleeding can lead to a medical emergency and should be treated right away.

External bleeding usually is the first sign of a low platelet count. External bleeding may cause purpura or petechiae. Purpura are purple, brown, and red bruises. This bruising may happen easily and often. Petechiae are small red or purple dots on your skin.

Purpura and Petechiae

Other signs of external bleeding include:

• Prolonged bleeding, even from minor cuts

• Bleeding or oozing from the mouth or nose, especially nosebleeds or bleeding from brushing your teeth

• Abnormal vaginal bleeding (especially heavy menstrual flow)

A lot of bleeding after surgery or dental work also might suggest a bleeding problem.

Heavy bleeding into the intestines or the brain (internal bleeding) is serious and can be fatal. Signs and symptoms include:

• Blood in the urine or stool or bleeding from the rectum. Blood in the stool can appear as red blood or as a dark, tarry color. (Taking iron supplements also can cause dark, tarry stools.)

- Headaches and other neurological symptoms. These problems are very rare, but you should discuss them with your doctor.

Living with Thrombocytopenia

If you have thrombocytopenia, watch for any signs and symptoms of bleeding. Report these signs and symptoms to your doctor right away.

Symptoms can appear suddenly or over time. Severe thrombocytopenia can cause bleeding in almost any part of the body. Bleeding can lead to a medical emergency and should be treated right away.

You can take steps to avoid health problems associated with thrombocytopenia. Be aware of the medicines you are taking, avoid injuries, and contact your doctor if you have a fever or other signs or symptoms of an infection.

Medicines

Avoid medicines that may affect your platelets and raise your risk of bleeding. Two examples of such medicines are aspirin and ibuprofen. These medicines may thin your blood too much. Be careful when using over-the-counter medicines—many contain aspirin or ibuprofen.

Tell your doctor about all of the medicines you take, including over-the-counter medicines, vitamins, supplements, and herbal remedies.

Injuries

Avoid injuries that can cause bruising and bleeding. Do not take part in contact sports, such as boxing, football, or karate. These sports are likely to lead to injuries that can cause bleeding.

Other sports, such as skiing or horseback riding, also put you at risk for injuries that can cause bleeding. Ask your doctor about physical activities that are safe for you.

Take safety precautions, such as using a seatbelt while riding in a car and wearing gloves when working with knives and other tools.

If your child has thrombocytopenia, try to protect her or him from injuries, especially from head injuries that can cause bleeding in the brain. Ask your child's doctor whether you need to restrict your child's activities.

Infection

If you have had your spleen removed, you may be more likely to become ill from certain types of infection. Watch for fever or other signs of infection, and report them to your doctor promptly. People who have had their spleens removed may need vaccines to prevent certain infections.

Chapter 28

Immune Thrombocytopenic Purpura

Immune thrombocytopenia (ITP) is a disorder characterized by a blood abnormality called "thrombocytopenia," which is a shortage of blood cell fragments called "platelets" that are needed for normal blood clotting.

Affected individuals can develop red or purple spots on the skin that are caused by bleeding just under the skin's surface. Small spots of bleeding under the skin are called "purpura" and larger spots are called "ecchymoses." People with immune thrombocytopenia can have significant bleeding episodes, such as nose bleeds (epistaxis) or bleeding in the moist lining (mucosae) of the mouth. In severe cases, individuals may have gastrointestinal (GI) bleeding or blood in the urine or stool, or heavy and prolonged menstrual bleeding (menorrhagia). In very rare instances, bleeding inside the skull (intracranial hemorrhage) can occur, which can be life-threatening. A greater reduction in platelet numbers is often associated with more frequent bleeding episodes and an increased risk of severe bleeding.

This chapter contains text excerpted from the following sources: Text in this chapter begins with excerpts from "Immune Thrombocytopenia," Genetics Home Reference (GHR), National Institutes of Health (NIH), June 2017; Text beginning with the heading "Risk Factors of Immune Thrombocytopenic Purpura" is excerpted from "Immune Thrombocytopenia," National Heart, Lung, and Blood Institute (NHLBI), January 31, 2008. Reviewed June 2019.

While immune thrombocytopenia can be diagnosed at any age, there are two periods when the condition is most likely to develop: early childhood and late adulthood. In children, the reduction in platelets is often sudden, but platelet levels usually return to normal levels within weeks to months. Immune thrombocytopenia in children is often preceded by a minor infection, such as an upper respiratory infection, but the relationship between the infection and immune thrombocytopenia is not clear. In adults, the development of immune thrombocytopenia is usually gradual and the condition tends to persist throughout life.

Frequency of Immune Thrombocytopenic Purpura

The incidence of immune thrombocytopenia is approximately 4 per 100,000 children and 3 per 100,000 adults. In adults with immune thrombocytopenia, women are affected more often than men.

It is likely that this condition is underdiagnosed because those with mild signs and symptoms often do not seek medical attention.

Causes of Immune Thrombocytopenic Purpura

The genetic cause of immune thrombocytopenia is unclear. This condition occurs when the body's own immune system malfunctions and attacks the body's tissues and organs (autoimmunity). Normally, the immune system produces proteins called "antibodies," which attach to specific foreign particles and germs, marking them for destruction. In immune thrombocytopenia, the immune system abnormally destroys platelets and makes fewer platelets than normal. People with immune thrombocytopenia produce antibodies that attack normal platelets. The platelets are destroyed and eliminated from the body, resulting in a shortage of these cells in affected individuals. Some of these antibodies also affect the cells in the bone marrow that produce platelets (known as "megakaryocytes"), which leads to a decrease in platelet production, further reducing the number of platelets in the blood.

In some people with immune thrombocytopenia, the abnormal immune reactions may coincide with an infection by certain viruses or bacteria. Exposure to these foreign invaders may trigger the body to fight the infection, but the immune system also mistakenly attacks platelets.

Genetic variations (polymorphisms) in a few genes have been found in some people with immune thrombocytopenia and may increase the risk of abnormal immune reactions. However, the contribution of these genetic changes to the development of immune thrombocytopenia is unclear.

When the condition is due to the targeted destruction of platelets by the body's own immune cells, it is known as "primary immune thrombocytopenia." Immune thrombocytopenia following bacterial or viral infection is considered primary because the infection triggers a platelet-specific immune reaction, typically without any other signs or symptoms. However, immune thrombocytopenia can be a feature of other immune disorders, such as common variable immune deficiency, which occurs when the immune system has a decreased ability to protect the body against foreign invaders, or other autoimmune disorders, such as systemic lupus erythematosus (SLE). Immune thrombocytopenia can also occur with other blood disorders, including a form of cancer of the blood-forming tissue known as "chronic lymphocytic leukemia" (CLL) and human immunodeficiency virus (HIV) infection. When immune thrombocytopenia is a feature of other disorders, the condition is known as "secondary immune thrombocytopenia."

Risk Factors of Immune Thrombocytopenic Purpura

Immune thrombocytopenia is a fairly common blood disorder. Both children and adults can develop ITP.

Children usually have the acute (short-term) type of ITP. Acute ITP often develops after a viral infection.

Adults tend to have the chronic (long-lasting) type of ITP. Women are two to three times more likely than men to develop chronic ITP.

The number of cases of ITP is rising because routine blood tests that can detect a low platelet count are being done more often.

Immune thrombocytopenia cannot be passed from one person to another.

Screening and Prevention of Immune Thrombocytopenic Purpura

You cannot prevent immune thrombocytopenia, but you can prevent its complications.

- **Talk with your doctor about which medicines are safe for you.** Your doctor may advise you to avoid medicines that can affect your platelets and increase your risk of bleeding. Examples of such medicines include aspirin and ibuprofen.

- **Protect yourself from injuries that can cause bruising or bleeding.**

- **Seek treatment right away if you develop any infections.** Report any symptoms of infection, such as a fever, to your doctor. This is very important for people who have ITP and have had their spleens removed.

Signs, Symptoms, and Complications of Immune Thrombocytopenic Purpura

Immune thrombocytopenia may not cause any signs or symptoms. However, ITP can cause bleeding inside the body (internal bleeding) or underneath or from the skin (external bleeding). Signs of bleeding may include:

- Bruising or purplish areas on the skin or mucous membranes (such as in the mouth). These bruises are called "purpura." They are caused by bleeding under the skin, and they may occur for no known reason.

- Pinpoint red spots on the skin called "petechiae." These spots often are found in groups and may look like a rash. Bleeding under the skin causes petechiae.

- A collection of clotted or partially clotted blood under the skin that looks or feels like a lump. This is called a "hematoma."

- Nosebleeds or bleeding from the gums (for example, during dental work)

- Blood in the urine or stool (bowel movement)

Any kind of bleeding that is hard to stop could be a sign of ITP. This includes menstrual bleeding that is heavier than normal. Bleeding in the brain is rare, and its symptoms may vary.

A low platelet count does not directly cause pain, problems concentrating, or other symptoms. However, a low platelet count might be associated with fatigue (tiredness).

Living with Immune Thrombocytopenic Purpura

If you have immune thrombocytopenia, you can take steps to prevent complications. Lifestyle changes and ongoing care can help you manage the condition.

Lifestyle Changes

Try to avoid injuries, especially head injuries, that can cause bleeding in the brain. For example, do not take part in contact sports, such as boxing, football, or karate. Other sports, such as skiing or horseback riding, also put you at risk for injuries that can cause bleeding.

Some safe activities are swimming, biking (with a helmet), and walking. Ask your doctor about physical activities that are safe for you.

Take precautions, such as regular use of seatbelts and wearing gloves while working with knives and other tools.

If your child has ITP, ask her or his doctor whether you need to restrict your child's activities.

Ongoing Care

You may want to find a doctor who is familiar with treating people who have ITP. For example, hematologists are doctors who specialize in diagnosing and treating blood disorders. Discuss with your doctor how to manage ITP and when to seek medical care.

Talk with your doctor before taking prescription medicines or over-the-counter medicines, supplements, vitamins, or herbal remedies. Some medicines and supplements can affect platelets and increase your chance of bleeding. Common examples are aspirin or ibuprofen. Your doctor may advise you to avoid these medicines.

Watch for symptoms of infection, such as a fever, and report them to your doctor promptly. If you have had your spleen removed, you may be more likely to become ill from certain infections.

Pregnancy

In women who are pregnant and have ITP, the ITP usually does not affect the fetus. However, some babies may be born with or develop low platelet counts soon after birth.

The babies' platelet counts almost always return to normal without any treatment. Treatment can speed up recovery in the babies whose platelet counts are very low.

Treatment for immune thrombocytopenia during pregnancy depends on a woman's platelet count. If treatment is needed, the doctor will take a close look at the possible effects of the treatment on the fetus.

Women who have mild cases of ITP usually can go through pregnancy without treatment. Pregnant women who have very low platelet counts or a lot of bleeding are more likely to have heavy bleeding during delivery or afterward. To prevent heavy bleeding, these women usually are treated.

Chapter 29

Thrombotic Thrombocytopenic Purpura

Acquired thrombotic thrombocytopenic purpura (TTP) is a blood disorder characterized by low platelets (i.e., thrombocytopenia), small areas of bleeding under the skin (i.e., purpura), low red blood cell count, and hemolytic anemia. TTP causes blood clots (thrombi) to form in small blood vessels throughout the body. These clots can cause serious medical problems if they block vessels and decrease or stop blood flow to organs, such as the brain, kidneys, and heart. Complications may include neurological problems (such as personality changes, headaches, confusion, and slurred speech), fever, abnormal kidney function, abdominal pain, and heart problems. Hemolytic anemia can lead to paleness, yellowing of the eyes and skin (jaundice), fatigue, shortness of breath, and a rapid heart rate. Acquired TTP usually begins in adulthood, but it can affect children. An episode of TTP usually occurs suddenly and lasts for days or weeks, but it may continue for months. Relapses (or flare-ups) can occur in up to 60 percent of people who have the acquired TTP. Acquired TTP is caused when a person's body

This chapter contains text excerpted from the following sources: Text in this chapter begins with excerpts from "Thrombotic Thrombocytopenic Purpura, Acquired," Genetic and Rare Diseases Information Center (GARD), National Center for Advancing Translational Sciences (NCATS), December 16, 2016; Text beginning with the heading "Risk Factors of Thrombotic Thrombocytopenic Purpura" is excerpted from "Thrombotic Thrombocytopenic Purpura," National Heart, Lung, and Blood Institute (NHLBI), August 29, 2011. Reviewed June 2019.

mistakenly makes antibodies that block the activity of the ADAMTS13 enzyme. The ADAMTS13 enzyme normally helps control the activity of certain blood-clotting factors. Treatment includes plasma exchange and in some cases may also include corticosteroid therapy or rituximab.

Risk Factors of Thrombotic Thrombocytopenic Purpura

Thrombotic thrombocytopenic purpura is a rare disorder. Most cases of TTP are acquired. Acquired thrombotic thrombocytopenic purpura mostly occurs in adults, but it can affect children. The condition occurs more often in women and in Black people than in other groups.

Inherited TTP mainly affects newborns and children. Most people who have inherited TTP begin to have symptoms soon after birth. Some, however, do not have symptoms until they are adults.

It is not clear what triggers inherited and acquired TTP, but some factors may play a role. These factors may include:

- Some diseases and conditions, such as pregnancy, cancer, human immunodeficiency virus (HIV), lupus, and infections

- Some medical procedures, such as surgery and blood and marrow stem cell transplant

- Some medicines, such as chemotherapy, ticlopidine, clopidogrel, cyclosporine A, and hormone therapy and estrogens

- Quinine, which is a substance often found in tonic water and nutritional health products

Screening and Prevention of Thrombotic Thrombocytopenic Purpura

Both inherited and acquired thrombotic thrombocytopenic purpura occur suddenly with no clear cause. You cannot prevent either type.

If you have had thrombotic thrombocytopenic purpura, watch for signs and symptoms of a relapse.

Ask your doctor about factors that may trigger TTP or a flare-up, including:

- Some diseases or conditions, such as pregnancy, cancer, HIV, lupus, or infections

- Some medical procedures, such as surgery and blood and marrow stem cell transplant

- Some medicines, such as ticlopidine, clopidogrel, cyclosporine A, chemotherapy, and hormone therapy and estrogens. If you take any of these medicines, your doctor may prescribe a different medicine.

- Quinine, which is a substance often found in tonic water and nutritional health products

Signs, Symptoms, and Complications of Thrombotic Thrombocytopenic Purpura

Blood clots, a low platelet count, and damaged red blood cells (RBCs) cause the signs and symptoms of thrombotic thrombocytopenic purpura.

The signs and symptoms include:

- Purplish bruises on the skin or mucous membranes (such as in the mouth). These bruises, called "purpura," are caused by bleeding under the skin.

- Pinpoint-sized red or purple dots on the skin. These dots called "petechiae," often are found in groups and may look like a rash. Bleeding under the skin causes petechiae.

- Paleness or jaundice (a yellowish color of the skin or whites of the eyes)

- Fatigue (feeling very tired and weak)

- Fever

- A fast heart rate or shortness of breath.

- Headache, speech changes, confusion, coma, stroke, or seizure.

- A low amount of urine, or protein or blood in the urine

If you have had TTP and have any of these signs or symptoms, you may be having a relapse. Ask your doctor when to call her or him or seek emergency care.

Living with Thrombotic Thrombocytopenic Purpura

Some people fully recover from thrombotic thrombocytopenic purpura. However, relapses can occur in many people who have acquired and inherited TTP.

If you have had TTP, call your doctor right away if you have signs or symptoms of a relapse.

If you have been treated for TTP, ask your doctor about medicines that may raise your risk of bleeding during a relapse, such as aspirin and ibuprofen.

Also, tell your doctor about all over-the-counter (OTC) medicines you take, including vitamins, supplements, and herbal remedies.

Your doctor may ask whether you are using any products that contain quinine. Quinine is a substance often found in tonic water and nutritional health products. Quinine may trigger TTP or a flare-up of the disorder.

If your child has inherited thrombotic thrombocytopenic purpura, ask the doctor whether you need to restrict your child's activities.

Report any symptoms of infection, such as a fever, to your doctor. This is very important for people who have had their spleens removed.

Talk with your doctor about changing medicines that may raise your risk of TTP, such as ticlopidine and clopidogrel.

Part Four

Circulatory Disorders

Chapter 30

Blood Pressure Disorders

Chapter Contents

Section 30.1

Hypertension

This section includes text excerpted from "High Blood Pressure,"
National Heart, Lung, and Blood Institute (NHLBI), July 25, 2018.

What Is Hypertension?

High blood pressure is a common disease in which blood flows
through blood vessels, or arteries, at higher than normal pressures.
Blood pressure is the force of blood pushing against the walls of your
arteries as the heart pumps blood. High blood pressure, sometimes
called "hypertension," is when this force against the artery walls is too
high. Your doctor may diagnose you with high blood pressure if you
have consistently high blood pressure readings.

To control or lower high blood pressure, your doctor may recommend
that you adopt heart-healthy lifestyle changes—such as heart-healthy
eating patterns, like the Dietary Approaches to Stop Hypertension
(DASH) eating plan—alone or with medicines. Controlling or lowering blood pressure can also help prevent or delay high blood pressure
complications, such as chronic kidney disease (CKD), heart attack,
heart failure, stroke, and possibly vascular dementia.

Causes of Hypertension

Eating too much sodium and having certain medical conditions can
cause high blood pressure. Taking certain medicines, including birth
control pills (BCPs) or over-the-counter (OTC) cold relief medicines,
can also make blood pressure rise.

Eating Too Much Sodium

Unhealthy eating patterns, particularly eating too much sodium,
are a common cause of high blood pressure in the United States.
Healthy lifestyle changes can help prevent or treat high blood pressure.

Other Medical Conditions

Other medical conditions change the way your body controls fluids,
sodium, and hormones in your blood. Other medical causes of high
blood pressure include:

- Certain tumors

- Chronic kidney disease

- Being overweight or obese

- Sleep apnea

- Thyroid problems

Risk Factors for Hypertension

There are many risk factors for high blood pressure. Some risk factors, such as unhealthy lifestyle habits, can be changed. Other risk factors, such as age, family history and genetics, race and ethnicity, and sex, cannot be changed. Healthy lifestyle changes can decrease your risk for developing high blood pressure.

Age

Blood pressure tends to increase with age. Our blood vessels naturally thicken and stiffen over time. These changes increase the risk for high blood pressure.

However, the risk of high blood pressure is increasing for children and teens, possibly due to the rise in the number of children and teens who are overweight or obese.

Family History and Genetics

High blood pressure often runs in families. Much of the understanding of the body systems involved in high blood pressure has come from genetic studies. Research has identified many gene variations associated with small increases in the risk of developing high blood pressure. Research suggests that certain deoxyribonucleic acid (DNA) changes during fetal development may also lead to the development of high blood pressure later in life.

Unhealthy Lifestyle Habits

Unhealthy lifestyle habits can increase the risk of high blood pressure. These habits include:

- Unhealthy eating patterns, such as eating too much sodium

- Drinking too much alcohol

- Being physically inactive

Race or Ethnicity

High blood pressure is more common in African American adults than in White, Hispanic, or Asian adults. Compared with other racial or ethnic groups, African Americans tend to have higher average blood pressure numbers and get high blood pressure earlier in life.

Sex

Before the age of 55, men are more likely than women to develop high blood pressure. After the age of 55, women are more likely than men to develop high blood pressure.

Screening and Prevention of Hypertension

Everyone three years of age or older should have their blood pressure checked by a healthcare provider at least once a year. Your doctor will use a blood pressure test to see if you have consistently high blood pressure readings. Even small increases in systolic blood pressure can weaken and damage your blood vessels. Your doctor will recommend heart-healthy lifestyle changes to help control your blood pressure and prevent you from developing high blood pressure.

Screening for Consistently High Blood Pressure Readings

Your doctor will use a blood pressure test to see if you have higher-than-normal blood pressure readings. The reading is made up of 2 numbers, with the systolic number above the diastolic number. These numbers are measures of pressure in millimeters of mercury (mmHg).

Your blood pressure is considered high when you have consistent systolic readings of 140 mmHg or higher, or diastolic readings of 90 mmHg or higher. Based on research, your doctor may also consider you to have high blood pressure if you are an adult or child 13 years of age or older who has consistent systolic readings of 130 to 139 mmHg or diastolic readings of 80 to 89 mmHg and you have other cardiovascular risk factors.

For children younger than 13 years of age, blood pressure readings are compared to readings common for children of the same, age, sex, and height.

Talk to your doctor if your blood pressure readings are consistently higher than normal.

A blood pressure test is easy and painless, and it can be done in a doctor's office or clinic. A healthcare provider will use a gauge, stethoscope, or electronic sensor and a blood pressure cuff to measure your blood pressure. To prepare, take the following steps:

- Do not exercise, drink coffee, or smoke cigarettes for 30 minutes before the test.

- Go to the bathroom before the test.

- For at least five minutes before the test, sit in a chair and relax.

- Make sure your feet are flat on the floor.

- Do not talk while you are relaxing or during the test.

- Uncover your arm for the cuff.

- Rest your arm on a table so it is supported and at the level of your heart.

If it is the first time your provider has measured your blood pressure, you may have readings taken on both arms.

Even after taking these steps, your blood pressure reading may not be accurate for other reasons.

- **You are excited or nervous.** The phrase "white coat hypertension" refers to blood pressure readings that are only high when taken in a doctor's office compared with readings taken in other places. Doctors can detect this type of high blood pressure by reviewing readings from the office and from other places.

- **If your blood pressure tends to be lower when measured at the doctor's office.** This is called "masked high blood pressure." When this happens, your doctor will have difficulty detecting high blood pressure.

- **The wrong blood pressure cuff was used.** Your readings can appear different if the cuff is too small or too large. It is important for your healthcare team to track your readings over time and ensure the correct pressure cuff is used for your sex and age.

Your doctor may run additional tests to confirm an initial reading. To gather more information about your blood pressure, your doctor may recommend wearing a blood pressure monitor to record readings over 24 hours. Your doctor may also teach you how to take blood pressure readings at home.

Healthy Lifestyle Changes to Prevent High Blood Pressure

Healthy lifestyle changes can help prevent high blood pressure from developing. Healthy lifestyle changes include choosing a heart-healthy eating patterns, such as the DASH eating plan, being physically active, aiming for a healthy weight, quitting smoking, and managing stress.

Signs, Symptoms, and Complications of Hypertension

It is important to have regular blood pressure readings taken and to know your numbers because high blood pressure usually does not cause symptoms until serious complications occur. Undiagnosed or uncontrolled high blood pressure can cause the following complications:

- Aneurysms
- Chronic kidney disease
- Eye damage
- Heart attack
- Heart failure
- Peripheral artery disease (PAD)
- Stroke
- Vascular dementia

Living with Hypertension

If you have been diagnosed with high blood pressure, it is important that you continue your treatment plan. Following your treatment plan, getting regular follow-up care, and learning how to monitor your condition at home are important. Let your doctor know if you are planning to become pregnant. These steps can help prevent or delay complications that high blood pressure can cause. Your doctor may adjust your treatment plan as needed to lower or control your high blood pressure.

Receive Routine Follow-Up Care

Check your blood pressure and have regular medical checkups or tests as your doctor advises. Your doctor may suggest ways for you to monitor your blood pressure at home. During checkups, talk to your doctor about these important topics:

- Blood pressure readings

- Your overall health

- Your treatment plan

Your doctor may need to change or add medicines to your treatment plan over time. To help control your blood pressure and prevent heart disease, keep up your healthy lifestyle changes. You can ask questions and discuss your progress as part of your follow-up.

Monitor Your Condition Yourself

Keeping track of your blood pressure is important. Your doctor can help you learn how to check your blood pressure at home. Each time you check your own blood pressure, record your numbers and the date. Send in or take the log of your blood pressure readings with you for appointments with your doctor.

Pregnancy Planning

High blood pressure can cause problems for a mother and her baby. High blood pressure can harm a mother's kidneys and other organs and can cause early birth and low birth weight. If you are thinking about having a baby and have high blood pressure, talk with your doctors so you can take steps to lower or control your high blood pressure before and during the pregnancy.

Some medicines used to treat high blood pressure are not recommended during pregnancy. If you are taking medicines to lower or control your high blood pressure, talk with your doctor about your choices for safely managing high blood pressure during pregnancy.

Some women with normal blood pressure develop high blood pressure during pregnancy. As part of your regular prenatal care, your doctor will measure your blood pressure at each visit. If you develop high blood pressure, your doctor will closely monitor you and the fetus and provide special care to lower the chance of complications. With such care, most women and babies have good outcomes.

Prevent Worsening High Blood Pressure or Complications over Your Lifetime

If you have high blood pressure, it is important to get routine medical care and to follow your prescribed treatment plan, which will include heart-healthy lifestyle changes and possibly medicines. Heart-healthy lifestyle changes can prevent high blood pressure; reduce elevated blood pressure; help control existing high blood pressure; and prevent complications, such as heart attack, heart failure, stroke, vascular dementia, or chronic kidney disease.

Learn the Warning Signs of Serious Complications and Have a Plan

High blood pressure can lead to serious complications, such as heart attack or stroke. Call 911 if you suspect any of the following in you or someone else:

- **Heart attack.** Signs of heart attack include mild or severe chest pain or discomfort in the center of the chest or upper abdomen that lasts for more than a few minutes or goes away and comes back. It can feel like pressure, squeezing, fullness, heartburn, or indigestion. There may also be pain down the left arm. Women may also have chest pain and pain down the left arm, but they are more likely to have less typical symptoms, such as shortness of breath; nausea; vomiting; unusual tiredness; and pain in the back, shoulders, or jaw.

- **Stroke.** If you think someone may be having a stroke, act F.A.S.T. and perform the following simple test:

  - **F—Face:** Ask the person to smile. Does one side of the face droop?

  - **A—Arms:** Ask the person to raise both arms. Does one arm drift downward?

  - **S—Speech:** Ask the person to repeat a simple phrase. Is their speech slurred or strange?

  - **T—Time:** If you observe any of these signs, call for help immediately. Early treatment is essential.

- **Dangerously high blood pressure.** Readings above 180 over 120 are dangerously high and require immediate medical attention.

Section 30.2

Pulmonary Hypertension

This section includes text excerpted from "Pulmonary Hypertension," National Heart, Lung, and Blood Institute (NHLBI), April 18, 2019.

What Is Pulmonary Hypertension?

Pulmonary hypertension occurs when the pressure in the blood vessels that carry blood from your heart to your lungs is higher than normal. One type of pulmonary hypertension is pulmonary arterial hypertension (PAH). Pulmonary hypertension can happen on its own or be caused by another disease or condition. In the United States, the most common cause of pulmonary hypertension is left heart disease. Other conditions that can cause pulmonary hypertension include sickle cell disease (SCD); pulmonary embolism (PE), which is a type of venous thromboembolism (VTE); and chronic obstructive pulmonary disease (COPD).

The increased pressure in the blood vessels of the lungs means that your heart has to work harder to pump blood into the lungs. This can cause symptoms, such as shortness of breath, chest pain, and light-headedness. If left untreated, the increased pressure can damage your heart. This may lead to serious or life-threatening complications, such as heart failure or arrhythmias, which are irregular heart rhythms.

Causes of Pulmonary Hypertension

Your genes or other medical conditions can cause pulmonary hypertension. Certain medical conditions can damage, change, or block the blood vessels of the pulmonary arteries. The cause of pulmonary hypertension is not always clear.

To understand pulmonary hypertension, it is helpful to understand the flow of blood through the heart and lungs. The right side of your heart receives oxygen-poor blood from your body's tissues. The pulmonary arteries connect your right heart and lungs. The heart pumps blood through the pulmonary arteries to the lungs to become oxygen-rich blood. The force or pressure of the blood against the walls of the pulmonary arteries is called the "pulmonary pressure."

Genes

Gene mutations are found in some people who have a family history of pulmonary arterial hypertension. Mutations are also found often in patients who do not have a family history of the condition.

Medical Conditions

Many medical conditions can cause pulmonary hypertension. Pulmonary arterial hypertension is caused by conditions that result in narrowing of the pulmonary arteries themselves, such as scleroderma or human immunodeficiency virus (HIV). Narrowed blood vessels can increase blood pressure in the lungs.

Medical conditions that can cause pulmonary hypertension include:

- **Blood clots** in the lungs, called "pulmonary embolism," a type of venous thromboembolism

- **Chronic exposure to high altitudes**

- **Chronic kidney failure**

- **Congenital heart defects** or congenital narrowing of the pulmonary arteries

- **Connective tissue diseases,** such as scleroderma

- **Human immunodeficiency virus**

- **Infection with parasites,** such as schistosomiasis or Echinococcus, which are tapeworms

- **Left heart diseases,** such as left heart failure, which may be caused by high blood pressure throughout your body or ischemic heart disease; and heart valve diseases, such as aortic stenosis and mitral valve disease

- **Liver diseases,** such as cirrhosis, that lead to higher-than-normal blood pressures in the liver

- **Lung diseases,** such as COPD, interstitial lung disease, or sleep apnea

- **Metabolic disorders,** such as thyroid disorders or Gaucher disease

- **Sarcoidosis**

- **Sickle cell disease**

- **Tumors** in the lungs

Risk Factors for Pulmonary Hypertension

You may have an increased risk for pulmonary hypertension because of your age, environment, family history, and genetics, lifestyle habits, medicines you are taking, other medical conditions, or sex.

Age

Your risk of pulmonary hypertension increases as you get older, although it may occur at any age. The condition is typically diagnosed between the ages of 30 and 60.

Environment

You may be at an increased risk of pulmonary hypertension if you have or are exposed to the following:

- **Asbestos** or silica

- **Infection** caused by parasites, such as schistosomiasis or Echinococcus

Family History and Genetics

Certain genetic disorders, such as Down syndrome, congenital heart disease (CHD), and Gaucher disease, can increase your risk of developing pulmonary hypertension.

A family history of blood clots or pulmonary embolism also increases your risk of developing pulmonary hypertension.

Lifestyle Habits

Unhealthy lifestyle habits can increase the risk of pulmonary hypertension. These habits include:

- **Illegal drugs,** such as cocaine and amphetamines
- **Smoking**

Medicines

Some medicines may increase your risk of pulmonary hypertension, including:

- **Chemotherapy medicines** to treat cancer, such as dasatinib, mitomycin C, and cyclophosphamide

- **Selective serotonin reuptake inhibitors (SSRIs)** to treat depression and anxiety. SSRIs may cause pulmonary arterial hypertension in newborns whose mothers have taken these medicines during pregnancy.

- **Weight-loss drugs,** such as fenfluramine and dexfenfluramine, which are no longer approved for weight loss in the United States

Other Medical Conditions

Certain medical conditions may increase your risk of developing pulmonary hypertension:

- **Blood clotting disorders,** such as blood clots in the lungs; a higher-than-normal platelet count in your blood; and conditions that make your blood more likely to clot, such as protein S and C deficiency, factor V Leiden thrombophilia, antithrombin III deficiency, and antiphospholipid syndrome (APS)

- **Chronic kidney disease**

- **Diseases that change the structure of the chest wall,** such as scoliosis

- **Infections,** such as hepatitis B or C

- **Liver disease,** such as cirrhosis

- **Surgical removal of the spleen**

- **Thyroid diseases**

Sex

Pulmonary hypertension is more common in women than in men. Pulmonary hypertension with certain types of heart failure is also more common in women.

Screening and Prevention of Pulmonary Hypertension

To screen for pulmonary hypertension, your doctor will determine whether you have any known risk factors and may have you undergo screening tests. Screening is not usually performed unless you have known risk factors, such as scleroderma. Your doctor may recommend prevention strategies to help you lower your risk of developing pulmonary hypertension.

Tests to Screen for Pulmonary Hypertension

Based on your symptoms or risk factors, your doctor may recommend the following tests to screen for changes in the heart or lungs that may be related to pulmonary hypertension.

- **Echocardiography (echo)** to look at your heart's function and structure and to estimate pulmonary artery pressure

- **Electrocardiography (ECG or EKG)** to look for signs of changes in your heart or abnormal rhythms in your heart's electrical activity

- **Pulmonary function tests** to look for changes in lung function for conditions, such as systemic sclerosis, COPD, or interstitial lung diseases

Based on the results of these screening tests, your doctor may do follow-up tests to see whether you have higher-than-normal pressures in the pulmonary arteries. These other tests can help diagnose pulmonary hypertension.

Prevention Strategies

To help prevent pulmonary hypertension, your doctor may recommend controlling certain medical conditions, avoiding certain medicines or illegal drugs, and protecting yourself against environmental hazards that are risk factors.

Signs, Symptoms, and Complications of Pulmonary Hypertension

Signs and symptoms of pulmonary hypertension are sometimes hard to recognize because they are similar to those of other medical conditions. People may have symptoms for years before being diagnosed with pulmonary hypertension. These symptoms may get worse over time and could eventually lead to serious complications, such as right heart failure.

Signs and Symptoms

Signs and symptoms of pulmonary hypertension may include the following:

- **Chest pain**

- **Cough** that is dry or may produce blood
- **Fatigue**
- **Hoarseness**
- **Light-headedness,** fainting, or dizziness
- **Nausea and vomiting**
- **Shortness of breath,** first with physical activity and then without it as the disease gets worse
- **Swelling** of your abdomen, legs, or feet caused by fluid buildup
- **Weakness**
- **Wheezing**

Complications

Complications of pulmonary hypertension may include the following:

- **Anemia**
- **Arrhythmias** and bundle branch blocks of the heart
- **Blood clots** in the pulmonary arteries
- **Bleeding in the lungs,** which may be life-threatening
- **Heart failure,** especially right ventricular failure
- **Liver damage** from increased pressure in the right heart
- **Pericardial effusion,** which is a collection of fluid in the sac-like structure around the heart
- **Pregnancy complications** that can be life-threatening for the mother and fetus

Living with Pulmonary Hypertension

After you are diagnosed with pulmonary hypertension, it is important to follow your treatment plan, get regular care, and learn how to monitor your condition. Taking these steps can slow down the progression of the disease and may improve your condition. Your specific treatment plan will depend on the cause of your pulmonary hypertension, as well as how advanced it is.

Receive Routine Follow-Up Care

Your follow-up care may include recommendations such as these:

- **Participate in support groups, counseling, and education efforts** that can help you manage the activities of daily living, experience a successful pregnancy, and generally improve the quality of your life.

- **Get the recommended vaccines,** which often include a vaccine for pneumococcus and an influenza, or flu, shot every year at the start of flu season.

Monitor Your Condition

Talk to your doctor about new or concerning symptoms. People who have pulmonary hypertension may need regular tests. Your doctor may recommend the following to monitor your condition and treatment response:

- **Six-minute walk test** to monitor your ability to exercise

- **Blood tests** to check hemoglobin, iron, and electrolyte levels; kidney, liver, and thyroid function; your blood's ability to clot; and signs of stress on the heart

- **Cardiac catheterization**

- **Cardiac magnetic resonance imaging (MRI)** to monitor your heart's size and how well it is working

- **Chest X-ray**

- **Echocardiography** to monitor your heart's size and how well it is working, and to measure the pressure in your right heart chambers

- **Electrocardiogram** to check for irregular heartbeats

- **Pulmonary function tests** to check for any change in your lung function

If your pulmonary hypertension is severe or does not respond to treatment, your doctor may talk to you about a lung transplant or a heart and lung transplant.

Prevent Complications over Your Lifetime

To help prevent some of the complications of pulmonary hypertension, your doctor may recommend the following.

- **Make heart-healthy lifestyle changes**, such as heart-healthy eating if your pulmonary hypertension is due to heart failure from ischemic heart disease or high blood pressure.

- **Engage in regular physical activity**. Before starting any exercise program, ask your doctor about what level of physical activity is right for you.

- **Avoid high altitudes** when possible and discuss with your doctor any plans for air travel or visits to places at high altitude.

- **Talk to your doctor** if you are planning to get pregnant, as there is an increased risk of pregnancy complications.

- **Treat other medical conditions**, such as COPD, heart conditions, and sleep apnea.

Learn the Warning Signs of Serious Complications and Have a Plan

Even with treatment, pulmonary hypertension may lead to serious complications, such as heart failure and arrhythmias. Know the signs and symptoms of pulmonary hypertension and how to recognize the possible complications.

If you are taking a blood thinner, this will increase your risk of bleeding. If you experience any abnormal bleeding, such as blood in your stool, black stool, or coughing up blood, contact your doctor right away. If you fall while taking a blood thinner, you are at a higher risk for bleeding inside your head. Let your doctor know if you have fallen while taking a blood thinner.

Some treatments for pulmonary hypertension must be given through a long-term intravenous (IV) line. Call your doctor right away if you have any signs of infection. Signs of infection include redness, swelling, or yellow discharge where the IV is inserted; a fever of 100.3°F or higher; and chills.

Section 30.3

Preeclampsia and Eclampsia

This section includes text excerpted from "About Preeclampsia and Eclampsia," *Eunice Kennedy Shriver* National Institute of Child Health and Human Development (NICHD), November 19, 2018.

Preeclampsia and eclampsia are part of the spectrum of high blood pressure, or hypertensive, disorders that can occur during pregnancy.

At the mild end of the spectrum is gestational hypertension, which occurs when a woman who previously had normal blood pressure develops high blood pressure when she is more than 20 weeks pregnant, and her blood pressure returns to normal within 12 weeks after delivery. This problem usually occurs without other symptoms. In many cases, gestational hypertension does not harm the mother or fetus. Severe gestational hypertension, however, may be associated with preterm birth and infants who are small for their age at birth. Some women who have gestational hypertension later develop preeclampsia.

Preeclampsia is similar to gestational hypertension because it also involves high blood pressure at or after 20 weeks of pregnancy in a woman whose blood pressure was normal before pregnancy. But, preeclampsia can also include blood pressure at or greater than 140/90 mmHg, increased swelling, and protein in the urine. The condition can be serious and is a leading cause of preterm birth (before 37 weeks of pregnancy). If it is severe enough to affect brain function, causing seizures or coma, it is called "eclampsia."

A serious complication of hypertensive disorders in pregnancy is HELLP syndrome, a situation in which a pregnant woman with preeclampsia or eclampsia suffers damage to the liver and blood cells. The letters in the name HELLP stand for the following problems:

- H—Hemolysis, in which oxygen-carrying red blood cells break down

- EL—Elevated Liver enzymes, showing damage to the liver

- LP—Low Platelet count, meaning that the cells responsible for stopping bleeding are low

Postpartum preeclampsia describes preeclampsia that develops after the baby is delivered, usually between 48 hours and 6 weeks after delivery. Symptoms can include high blood pressure, severe headache, visual changes, upper abdominal pain, and nausea or vomiting.

Postpartum preeclampsia can occur regardless of whether a woman had high blood pressure or preeclampsia during pregnancy.

Postpartum eclampsia refers to seizures that occur between 48 and 72 hours after delivery. Symptoms also include high blood pressure and difficulty breathing. About one-third of eclampsia cases occur after delivery, and nearly half of those are more than 48 hours after the birth.

Postpartum preeclampsia and eclampsia can be serious and, if not treated quickly, may result in death.

What Causes Preeclampsia and Eclampsia

The causes of preeclampsia and eclampsia are not known. These disorders previously were believed to be caused by a toxin, called "toxemia," in the blood, but healthcare providers now know that is not true. Nevertheless, preeclampsia is sometimes still referred to as "toxemia."

To learn more about preeclampsia and eclampsia, scientists are investigating many factors that could contribute to the development and progression of these diseases, including:

- Placental abnormalities, such as insufficient blood flow
- Genetic factors
- Environmental exposures
- Nutritional factors
- Maternal immunology and autoimmune disorders
- Cardiovascular and inflammatory changes
- Hormonal imbalances

What Are the Risks of Preeclampsia and Eclampsia to the Mother?

Risks during Pregnancy

Preeclampsia during pregnancy is mild in the majority of cases. However, a woman can progress from mild to severe preeclampsia or to full eclampsia very quickly? even in a matter of days. Both preeclampsia and eclampsia can cause serious health problems for the mother and infant.

Women with preeclampsia are at increased risk for damage to the kidneys, liver, brain, and other organ and blood systems. Preeclampsia may also affect the placenta. The condition could lead to a separation of the placenta from the uterus (referred to as "placental abruption"), preterm birth, and pregnancy loss or stillbirth. In some cases, preeclampsia can lead to organ failure or stroke.

In severe cases, preeclampsia can develop into eclampsia, which includes seizures. Seizures in eclampsia may cause a woman to lose consciousness and twitch uncontrollably. If the fetus is not delivered, these conditions can cause the death of the mother and/ or the fetus.

Although most pregnant women in developed countries survive preeclampsia, it is still a major cause of illness and death globally. According to the World Health Organization (WHO), preeclampsia and eclampsia cause 14 percent of maternal deaths each year, or about 50,000 to 75,000 women worldwide.

Risks after Pregnancy

In uncomplicated preeclampsia, the mother's high blood pressure and other symptoms usually go back to normal within six weeks of the infant's birth. However, studies have shown that women who had preeclampsia are four times more likely than women who did not have preeclampsia to later develop hypertension (high blood pressure) and are twice as likely to later develop ischemic heart disease (reduced blood supply to the heart muscle, which can cause heart attacks), a blood clot in a vein, and stroke.

Less commonly, mothers who had preeclampsia can experience permanent damage to their organs, such as their kidneys and liver. They can also experience fluid in the lungs. In the days following birth, women with preeclampsia remain at an increased risk for developing eclampsia and seizures.

In some women, preeclampsia develops between 48 hours and 6 weeks after they deliver their baby—a condition called "postpartum preeclampsia." Postpartum preeclampsia can occur in women who had preeclampsia during pregnancy and among those who did not. One study found that slightly more than one-half of women who had postpartum preeclampsia did not have preeclampsia during pregnancy. If a woman has seizures within 72 hours of delivery, she may have postpartum eclampsia. It is important to recognize and treat postpartum preeclampsia and eclampsia because the risk of complications may be higher than if the conditions had occurred during pregnancy.

Postpartum preeclampsia and eclampsia can progress very quickly if not treated and may lead to stroke or death.

What Are the Risks of Preeclampsia and Eclampsia to the Fetus?

Preeclampsia may be related to problems with the placenta early in the pregnancy. Such problems pose risks to the fetus, including:

- Lack of oxygen and nutrients, which can impair fetal growth
- Preterm birth
- Stillbirth if placental abruption leads to heavy bleeding in the mother
- Infant death

Stillbirths are more likely to occur when the mother has a more severe form of preeclampsia, including HELLP syndrome.

Infants whose mothers had preeclampsia are also at increased risk for later problems, even if they were born at full term (39 weeks of pregnancy). Infants born preterm due to preeclampsia face a higher risk of some long-term health issues, mostly related to being born early, including learning disorders, cerebral palsy, epilepsy, deafness, and blindness. Infants born preterm may also have to be hospitalized for a long time after birth and may be smaller than infants born full term. Infants who experienced poor growth in the uterus may later be at a higher risk of diabetes, congestive heart failure, and high blood pressure.

How Many Women Are Affected by or at Risk of Preeclampsia?

Although preeclampsia occurs primarily in first pregnancies, a woman who had preeclampsia in a previous pregnancy is seven times more likely to develop preeclampsia in a later pregnancy.

Other factors that can increase a woman's risk include:

- Chronic high blood pressure or kidney disease before pregnancy
- High blood pressure or preeclampsia in an earlier pregnancy
- Obesity. Overweight or obese women are also more likely to have preeclampsia in more than one pregnancy.
- Age. Women older than 40 years of age are at a higher risk.

- Multiple gestation (being pregnant with more than one fetus)

- African American ethnicity. Also, among women who have had preeclampsia before, non-White women are more likely than White women to develop preeclampsia again in a later pregnancy.

- Family history of preeclampsia. According to the World Health Organization, among women who have had preeclampsia, about 20 to 40 percent of their daughters and 11 to 37 percent of their sisters also will get the disorder.

Preeclampsia is also more common among women who have histories of certain health conditions, such as migraines, diabetes, rheumatoid arthritis (RA), lupus, scleroderma, urinary tract infections (UTIs), gum disease, polycystic ovary syndrome (PCOS), multiple sclerosis (MS), gestational diabetes, and sickle cell disease (SCD).

Preeclampsia is also more common in pregnancies resulting from egg donation, donor insemination, or in vitro fertilization.

The U.S. Preventive Services Task Force (USPSTF) recommends that women who are at a high risk for preeclampsia take low-dose aspirin starting after 12 weeks of pregnancy to prevent preeclampsia. Women who are pregnant or who are thinking about getting pregnant should talk with their healthcare provider about preeclampsia risk and ways to reduce the risk.

What Are the Symptoms of Preeclampsia, Eclampsia, and Hemolysis Elevated Liver Enzymes Low Platelet Count Syndrome?

Preeclampsia

Possible symptoms of preeclampsia include:

- High blood pressure

- Too much protein in the urine

- Swelling in a woman's face and hands (a woman's feet might swell too, but swollen feet are common during pregnancy and may not signal a problem)

- Systemic problems, such as headache, blurred vision, and right upper quadrant abdominal pain

Eclampsia

The following symptoms are cause for immediate concern:

- Seizures

- Severe headache

- Vision problems, such as temporary blindness

- Abdominal pain, especially in the upper right area of the belly

- Nausea and vomiting

- Smaller urine output or not urinating very often

Hemolysis Elevated Liver Enzymes Low Platelet Count

HELLP syndrome can lead to serious complications, including liver failure and death.

A pregnant woman with HELLP syndrome might bleed or bruise easily and/or experience abdominal pain, nausea or vomiting, headache, or extreme fatigue. Although most women who develop HELLP syndrome already have high blood pressure and preeclampsia, sometimes the syndrome is the first sign. In addition, HELLP syndrome can occur without a woman having either high blood pressure or protein in her urine.

Section 30.4

Hypotension

This section contains text excerpted from the following sources: Text under the heading "What Is Hypotension?" is excerpted from "Low Blood Pressure," MedlinePlus, National Institutes of Health (NIH), January 28, 2019; Text beginning with the heading "Causes of Hypotension" is excerpted from "Hypotension," National Heart, Lung, and Blood Institute (NHLBI), August 29, 2011. Reviewed June 2019.

What Is Hypotension?

You have probably heard that high blood pressure is a problem. Sometimes, blood pressure that is too low can also cause problems.

Hypotension is abnormally low blood pressure.

Blood pressure is the force of your blood pushing against the walls of your arteries. Each time your heart beats, it pumps out blood into the arteries. Your blood pressure is highest when your heart beats, pumping the blood. This is called "systolic pressure." When your heart is at rest, between beats, your blood pressure falls. This is the "diastolic pressure." Your blood pressure reading uses these 2 numbers. Usually, they are written one above or before the other, such as 120/80. If your blood pressure reading is 90/60 or lower, you have low blood pressure.

Some people have low blood pressure all the time. They have no symptoms, and their low readings are normal for them. In other people, blood pressure drops below normal because of a medical condition or certain medicines. Some people may have symptoms of low blood pressure when standing up too quickly. Low blood pressure is a problem only if it causes dizziness, fainting, or, in extreme cases, shock.

Causes of Hypotension

Conditions or factors that disrupt the body's ability to control blood pressure cause hypotension. The different types of hypotension have different causes.

Orthostatic Hypotension

Orthostatic hypotension has many causes. Sometimes, two or more factors combine to cause this type of low blood pressure.

Dehydration is the most common cause of orthostatic hypotension. Dehydration occurs if the body loses more water than it takes in.

You may become dehydrated if you do not drink enough fluids or if you sweat a lot during physical activity. Fever, vomiting, and severe diarrhea also can cause dehydration.

Orthostatic hypotension also may occur during pregnancy, but it usually goes away after birth.

Because an older body does not manage changes in blood pressure as well as a younger body, getting older also can lead to this type of hypotension.

Postprandial hypotension (a type of orthostatic hypotension) mostly affects older adults. Postprandial hypotension is a sudden drop in blood pressure after a meal.

Certain medical conditions can raise your risk of orthostatic hypotension, including:

- Heart conditions, such as heart attack, heart valve disease, bradycardia (a very low heart rate), and heart failure. These conditions prevent the heart from pumping enough blood to the body.

- Anemia

- Severe infections

- Endocrine conditions, such as thyroid disorders, Addison disease, low blood sugar, and diabetes

- Central nervous system disorders, such as Parkinson disease (PD)

- Pulmonary embolism (PE)

Some medicines for high blood pressure and heart disease can raise your risk of orthostatic hypotension. These medicines include:

- Diuretics, also called "water pills"

- Calcium channel blockers

- Angiotensin-converting enzyme (ACE) inhibitors

- Angiotensin II receptor blockers (ARBs)

- Nitrates

- Beta-blockers

Medicines for conditions, such as anxiety, depression, erectile dysfunction, and central nervous system disorders, also can increase your risk of orthostatic hypotension.

Other substances, when taken with high blood pressure medicines, also can lead to orthostatic hypotension. These substances include alcohol, barbiturates, and some prescription and over-the-counter (OTC) medicines.

Finally, other factors or conditions that can trigger orthostatic hypotension include being out in the heat or being immobile for a long time. Immobile means you cannot move around very much.

Neurally Mediated Hypotension

Neurally mediated hypotension (NMH) occurs when the brain and heart do not communicate with each other properly.

For example, when you stand for a long time, blood begins to pool in your legs. This causes your blood pressure to drop. In NMH, the body mistakenly tells the brain that blood pressure is high. In response, the brain slows the heart rate. This makes blood pressure drop even more, causing dizziness and other symptoms.

Severe Hypotension Linked to Shock

Many factors and conditions can cause severe hypotension linked to shock. Some of these factors also can cause orthostatic hypotension. In shock, though, blood pressure drops very low and does not return to normal on its own.

Shock is an emergency and must be treated right away. If a person has signs or symptoms of shock, call 911.

Some severe infections can cause shock. This is known as "septic shock." It can occur if bacteria enter the bloodstream. The bacteria release a toxin (poison) that leads to a dangerous drop in blood pressure.

A severe loss of blood or fluids from the body also can cause shock. This is known as "hypovolemic shock." Hypovolemic shock can happen as a result of:

- Major external bleeding (for example, from a severe cut or injury)

- Major internal bleeding (for example, from a ruptured blood vessel or injury that causes bleeding inside the body)

- Major loss of body fluids from severe burns

- Severe swelling of the pancreas (an organ that produces enzymes and hormones, such as insulin)

- Severe diarrhea

- Severe kidney disease

- Overuse of diuretics

A major decrease in the heart's ability to pump blood also can cause shock. This is known as "cardiogenic shock."

A heart attack, pulmonary embolism, or an ongoing arrhythmia that disrupts heart function can cause this type of shock.

A sudden and extreme relaxation of the arteries linked to a drop in blood pressure also can cause shock. This is known as "vasodilatory shock." It can occur due to:

- A severe head injury

- A reaction to certain medicines

- Liver failure

- Poisoning

- A severe allergic reaction (called "anaphylactic shock")

Risk Factors for Hypotension

Hypotension can affect people of all ages. However, people in certain age groups are more likely to have certain types of hypotension.

Older adults are more likely to have orthostatic and postprandial hypotension. Children and young adults are more likely to have neurally mediated hypotension.

People who take certain medicines—such as diuretics or other high blood pressure medicines—are at an increased risk for hypotension. Certain conditions also increase the risk for hypotension. Examples include central nervous system disorders (such as Parkinson disease) and some heart conditions.

Other risk factors for hypotension include being immobile for long periods, being out in the heat for a long time, and pregnancy. Hypotension during pregnancy is normal and usually goes away after birth.

Signs, Symptoms, and Complications of Hypotension
Orthostatic Hypotension and Neurally Mediated Hypotension

The signs and symptoms of orthostatic hypotension and neurally mediated hypotension are similar. They include:

- Dizziness or light-headedness

- Blurry vision

- Confusion

- Weakness

- Fatigue (feeling tired)

- Nausea (feeling sick to your stomach)

Orthostatic hypotension may happen within a few seconds or minutes of standing up after you have been sitting or lying down.

You may feel that you are going to faint, or you may actually faint. These signs and symptoms go away if you sit or lie down for a few minutes until your blood pressure adjusts to normal.

The signs and symptoms of NMH occur after standing for a long time or in response to an unpleasant, upsetting, or scary situation. The drop in blood pressure with NMH does not last long and often goes away after sitting down.

Severe Hypotension Linked to Shock

In shock, not enough blood and oxygen flow to the body's major organs, including the brain. The early signs and symptoms of reduced blood flow to the brain include light-headedness, sleepiness, and confusion.

In the earliest stages of shock, it may be hard to detect any signs or symptoms. In older people, the first symptom may only be confusion.

Over time, as shock worsens, a person will not be able to sit up without passing out. If the shock continues, the person will lose consciousness. Shock often is fatal if not treated right away.

Other signs and symptoms of shock vary, depending on what is causing the shock. When low blood volume (from major blood loss, for example) or poor pumping action in the heart (from heart failure, for example) causes shock:

- The skin becomes cold and sweaty. It often looks blue or pale. If pressed, the color returns to normal more slowly than usual. A bluish network of lines appears under the skin.

- The pulse becomes weak and rapid.

- The person begins to breathe very quickly.

When extreme relaxation of blood vessels causes shock (such as in vasodilatory shock), a person feels warm and flushed at first.

Later, the skin becomes cold and sweaty, and the person feels very sleepy.

Shock is an emergency and must be treated right away. If a person has signs or symptoms of shock, call 911.

Living with Hypotension

Doctors can successfully treat hypotension. Many people who had the condition and were successfully treated live normal, healthy lives.

If you have hypotension, you can take steps to prevent or limit symptoms, such as dizzy spells and fainting.

If you have orthostatic hypotension, get up slowly after sitting or lying down, or move your legs before changing your position. Eat small, low-carbohydrate meals if you have postprandial hypotension (a form of orthostatic hypotension).

If you have neurally mediated hypotension, try not to stand for long periods. If you do have to stand for a long time, move around and wear compression stockings. These stockings apply pressure to your lower legs. The pressure helps move blood throughout your body.

Drink plenty of fluids, such as water or sports drinks that contain nutrients, such as sodium and potassium. Also, try to avoid unpleasant, upsetting, or scary situations. Learn to recognize symptoms and take action to raise your blood pressure. Children who have NMH often outgrow it.

Other lifestyle changes also can help you control hypotension.

Ask your doctor about learning how to measure your own blood pressure. This will help you find out what a normal blood pressure reading is for you. Keeping a record of blood pressure readings done by healthcare providers also can help you learn more about your blood pressure.

Severe hypotension linked to shock is an emergency. Shock can lead to death if it is not treated right away. If you see someone having signs or symptoms of shock, call 911.

Section 30.5

Shock

This section includes text excerpted from "Shock," MedlinePlus, National Institutes of Health (NIH), October 11, 2016.

Shock happens when not enough blood and oxygen can get to your organs and tissues. It causes very low blood pressure and may be life-threatening. It often happens along with a serious injury.

There are several kinds of shock. Hypovolemic shock happens when you lose a lot of blood or fluids, and its causes include internal or external bleeding, dehydration, burns, and severe vomiting and/or diarrhea. Septic shock is caused by infections in the bloodstream. A severe allergic reaction can cause anaphylactic shock. An insect bite or sting might cause it. Cardiogenic shock happens when the heart cannot pump blood effectively. This may happen after a heart attack. Neurogenic shock is caused by damage to the nervous system.

Symptoms of shock include:

- Confusion or lack of alertness

- Loss of consciousness

- Sudden and ongoing rapid heartbeat

- Sweating

- Pale skin

- A weak pulse

- Rapid breathing

- Decreased or no urine output

- Cool hands and feet

Shock is a life-threatening medical emergency, and it is important to get help right away. Treatment of shock depends on the cause.

Section 30.6

Syncope

> This section contains text excerpted from the following sources: Text
> under the heading "What Is Syncope?" is excerpted from "Syncope
> Information Page," National Institute of Neurological Disorders and
> Stroke (NINDS), March 27, 2019; Text beginning with the heading
> "What Causes Syncope" is excerpted from "Fainting," MedlinePlus,
> National Institutes of Health (NIH), August 4, 2016.

What Is Syncope?

"Syncope" is a medical term used to describe a temporary loss of consciousness due to the sudden decline of blood flow to the brain. Syncope is commonly called "fainting" or "passing out." If an individual is about to faint, she or he will feel dizzy, light-headed, or nauseous and their field of vision may "white out" or "black out." The skin may be cold and clammy. The person drops to the floor as she or he loses consciousness. After fainting, an individual may be unconscious for a minute or two, but will revive and slowly return to normal. Syncope can occur in otherwise healthy people, and it affects all age groups but occurs more often in the elderly.

There are several types of syncope. Vasovagal syncope usually has an easily identified triggering event, such as emotional stress, trauma, pain, the sight of blood, or prolonged standing. Carotid sinus syncope (CSS) happens because of constriction of the carotid artery in the neck and can occur after turning the head, while shaving, or when wearing a tight collar. Situational syncope happens during urination, defecation, coughing, or as a result of gastrointestinal (GI) stimulation. Syncope can also be a symptom of heart disease or abnormalities that create an uneven heart rate or rhythm that temporarily affects blood volume and its distribution in the body. Syncope is not normally a primary sign of a neurological disorder, but it may indicate an increased risk for neurologic disorders, such as Parkinson disease (PD), postural orthostatic tachycardia syndrome (POTS), diabetic neuropathy, and other types of neuropathy. Certain classes of drugs are associated with an increased risk of syncope, including diuretics, calcium antagonists, Angiotensin-converting enzyme (ACE) inhibitors, nitrates, antipsychotics, antihistamines, levodopa, narcotics, and alcohol.

What Causes Syncope

Fainting usually happens when your blood pressure drops suddenly, causing a decrease in blood flow to your brain. It is more common in older people. Some causes of fainting include:

- Heat or dehydration
- Emotional distress
- Standing up too quickly
- Certain medicines
- Drop in blood sugar
- Heart problems

What You Should Do When Someone Faints

When someone faints, make sure that the airway is clear and check for breathing. The person should stay lying down for 10 to 15 minutes. Most people recover completely. Fainting is usually nothing to worry about, but it can sometimes be a sign of a serious problem. If you faint, it is important to see your healthcare provider and find out why it happened.

Chapter 31

Carotid Artery Disease

What Is Carotid Artery Disease?

Carotid artery disease is a disease in which a waxy substance called "plaque" builds up inside the carotid arteries. You have two common carotid arteries, one on each side of your neck. They each divide into internal and external carotid arteries.

The internal carotid arteries supply oxygen-rich blood to your brain. The external carotid arteries supply oxygen-rich blood to your face, scalp, and neck.

Carotid artery disease is serious because it can cause a stroke, also called a "brain attack." A stroke occurs if blood flow to your brain is cut off.

If blood flow is cut off for more than a few minutes, the cells in your brain start to die. This impairs the parts of the body that the brain cells control. A stroke can cause lasting brain damage; long-term disability, such as vision or speech problems or paralysis (an inability to move); or death.

Causes of Carotid Artery Disease

Carotid artery disease seems to start when damage occurs to the inner layers of the carotid arteries. Major factors that contribute to damage include:

This chapter includes text excerpted from "Carotid Artery Disease," National Heart, Lung, and Blood Institute (NHLBI), December 26, 2011. Reviewed June 2019.

- Smoking

- High levels of certain fats and cholesterol in the blood

- High blood pressure

- High levels of sugar in the blood due to insulin resistance or diabetes

When damage occurs, your body starts a healing process. The healing may cause plaque to build up where the arteries are damaged.

The plaque in an artery can crack or rupture. If this happens, blood cell fragments called "platelets" will stick to the site of the injury and may clump together to form blood clots.

The buildup of plaque or blood clots can severely narrow or block the carotid arteries. This limits the flow of oxygen-rich blood to your brain, which can cause a stroke.

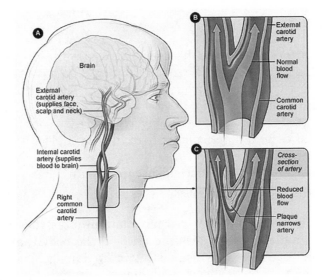

Figure 31.1. *Carotid Arteries*

Figure A shows the location of the right carotid artery in the head and neck. Figure B shows the inside of a normal carotid artery that has normal blood flow. Figure C shows the inside of a carotid artery that has plaque buildup and reduced blood flow.

Risk Factors of Carotid Artery Disease

The major risk factors for carotid artery disease, listed below, also are the major risk factors for coronary heart disease (also called "coronary artery disease") and peripheral artery disease.

- **Diabetes.** With this disease, the body's blood sugar level is too high because the body does not make enough insulin or does not use its insulin properly. People who have diabetes are four times more likely to have carotid artery disease than are people who do not have diabetes.

- **Family history of atherosclerosis.** People who have a family history of atherosclerosis are more likely to develop carotid artery disease.

- **High blood pressure (hypertension).** Blood pressure is considered high if it stays at or above 140/90 mmHg over time. If you have diabetes or chronic kidney disease, high blood pressure is defined as 130/80 mmHg or higher. (The mmHg is millimeters of mercury—the units used to measure blood pressure.)

- **Lack of physical activity.** Too much sitting (sedentary lifestyle) and a lack of aerobic activity can worsen other risk factors for carotid artery disease, such as unhealthy blood cholesterol levels, high blood pressure, diabetes, and being overweight or obese.

- **Metabolic syndrome.** Metabolic syndrome is the name for a group of risk factors that raise your risk for stroke and other health problems, such as diabetes and heart disease. The five metabolic risk factors are a large waistline (abdominal obesity), a high triglyceride level (a type of fat found in the blood), a low high-density (HDL) cholesterol level, high blood pressure, and high blood sugar. Metabolic syndrome is diagnosed if you have at least three of these metabolic risk factors.

- **Older age.** As you age, your risk for atherosclerosis increases. The process of atherosclerosis begins in youth and typically progresses over many decades before diseases develop.

- **Being overweight or obese.** The terms "overweight" and "obesity" refer to body weight that is greater than what is considered healthy for a certain height.

- **Smoking.** Smoking can damage and tighten blood vessels, lead to unhealthy cholesterol levels, and raise blood pressure. Smoking also can limit how much oxygen reaches the body's tissues.

- **Unhealthy blood cholesterol levels.** This includes high low-density lipoprotein (LDL) ("bad") cholesterol) and low HDL ("good") cholesterol.

- **Unhealthy diet.** An unhealthy diet can raise your risk for carotid artery disease. Foods that are high in saturated and trans fats, cholesterol, sodium, and sugar can worsen other risk factors for carotid artery disease.

Having any of these risk factors does not guarantee that you will develop carotid artery disease. However, if you know that you have one or more risk factors, you can take steps to help prevent or delay the disease.

If you have plaque buildup in your carotid arteries, you also may have plaque buildup in other arteries. People who have carotid artery disease also are at an increased risk for coronary heart disease.

Screening and Prevention of Carotid Artery Disease

Taking action to control your risk factors can help prevent or delay carotid artery disease and stroke. Your risk for carotid artery disease increases with the number of risk factors you have.

One step you can take is to make heart-healthy lifestyle changes, which can include:

- **Heart-healthy eating.** Following heart-healthy eating is an important part of a healthy lifestyle. Dietary Approaches to Stop Hypertension (DASH) is a program that promotes heart-healthy eating.

- **Aiming for a healthy weight.** If you are overweight or obese, work with your doctor to create a reasonable plan for weight loss. Controlling your weight helps you control risk factors for carotid artery disease.

- **Physical activity.** Be as physically active as you can. Physical activity can improve your fitness level and your health. Ask your doctor what types and amounts of activity are safe for you.

- **Quit smoking.** If you smoke, quit. Talk with your doctor about programs and products that can help you quit.

Other steps that can prevent or delay carotid artery disease include knowing your family history of carotid artery disease. If you or someone in your family has carotid artery disease, be sure to tell your doctor.

If lifestyle changes are not enough, your doctor may prescribe medicines to control your carotid artery disease risk factors. Take all of your medicines as your doctor advises.

Signs, Symptoms, and Complications of Carotid Artery Disease

Carotid artery disease may not cause signs or symptoms until it severely narrows or blocks a carotid artery. Signs and symptoms may include a bruit, a transient ischemic attack (TIA), or a stroke.

Bruit

During a physical exam, your doctor may listen to your carotid arteries with a stethoscope. She or he may hear a whooshing sound called a "bruit." This sound may suggest changed or reduced blood flow due to plaque buildup. To find out more, your doctor may recommend tests.

Not all people who have carotid artery disease have bruits.

Transient Ischemic Attack

For some people, having a transient ischemic attack, or "mini-stroke," is the first sign of carotid artery disease. During a mini-stroke, you may have some or all of the symptoms of a stroke. However, the symptoms usually go away on their own within 24 hours.

Stroke and mini-stroke symptoms may include:

- A sudden, severe headache with no known cause

- Dizziness or loss of balance

- Inability to move one or more of your limbs

- Sudden trouble seeing in one or both eyes

- Sudden weakness or numbness in the face or limbs, often on just one side of the body

- Trouble speaking or understanding speech

Even if the symptoms stop quickly, call 911 for emergency help. Do not drive yourself to the hospital. It is important to get checked and to get treatment started as soon as possible.

A mini-stroke is a warning sign that you are at high risk of having a stroke. You should not ignore these symptoms. Getting medical care can help find possible causes of a mini-stroke and help you manage risk factors. These actions might prevent a future stroke.

Although a mini-stroke may warn of a stroke, it does not predict when a stroke will happen. A stroke may occur days, weeks, or even months after a mini-stroke.

Stroke

The symptoms of a stroke are the same as those of a mini-stroke, but the results are not. A stroke can cause lasting brain damage; long-term disability, such as vision or speech problems or paralysis (an inability to move); or death. Most people who have strokes have not previously had warning mini-strokes.

Getting treatment for a stroke right away is very important. You have the best chance for full recovery if treatment to open a blocked artery is given within 4 hours of symptom onset. The sooner treatment occurs, the better your chances of recovery.

Call 911 for emergency help as soon as symptoms occur. Do not drive yourself to the hospital. It is very important to get checked and to get treatment started as soon as possible.

Make those close to you aware of stroke symptoms and the need for urgent action. Learning the signs and symptoms of a stroke will allow you to help yourself or someone close to you lower the risk of brain damage or death due to a stroke.

Diagnosis of Carotid Artery Disease

Your doctor will diagnose carotid artery disease based on your medical history, a physical exam, and test results.

Medical History

Your doctor will find out whether you have any of the major risk factors for carotid artery disease. She or he also will ask whether you have had any signs or symptoms of a mini-stroke or stroke.

Physical Exam

To check your carotid arteries, your doctor will listen to them with a stethoscope. She or he will listen for a bruit. This sound may indicate changed or reduced blood flow due to plaque buildup. To find out more, your doctor may recommend tests.

Diagnostic Tests

The following tests are common for diagnosing carotid artery disease. If you have symptoms of a mini-stroke or stroke, your doctor may use other tests as well.

Carotid Ultrasound

Carotid ultrasound (also called "sonography") is the most common test for diagnosing carotid artery disease. It is a painless, harmless test that uses sound waves to create pictures of the insides of your carotid arteries. This test can show whether plaque has narrowed your carotid arteries and how narrow they are.

A standard carotid ultrasound shows the structure of your carotid arteries. A Doppler carotid ultrasound shows how blood moves through your carotid arteries.

Carotid Angiography

Carotid angiography is a special type of X-ray. This test may be used if the ultrasound results are unclear or do not give your doctor enough information.

For this test, your doctor will inject a substance (called "contrast dye") into a vein, most often in your leg. The dye travels to your carotid arteries and highlights them on X-ray pictures.

Magnetic Resonance Angiography

Magnetic resonance angiography (MRA) uses a large magnet and radio waves to take pictures of your carotid arteries. Your doctor can see these pictures on a computer screen.

For this test, your doctor may give you contrast dye to highlight your carotid arteries on the pictures.

Computed Tomography Angiography

Computed tomography angiography, or CT angiography, takes X-ray pictures of the body from many angles. A computer combines the pictures into two- and three-dimensional images.

For this test, your doctor may give you contrast dye to highlight your carotid arteries on the pictures.

Treatment of Carotid Artery Disease

Treatments for carotid artery disease may include heart-healthy lifestyle changes, medicines, and medical procedures. The goals of treatment are to stop the disease from getting worse and to prevent a stroke. Your treatment will depend on your symptoms, how severe the disease is, and your age and overall health.

Heart-Healthy Lifestyle Changes

Your doctor may recommend heart-healthy lifestyle changes if you have carotid artery disease. Heart-healthy lifestyle changes include:

- Heart-healthy eating
- Aiming for a healthy weight
- Managing stress
- Physical activity
- Quitting smoking

Medicines

If you have a stroke caused by a blood clot, you may be given a clot-dissolving, or clot-busting, medication. This type of medication must be given within four hours of symptom onset. The sooner treatment occurs, the better your chances of recovery. If you think you are having a stroke, call 911 right away for emergency care.

Medicines to prevent blood clots are the mainstay treatment for people who have carotid artery disease. They prevent platelets from clumping together and forming blood clots in your carotid arteries, which can lead to a stroke. Two common medications are:

- Aspirin
- Clopidogrel

Sometimes, lifestyle changes alone are not enough to control your cholesterol levels. For example, you also may need statin medications to control or lower your cholesterol. By lowering your blood cholesterol level, you can decrease your chance of having a heart attack or stroke. Doctors usually prescribe statins for people who have:

- Diabetes
- Heart disease or have had a stroke
- High LDL cholesterol levels

Doctors may discuss beginning statin treatment with those who have an elevated risk for developing heart disease or having a stroke.

You may need other medications to treat diseases and conditions that damage the carotid arteries. Your doctor also may prescribe medications to:

- Lower your blood pressure
- Lower your blood sugar level

- Prevent blood clots from forming, which can lead to stroke

- Prevent or reduce inflammation

Take all medicines regularly, as your doctor prescribes. Do not change the amount of your medicine or skip a dose unless your doctor tells you to. Your healthcare team will help find a treatment plan that is right for you.

Medical Procedures

You may need a medical procedure if you have symptoms caused by the narrowing of the carotid artery. Doctors use one of two methods to open narrowed or blocked carotid arteries: carotid endarterectomy and carotid artery angioplasty and stenting.

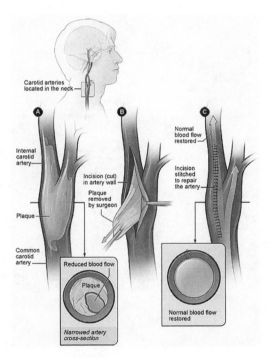

Figure 31.2. *Carotid Endarterectomy*

The illustration shows the process of carotid endarterectomy. Figure A shows a carotid artery with plaque buildup. The inset image shows a cross-section of the narrowed carotid artery. Figure B shows how the carotid artery is cut and how the plaque is removed. Figure C shows the artery stitched up and normal blood flow restored. The inset image shows a cross-section of the artery with plaque removed and normal blood flow restored.

Carotid Endarterectomy

Carotid endarterectomy is mainly for people whose carotid arteries are blocked 50 percent or more.

For the procedure, a surgeon will make a cut in your neck to reach the narrowed or blocked carotid artery. Next, she or he will make a cut in the blocked part of the artery and remove the artery's inner lining that is blocking the blood flow.

Finally, your surgeon will close the artery with stitches and stop any bleeding. She or he will then close the cut in your neck.

Carotid Artery Angioplasty and Stenting

Doctors use a procedure called "angioplasty" to widen the carotid arteries and restore blood flow to the brain.

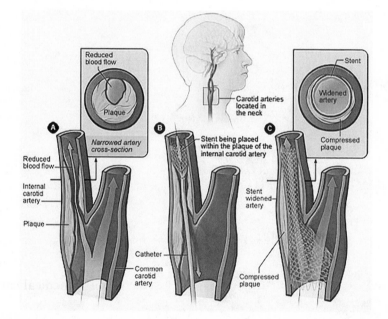

Figure 31.3. *Carotid Artery Stenting*

The illustration shows the process of carotid artery stenting. Figure A shows an internal carotid artery that has plaque buildup and reduced blood flow. The inset image shows a cross-section of the narrowed carotid artery. Figure B shows a stent being placed in the carotid artery to support the inner artery wall and keep the artery open. Figure C shows normal blood flow restored in the stent-widened artery. The inset image shows a cross-section of the stent-widened artery.

A thin tube with a deflated balloon on the end is threaded through a blood vessel in your neck to the narrowed or blocked carotid artery. Once in place, the balloon is inflated to push the plaque outward against the wall of the artery.

A stent (a small mesh tube) is then put in the artery to support the inner artery wall. The stent also helps prevent the artery from becoming narrowed or blocked again.

Living with Carotid Artery Disease

If you have carotid artery disease, you can take steps to manage the condition, reduce risk factors, and prevent complications. These steps include making heart-healthy lifestyle changes, following your treatment plan, and getting ongoing care.

Having carotid artery disease raises your risk of having a stroke. Know the warning signs of a stroke—such as weakness and trouble speaking—and what to do if they occur. Call 911 as soon as symptoms start (do not drive yourself to the hospital).

Treatment Plan

Following your treatment plan may help prevent your carotid artery disease from getting worse. It also can lower your risk for stroke and other health problems.

You may need to take medicines to control certain risk factors and to prevent blood clots that could cause a stroke. Taking prescribed medicines and following a healthy lifestyle can help control carotid artery disease. However, they do not cure the disease. You will likely have to stick with your treatment plan for life.

Ongoing Care

If you have carotid artery disease, having ongoing medical care is important.

Most people who have the disease will need to have their blood pressure checked regularly and their blood sugar and blood cholesterol levels tested one or more times a year. If you have diabetes, you will need routine blood sugar tests and other tests.

Testing shows whether these conditions are under control or whether your doctor needs to adjust your treatment for better results.

If you have had a stroke or procedures to restore blood flow in your carotid arteries, you will likely need a yearly carotid Doppler ultrasound test. This test shows how well blood flows through your carotid arteries.

Repeating this test over time will show whether the narrowing in your carotid arteries is getting worse. Results also can show how well procedures to treat your arteries have worked.

Follow up with your doctor regularly. The sooner your doctor spots problems, the sooner she or he can prescribe treatment.

Stroke Warning Signs

The signs and symptoms of stroke may include:

- Sudden weakness or numbness in the face or limbs, often on only one side of the body

- The inability to move one or more of your limbs

- Trouble speaking or understanding speech

- Sudden trouble seeing in one or both eyes

- Dizziness or loss of balance

- A sudden, severe headache with no known cause

Call 911 for help as soon as symptoms start. Do not drive yourself to the hospital. It is very important to get checked and treated as soon as possible.

If you are a candidate for clot-busting therapy, you have the best chance for a full recovery if treatment to open a blocked artery is given within four hours of symptom onset. The sooner treatment occurs, the better your chances of recovery.

Make those close to you aware of stroke symptoms and the need for urgent action. Learning the signs and symptoms of a stroke will allow you to help yourself or someone close to you lower the risk of damage or death due to a stroke.

Chapter 32

Coronary Artery and Heart Disease

Chapter Contents

Section 32.1

Coronary Artery Disease

This section contains text excerpted from the following sources: Text under the heading "What Is Coronary Artery Disease?" is excerpted from "Coronary Artery Disease," MedlinePlus, National Institutes of Health (NIH), November 1, 2016; Text beginning with the heading "Causes of Coronary Artery Disease" is excerpted from "Coronary Artery Disease (CAD)," Centers for Disease Control and Prevention (CDC), August 10, 2015. Reviewed June 2019.

What Is Coronary Artery Disease?

Coronary artery disease (CAD) is the most common type of heart disease. It is the leading cause of death in the United States in both men and women.

Coronary artery disease happens when the arteries that supply blood to heart muscle become hardened and narrowed. This is due to the buildup of cholesterol and other material, called "plaque," on their inner walls. This buildup is called "atherosclerosis." As it grows, less blood can flow through the arteries. As a result, the heart muscle cannot get the blood or oxygen it needs. This can lead to chest pain (angina) or a heart attack. Most heart attacks happen when a blood clot suddenly cuts off the hearts' blood supply, causing permanent heart damage.

Over time, CAD can also weaken the heart muscle and contribute to heart failure and arrhythmias. Heart failure means that the heart cannot pump blood well to the rest of the body. Arrhythmias are changes in the normal beating rhythm of the heart.

Causes of Coronary Artery Disease

Coronary artery disease is caused by plaque buildup in the walls of the arteries that supply blood to the heart (called "coronary arteries") and other parts of the body. Plaque is made up of deposits of cholesterol and other substances in the artery. Plaque buildup causes the inside of the arteries to narrow over time, which could partially or totally block the blood flow. This process is called "atherosclerosis."

Too much plaque buildup and narrowed artery walls can make it harder for blood to flow through your body. When your heart muscle does not get enough blood, you may have chest pain or discomfort, called "angina." Angina is the most common symptom of CAD.

Over time, coronary artery disease can weaken the heart muscle. This may lead to heart failure, a serious condition where the heart cannot pump blood the way that it should. An irregular heartbeat, or arrhythmia, also can develop.

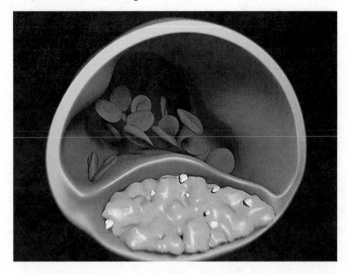

Figure 32.1. *Coronary Artery Disease Caused by Plaque*

Coronary artery disease is caused by plaque buildup in the wall of the arteries that supply blood to the heart (called coronary arteries). Plaque is made up of cholesterol deposits. Plaque buildup causes the inside of the arteries to narrow over time. This process is called atherosclerosis.

Reducing Your Risk for Coronary Artery Disease

If you have CAD, your healthcare team may suggest the following steps to help lower your risk for heart attack or worsening heart disease:

- Lifestyle changes, such as eating a healthier (lower sodium, lower fat) diet, increasing physical activity, and quitting smoking

- Medications to treat the risk factors for CAD, such as high cholesterol, high blood pressure, an irregular heartbeat, and low blood flow

- Surgical procedures to help restore blood flow to the heart

Section 32.2

Angina

This section includes text excerpted from "Angina," National Heart, Lung, and Blood Institute (NHLBI), December 10, 2018.

What Is Angina?

Angina is chest pain or discomfort that occurs if an area of your heart muscle does not get enough oxygen-rich blood. It is a common symptom of ischemic heart disease, which limits or cuts off blood flow to the heart.

There are several types of angina, and the signs and symptoms depend on which type you have. Angina chest pain, called an "angina event," can happen when your heart is working hard. It can go away when you stop to rest again, or it can happen at rest. This pain can feel like pressure or squeezing in your chest. It also can spread to your shoulders, arms, neck, jaw, or back, similar to a heart attack. Angina pain can even feel like an upset stomach. Symptoms can be different for women and men.

Angina can be a warning sign that you are at an increased risk for a heart attack. If you have chest pain that does not go away, call 911 immediately.

To diagnose angina, your doctor will ask you about your signs and symptoms and may run blood tests; take an X-ray; or order tests, such as an electrocardiogram (EKG), an exercise stress test, or cardiac catheterization, to determine how well your heart is working. With some types of angina, you may need emergency medical treatment to try to prevent a heart attack. To control your condition, your doctor may recommend heart-healthy lifestyle changes, medicines, medical procedures, and cardiac rehabilitation.

Causes of Angina

Angina happens when your heart muscle does not get enough oxygen-rich blood. Medical conditions, particularly ischemic heart disease, or lifestyle habits can cause angina. To understand the causes of angina, it helps to understand how the heart works.

Ischemic Heart Disease

Two types of ischemic heart disease can cause angina.

- Coronary artery disease happens when plaque builds up inside the large arteries that supply blood to the heart. This is called "atherosclerosis." Plaque narrows or blocks the arteries, reducing blood flow to the heart muscle. Sometimes, plaque breaks open and causes blood clots to form. Blood clots can partially or totally block the coronary arteries.

- Coronary microvascular disease affects the tiny arteries that branch off the larger coronary arteries. Reduced blood flow in these arteries causes microvascular angina. The arteries may be damaged and unable to expand as usual when the heart needs more oxygen-rich blood.

Spasm of the Coronary Arteries

A spasm that tightens your coronary arteries can cause angina. Spasms can occur whether or not you have ischemic heart disease and can affect large or small coronary arteries. Damage to your heart's arteries may cause them to narrow instead of widen when the heart needs more oxygen-rich blood.

In one day, your heart beats about 100,000 times and pumps about 2,400 gallons of blood throughout your body. To meet this demand, your heart's cells need a great deal of oxygen, which is supplied by the large coronary arteries and the tiny arteries that branch off the large arteries. When your heart is working hard, such as during physical activity or emotional stress, its demand for oxygen increases. Angina occurs when there is an imbalance between the heart's need for oxygen-rich blood and the ability of the arteries to deliver blood to all areas of the heart.

Risk Factors of Angina

You may have an increased risk for angina because of your age, environment or occupation, family history and genetics, lifestyle, other medical conditions, race, or sex.

Age

Genetic or lifestyle factors can cause plaque to build up in your arteries as you age. This means that your risk for ischemic heart disease and angina increases as you get older.

Variant angina is rare, but people who have variant angina often are younger than those who have other types of angina.

Environment or Occupation

Angina may be linked to a type of air pollution called "particle pollution." Particle pollution can include dust from roads, farms, dry riverbeds, construction sites, and mines.

Your work life can increase your risk of angina. Examples include work that limits your time available for sleep; involves high stress; requires long periods of sitting or standing; is noisy; or exposes you to potential hazards, such as radiation.

Family History and Genetics

Ischemic heart disease often runs in families. Also, people who have no lifestyle-related risk factors can develop ischemic heart disease. These factors suggest that genes are involved in ischemic heart disease and can influence a person's risk of developing angina.

Variant angina has also been linked to specific DNA changes.

Lifestyle Habits

The more heart disease risk factors you have, the greater your risk of developing angina. The main lifestyle risk factors for angina include:

- Alcohol use, for variant angina

- Illegal drug use

- Lack of physical activity

- Smoking tobacco or long-term exposure to secondhand smoke

- Stress

- Unhealthy eating patterns

Other Medical Conditions

Medical conditions in which your heart needs more oxygen-rich blood than your body can supply increase your risk for angina. They include:

- Anemia

- A racing heart rate or blood vessel damage due to cocaine or methamphetamine use

- Cardiomyopathy, or disease of the heart muscle

- Damage to the heart caused by injury
- Heart failure
- Heart valve disease
- High blood pressure
- Inflammation
- Insulin resistance or diabetes
- Low blood pressure
- Metabolic syndrome
- Overweight or obesity
- Unhealthy cholesterol levels

Medical Procedures

Heart procedures, such as stent placement, percutaneous coronary intervention (PCI), or coronary artery bypass grafting (CABG), can trigger coronary spasms and angina. Although rare, noncardiac surgery can also trigger unstable angina or variant angina.

Race or Ethnicity

Some groups of people are at a higher risk for developing ischemic heart disease and one of its main symptoms, angina. African Americans who have already had a heart attack are more likely than Whites to develop angina.

Variant angina is more common among people living in Japan, especially men, than among people living in Western countries.

Sex

Angina affects both men and women, but at different ages, based on men and women's risk of developing ischemic heart disease. In men, ischemic heart disease risk starts to increase at 45 years of age. Before the age of 55, women have a lower risk for heart disease than men. After the age of 55, the risk rises in both women and men. Women who have already had a heart attack are more likely to develop angina when compared with men.

Microvascular angina most often begins in women around the time of menopause.

Screening and Prevention of Angina

Typically, doctors screen for angina only when you have symptoms. However, your doctor may assess your risk factors for ischemic heart disease every few years as part of your regular office visits. If you have 2 or more risk factors, then your doctor may estimate the chance that you will develop ischemic heart disease, which may include angina, over the next 10 years.

Prevention Strategies

To prevent angina, your doctor may recommend that you adopt heart-healthy lifestyle changes to lower your risk of ischemic heart disease. Heart-healthy lifestyle changes include choosing a heart-healthy eating pattern, such as the Dietary Approaches to Stop Hypertension (DASH) eating plan; being physically active; aiming for a healthy weight; quitting smoking; and managing stress. You should also avoid using illegal drugs.

Signs, Symptoms, and Complications of Angina

Signs and symptoms vary based on the type of angina you have and on whether you are a man or a woman. Angina symptoms can differ in severity, location in the body, timing, and how much relief you may feel with rest or medicines. Since symptoms of angina and of heart attack can be the same, call 911 if you feel chest discomfort that does not go away with rest or medicine. Angina can also lead to a heart attack and other complications that can be life-threatening.

Signs and Symptoms

Pain and discomfort are the main symptoms of angina. Angina is often described as pressure, squeezing, burning, indigestion, or tightness in the chest. The pain or discomfort usually starts behind the breastbone. Some people say that angina pain is hard to describe or that they cannot tell exactly where the pain is coming from.

Other symptoms include:

- Fatigue

- Light-headedness or fainting

- Nausea, or feeling sick in the stomach

- Shortness of breath

- Sweating

- Weakness

Symptoms of angina can be different for women and men. Instead of chest pain, or in addition to it, women may feel pain in the neck, jaw, throat, abdomen, or back. Sometimes, this pain is not recognized as a symptom of a heart condition. As a result, treatment for women can be delayed.

Because angina has so many possible symptoms and causes, all chest pain should be checked by a doctor.

Each type of angina has certain typical symptoms. Learn more about the symptoms that are characteristic of each type.

Stable Angina

- Discomfort that feels similar to gas or indigestion

- Pain during physical exertion or mental stress

- Pain that spreads from your breastbone to your arms or back

- Pain that is relieved by medicines

- Pattern of symptoms that has not changed in the last two months

- Symptoms that go away within five minutes

Unstable Angina

- Changes in your stable angina symptoms

- Pain that grows worse

- Pain that is not relieved by rest or medicines

- Pain that lasts longer than 20 minutes or goes away and then comes back

- Pain while you are resting or sleeping

- Severe pain

- Shortness of breath

Microvascular Angina

- Pain after physical or emotional stress

- Pain that is not immediately relieved by medicines
- Pain that lasts a long time
- Pain that you feel while doing regular daily activities
- Severe pain
- Shortness of breath

Variant Angina

- Cold sweats
- Fainting
- Numbness or weakness of the left shoulder and upper arm
- Pain that is relieved by medicines
- Pain that occurs during rest or while sleeping
- Pain that starts in the early morning hours
- Severe pain
- Vague pain with a feeling of pressure in the lower chest, perhaps spreading to the neck, jaw, or left shoulder

Complications

Angina is not a heart attack, but it suggests that a heart attack or other life-threatening complications are more likely to happen in the future.

The following are other possible complications of angina:

- Arrhythmia
- Cardiomyopathy
- Sudden cardiac arrest

Living with Angina

Angina is not a heart attack, but it is a signal that you are at greater risk of having a heart attack. The risk is higher if you have unstable angina. For this reason, it is important that you receive follow-up care, monitor your condition, and understand your condition so that you know when to get medical help. Your doctor may recommend heart-healthy lifestyle changes and cardiac rehabilitation to help manage angina.

Receive Routine Follow-Up Care

You may need follow-up visits every 4 to 6 months for the first year after diagnosis of angina and every 6 to 12 months as long as your condition is stable. Your care plan may be changed if your angina worsens or if stable angina becomes unstable. Unstable angina is a medical emergency.

- Your doctor may recommend cholesterol-lowering statins as part of your long-term treatment, especially if you have had a heart attack.

- Ask your doctor about when you can resume normal physical activity, such as climbing stairs.

- Ask your doctor whether sexual activity is safe for you. People who have unstable angina or angina that does not respond well to treatment should not engage in sexual activity until their heart condition and angina are stable and well managed.

- Talk to your medical team about vaccinations to prevent the flu and pneumonia.

Monitor Your Condition

To monitor your condition, your doctor may recommend the following tests or procedures:

- Blood pressure checks to ensure that your blood pressure is in a healthy range. Keeping your blood pressure under control can help your angina.

- EKGs to detect changes in heart health after treatment or for monitoring the heart during exercise as part of cardiac rehabilitation

- Repeat lipid panels to see if blood cholesterol levels are at healthy levels. A lipid panel should be done every year and also two to three months after any change in treatment.

- Stress testing to assess your risk for complications either before or after starting angina medicines. Stress tests can also make sure your heart is strong enough for physical and sexual activity.

Adopt Heart-Healthy Lifestyle Changes

Angina is a symptom of ischemic heart disease. Your doctor may recommend the following heart-healthy lifestyle changes to help you manage angina:

- **Heart-healthy eating.** Following a healthy eating plan, including limiting alcohol, can prevent or reduce high blood pressure and high blood cholesterol, helping you reduce angina symptoms and maintain a healthy weight. You should avoid large meals and rich foods if heavy meals trigger your angina. If you have variant angina, drinking alcohol can also be a trigger.

- **Aiming for a healthy weight.** If you are overweight or obese, work with your doctor to create a reasonable weight-loss plan. Controlling your weight helps you manage the risk factors for angina.

- **Being physically active.** Before starting any exercise program, ask your doctor about what level of physical activity is right for you. Slow down or take rest breaks if physical exertion triggers angina.

- **Managing stress.** If emotional stress triggers your angina, try to avoid situations that make you upset or stressed.

- **Quitting smoking.** Smoking can damage and tighten blood vessels, make angina worse, and raise the risk of life-threatening complications. For free help and support to quit smoking, you may call the National Cancer Institute's (NCI) Smoking Quitline at 877-44U-QUIT (877-448-7848).

Your doctor may recommend these heart-healthy lifestyle changes as part of a larger cardiac rehabilitation program that your doctors oversee.

Prevent Repeat Angina Events

Stable angina usually occurs in a pattern. After several events, you will learn what causes the pain to occur, what the pain feels like, and how long the pain usually lasts. To help learn your angina's pattern and triggers, keep a log of when you feel pain. The log helps your doctor regulate your medicines and evaluate your need for future treatments. When you know what triggers your angina, you can take steps to prevent or lessen the severity of events.

- Know the limits of your physical activity. Most people who have stable angina can continue their normal activities. This includes work, hobbies, and sexual relations. Learn how much exertion triggers your angina so you can try to stop and rest before the chest pain starts.

- Learn how to reduce and manage stress. Try to avoid or limit situations that cause anger, arguments, and worry. Exercise and relaxation can help relieve stress. Alcohol and drug use play a part in causing stress and do not relieve it. If stress is a problem for you, talk with your doctor about getting help.

- Avoid exposure to very hot or cold conditions because temperature extremes strain the heart.

- Eat smaller meals if large meals lead to chest pain.

Tell your doctor right away if your pattern changes. Pattern changes may include angina that occurs more often, lasts longer, is more severe, occurs without physical exertion, or does not go away with rest or medicines. These changes may be a sign that your symptoms are getting worse or becoming unstable.

Seek Help for Angina That Does Not Improve

Not all angina improves with medicines or medical procedures. If your symptoms continue, your doctor may change your medicines or therapies to help relieve your chest pain. Additional treatments for hard-to-treat angina include:

- **Enhanced external counterpulsation therapy (EECP)** to improve the flow of oxygen-rich blood to your heart muscle, which may help relieve angina. EECP uses large cuffs, similar to blood pressure cuffs, on your legs. The cuffs inflate and deflate in sync with your heartbeat. You typically get five one-hour treatments per week for seven weeks. Side effects may include back or neck pain and skin abrasions.

- **Spinal cord stimulators** to block the sensation of pain. Emerging research suggests that this technology can help people be more physically active, feel angina less often, and have a better quality of life.

- **Transmyocardial laser therapy** to stimulate growth of new blood vessels or improve blood flow in the heart muscle. It can relieve angina pain and increase your ability to exercise without discomfort. This laser-based treatment is done during open-heart surgery or through cardiac catheterization. Rarely, your doctor may recommend this treatment in combination with CABG.

Know Your Medicines

You should know what medicines you are taking, the purpose of each, how and when to take them, and possible side effects. Learn exactly when and how to take nitroglycerin or other short-acting nitrates to relieve chest pain. Then talk to your doctor about the following:

- Any other medicines you are taking, including vitamins and nutritional supplements. Some medicines can cause serious or life-threatening problems if they are taken with nitrates or other angina medicines. For example, men who take nitrates, including nitroglycerin, for their angina should not take medicines for erectile dysfunction without checking with their doctor first.

- Any side effects you may experience. Do not stop taking your medicines without talking to your doctor first.

- How to store your medicines correctly and when to replace them.

What is the safest and most effective way to use short-acting nitrates, such as nitroglycerin, to treat stable angina events? The following are some tips for taking short-acting nitrates.

- Use the short-acting nitrate immediately before any planned exercise or physical exertion.

- Watch for side effects, such as flushing, headache, or dizziness. Find a place to sit down or something to hold on to if you feel dizzy.

- After five minutes, if the pain has not gone away, take another dose.

- Call 911 if the pain continues after taking a second dose. This could be a symptom of unstable angina, which is a medical emergency.

Learn the Warning Signs of Serious Complications and Have a Plan

Sometimes, it is hard to tell the difference between unstable angina and a heart attack. Angina can be a sign of increased risk of stroke.

Angina can also trigger sudden cardiac arrest. These are medical emergencies.

If you think that you or someone else is having the following symptoms, call 911 immediately. Every minute matters.

Heart Attack

Signs of heart attack include mild or severe chest pain or discomfort in the center of the chest or upper abdomen that lasts for more than a few minutes, or goes away and comes back. It can feel like pressure, squeezing, fullness, heartburn, or indigestion. There may also be pain down the left arm. Women may also have chest pain and pain down the left arm, but they are more likely to have symptoms, such as shortness of breath, nausea, vomiting, unusual tiredness, and pain in the back, shoulders, or jaw.

Stroke

If you think someone may be having a stroke, act F.A.S.T. and do the following simple test.

F—Face: Ask the person to smile. Does one side of the face droop?

A—Arms: Ask the person to raise both arms. Does one arm drift downward?

S—Speech: Ask the person to repeat a simple phrase. Is her or his speech slurred or strange?

T—Time: If you observe any of these signs, call 911 immediately. Early treatment is essential.

Sudden Cardiac Arrest

It is possible for a spasm causing angina to trigger arrhythmia. This can lead to sudden cardiac arrest. Fainting is usually the first sign of sudden cardiac arrest. If you think someone may be in cardiac arrest, try the following steps.

- If you see a person faint or if you find a person already unconscious, first confirm that the person cannot respond. The person may not move, or her or his movements may be seizure-like.

- You can shout at or gently shake the person to make sure she or he is not sleeping, but never shake an infant or young child.

Instead, you can gently pinch the child to try to wake her or him up.

• Check the person's breathing and pulse. If the person is not breathing and has no pulse or has an irregular heartbeat, prepare to use an automated external defibrillator (AED) as soon as possible.

Section 32.3

Heart Attack

This section includes text excerpted from "Heart Attack," National Heart, Lung, and Blood Institute (NHLBI), June 12, 2017.

What Is Heart Attack?

A heart attack happens when the flow of oxygen-rich blood to a section of heart muscle suddenly becomes blocked, and the heart cannot get oxygen. If blood flow is not restored quickly, the section of heart muscle begins to die.

Heart attack treatment works best when it is given right after symptoms occur. If you think you or someone else is having a heart attack, even if you are not sure, call 911 right away.

Causes of Heart Attack
Coronary Heart Disease

A heart attack happens if the flow of oxygen-rich blood to a section of heart muscle suddenly becomes blocked and the heart cannot get oxygen. Most heart attacks occur as a result of ischemic heart disease.

Ischemic heart disease is a condition in which a waxy substance called "plaque" builds up inside of the coronary arteries. These arteries supply oxygen-rich blood to your heart.

When plaque builds up in the arteries, the condition is called "atherosclerosis." The buildup of plaque occurs over many years.

Eventually, an area of plaque can rupture (break open) inside of an artery. This causes a blood clot to form on the plaque's surface. If the clot becomes large enough, it can mostly or completely block blood flow through a coronary artery.

If the blockage is not treated quickly, the portion of heart muscle fed by the artery begins to die. Healthy heart tissue is replaced with scar tissue. This heart damage may not be obvious, or it may cause severe or long-lasting problems.

Coronary Artery Spasm

A less common cause of heart attack is a severe spasm (tightening) of a coronary artery. The spasm cuts off blood flow through the artery. Spasms can occur in coronary arteries that are not affected by atherosclerosis.

What causes a coronary artery to spasm is not always clear. A spasm may be related to:

- Taking certain drugs, such as cocaine

- Emotional stress or pain

- Exposure to extreme cold

- Cigarette smoking

Risk Factors of Heart Attack

Certain risk factors make it more likely that you will develop ischemic heart disease and have a heart attack. You can control many of these risk factors.

Risk Factors You Can Control

The major risk factors for a heart attack that you can control include:

- Smoking

- High blood pressure

- High blood cholesterol

- Being overweight or obese

- An unhealthy diet (for example, a diet high in saturated fat, trans fat, cholesterol, and sodium)

- Lack of routine physical activity

- High blood sugar due to insulin resistance or diabetes

Some of these risk factors—such as obesity, high blood pressure, and high blood sugar—tend to occur together. When they do, it is called "metabolic syndrome."

In general, a person who has metabolic syndrome is twice as likely to develop heart disease and five times as likely to develop diabetes as someone who does not have metabolic syndrome.

Risk Factors You Cannot Control

Risk factors that you cannot control include:

- Age. The risk of heart disease increases for men after the age of 45 and for women after the age of 55 (or after menopause).

- Family history of early heart disease. Your risk increases if your father or a brother was diagnosed with heart disease before 55 years of age, or if your mother or a sister was diagnosed with heart disease before 65 years of age.

- Preeclampsia. This condition can develop during pregnancy. The two main signs of preeclampsia are a rise in blood pressure and excess protein in the urine. Preeclampsia is linked to an increased lifetime risk of heart disease, including CHD, heart attack, heart failure, and high blood pressure.

Screening and Prevention of Heart Attack

Lowering your risk factors for ischemic heart disease can help you prevent a heart attack. Even if you already have heart disease, you still can take steps to lower your risk for a heart attack. These steps involve making heart-healthy lifestyle changes and getting ongoing medical care for related conditions that make a heart attack more likely. Talk to your doctor about whether you may benefit from aspirin primary prevention or from using aspirin to help prevent your first heart attack.

Heart-Healthy Lifestyle Changes

A heart-healthy lifestyle can help prevent a heart attack and includes heart-healthy eating, being physically active, quitting smoking, managing stress, and managing your weight.

Ongoing Care
Treat Related Conditions

Treating conditions that make a heart attack more likely also can help lower your risk for a heart attack. These conditions may include:

- **Diabetes (high blood sugar).** If you have diabetes, try to control your blood sugar level through diet and physical activity (as your doctor recommends). If needed, take medicine as prescribed.

- **High blood cholesterol.** Your doctor may prescribe a statin medicine to lower your cholesterol if diet and exercise are not enough.

- **High blood pressure.** Your doctor may prescribe medicine to keep your blood pressure under control.

- **Chronic kidney disease (CKD).** Your doctor may prescribe medicines to control your high blood pressure or high blood sugar levels.

- **Peripheral artery disease (PAD).** Your doctor may recommend surgery or procedures to unblock the affected arteries.

Have an Emergency Action Plan

Make sure that you have an emergency action plan in case you or someone in your family has a heart attack. This is very important if you are at high risk for, or have already had, a heart attack.

Write down a list of medicines you are taking, medicines you are allergic to, your healthcare provider's phone numbers (both during and after office hours), and contact information for a friend or relative. Keep the list in a handy place to share in a medical emergency.

Talk with your doctor about the signs and symptoms of a heart attack, when you should call 911, and steps you can take while waiting for medical help to arrive.

Signs, Symptoms, and Complications of Heart Attack

Not all heart attacks begin with the sudden, crushing chest pain that often is shown on TV or in the movies. In one study, for example, one-third of the patients who had heart attacks had no chest pain. These patients were more likely to be older, female, or diabetic.

The symptoms of a heart attack can vary from person to person. Some people can have few symptoms and are surprised to learn they have had a heart attack. If you have already had a heart attack, your symptoms may not be the same for another one. It is important for you to know the most common symptoms of a heart attack and also remember these facts:

- Heart attacks can start slowly and cause only mild pain or discomfort. Symptoms can be mild or more intense and sudden. Symptoms also may come and go over several hours.

- People who have high blood sugar (diabetes) may have no symptoms or very mild ones.

- The most common symptom, in both men and women, is chest pain or discomfort.

- Women are somewhat more likely to have shortness of breath, nausea and vomiting, unusual tiredness (sometimes for days), and pain in the back, shoulders, and jaw.

Some people do not have symptoms at all. Heart attacks that occur without any symptoms or with very mild symptoms are called silent heart attacks.

Most Common Symptoms

The most common warning symptoms of a heart attack for both men and women are:

- **Chest pain or discomfort.** Most heart attacks involve discomfort in the center or left side of the chest. The discomfort usually lasts for more than a few minutes or goes away and comes back. It can feel like pressure, squeezing, fullness, or pain. It also can feel like heartburn or indigestion. The feeling can be mild or severe.

- **Upper body discomfort.** You may feel pain or discomfort in one or both arms, the back, shoulders, neck, jaw, or upper part of the stomach (above the belly button).

- **Shortness of breath.** This may be your only symptom, or it may occur before or along with chest pain or discomfort. It can occur when you are resting or doing a little bit of physical activity.

The symptoms of angina can be similar to the symptoms of a heart attack. Angina is chest pain that occurs in people who have ischemic heart disease, usually when they are active. Angina pain usually lasts for only a few minutes and goes away with rest.

Chest pain or discomfort that does not go away or changes from its usual pattern (for example, occurs more often or while you are resting) can be a sign of a heart attack.

All chest pain should be checked by a doctor.

Other Common Signs and Symptoms of Heart Attack

Pay attention to these other possible symptoms of a heart attack:

- Breaking out in a cold sweat

- Feeling unusually tired for no reason, sometimes for days (especially if you are a woman)

- Nausea (feeling sick to the stomach) and vomiting

- Light-headedness or sudden dizziness

- Any sudden, new symptoms or a change in the pattern of symptoms you already have (for example, if your symptoms become stronger or last longer than usual)

Not everyone having a heart attack has typical symptoms. If you have already had a heart attack, your symptoms may not be the same for another one. However, some people may have a pattern of symptoms that recur.

The more signs and symptoms you have, the more likely it is that you are having a heart attack.

Quick Action Can Save Your Life: Call 911

The signs and symptoms of a heart attack can develop suddenly. However, they also can develop slowly—sometimes within hours, days, or weeks of a heart attack.

Any time you think you might be having heart attack symptoms or a heart attack, do not ignore it or feel embarrassed to call for help. Call 911 for emergency medical care, even if you are not sure whether you are having a heart attack. Here is why:

- Acting fast can save your life.

- An ambulance is the best and safest way to get to the hospital. Emergency medical services (EMS) personnel can check how you are doing and start life-saving medicines and other treatments right away. People who arrive by ambulance often receive faster treatment at the hospital.

• The 911 operator or EMS technician can give you advice. You might be told to crush or chew an aspirin if you are not allergic, unless there is a medical reason for you not to take one. Aspirin taken during a heart attack can limit the damage to your heart and save your life.

Every minute matters. Never delay calling 911 to take aspirin or do anything else you think might help.

Life after a Heart Attack

Many people survive heart attacks and live active, full lives. If you get help quickly, treatment can limit damage to your heart muscle. Less heart damage improves your chances for a better quality of life after a heart attack.

Medical Follow-Up

After a heart attack, you will need treatment for ischemic heart disease. This will help prevent another heart attack. Your doctor may recommend:

• Lifestyle changes, such as following a healthy diet, being physically active, maintaining a healthy weight, and quitting smoking

• Medicines to control chest pain or discomfort, high blood cholesterol, high blood pressure, and your heart's workload. Some of these medicines can help you prevent another heart attack.

• Anticlotting medicines, such as aspirin, that your doctor may prescribe to help you prevent another heart attack

• A cardiac rehabilitation program

If you find it hard to get your medicines or to complete your cardiac rehabilitation program, talk with your doctor. Do not stop the medicines or program because it can help you prevent another heart attack.

Returning to Normal Activities

After a heart attack, most people who do not have chest pain or discomfort or other problems can safely return to most of their normal activities within a few weeks. Most can begin walking right away.

Sexual activity also can begin within a few weeks for most patients. Talk with your doctor about a safe schedule for returning to your normal routine.

If allowed by state law, driving usually can begin within a week for most patients who do not have chest pain or discomfort or other disabling problems. Each state has rules about driving a motor vehicle following a serious illness. People who have complications should not drive until their symptoms have been stable for a few weeks.

Anxiety and Depression after a Heart Attack

After a heart attack, many people worry about having another heart attack. Sometimes, they feel depressed and have trouble adjusting to new lifestyle changes.

Talk about how you feel with your healthcare team. Talking to a professional counselor also can help. If you are very depressed, your doctor may recommend medicines or other treatments that can improve your quality of life.

Joining a patient support group may help you adjust to life after a heart attack. You can see how other people who have the same symptoms have coped with them. Talk with your doctor about local support groups or check with an area medical center.

Support from family and friends also can help relieve stress and anxiety. Let your loved ones know how you feel and what they can do to help you.

Risk of a Repeat Heart Attack

Once you have had a heart attack, you are at higher risk for another one. Knowing the difference between angina and a heart attack is important.

The pain from angina usually occurs after physical exertion and goes away in a few minutes when you rest or take medicine as directed.

The pain from a heart attack usually is more severe than the pain from angina. Heart attack pain does not go away when you rest or take medicine.

If you do not know whether your chest pain is angina or a heart attack, call 911.

The symptoms of a second heart attack may not be the same as those of a first heart attack. Do not take a chance if you are in doubt. Always call 911 right away if you or someone else has heart attack symptoms.

Unfortunately, most heart attack victims wait two hours or more after their symptoms start before they seek medical help. This delay can result in lasting heart damage or death.

Chapter 33

Stroke

What Is a Stroke?

A stroke occurs if the flow of oxygen-rich blood to a portion of the brain is blocked. Without oxygen, brain cells start to die after a few minutes. Sudden bleeding in the brain also can cause a stroke if it damages brain cells.

If brain cells die or are damaged because of a stroke, symptoms occur in the parts of the body that these brain cells control. Examples of stroke symptoms include sudden weakness; paralysis (an inability to move) or numbness of the face, arms, or legs; trouble speaking or understanding speech; and trouble seeing.

A stroke is a serious medical condition that requires emergency care. A stroke can cause lasting brain damage, long-term disability, or even death.

If you think you or someone else is having a stroke, call 911 right away. Do not drive to the hospital or let someone else drive you. Call an ambulance so that medical personnel can begin life-saving treatment on the way to the emergency room. During a stroke, every minute counts.

Causes of a Stroke
Ischemic Stroke and Transient Ischemic Attack

An ischemic stroke or transient ischemic attack (TIA) occurs if an artery that supplies oxygen-rich blood to the brain becomes blocked.

This chapter includes text excerpted from "Stroke," National Heart, Lung, and Blood Institute (NHLBI), August 14, 2018.

Many medical conditions can increase the risk of an ischemic stroke or TIA.

For example, atherosclerosis is a disease in which a fatty substance called "plaque" builds up on the inner walls of the arteries. Plaque hardens and narrows the arteries, which limits the flow of blood to tissues and organs (such as the heart and brain).

Plaque in an artery can crack or rupture (break open). Blood platelets, which are disc-shaped cell fragments, stick to the site of the plaque injury and clump together to form blood clots. These clots can partly or fully block an artery.

Plaque can build up in any artery in the body, including arteries in the heart, brain, and neck. The two main arteries on each side of the neck are called the "carotid arteries." These arteries supply oxygen-rich blood to the brain, face, scalp, and neck.

When plaque builds up in the carotid arteries, the condition is called "carotid artery disease." Carotid artery disease causes many of the ischemic strokes and TIAs that occur in the United States.

An embolic stroke (a type of ischemic stroke) or TIA also can occur if a blood clot or piece of plaque breaks away from the wall of an artery. The clot or plaque can travel through the bloodstream and get stuck in one of the brain's arteries. This stops blood flow through the artery and damages brain cells.

Heart conditions and blood disorders also can cause blood clots that can lead to a stroke or TIA. For example, atrial fibrillation, or AF, is a common cause of embolic stroke.

In atrial fibrillation, the upper chambers of the heart contract in a very fast and irregular way. As a result, some blood pools in the heart. The pooling increases the risk of blood clots forming in the heart chambers.

An ischemic stroke or TIA also can occur because of lesions caused by atherosclerosis. These lesions may form in the small arteries of the brain, and they can block blood flow to the brain.

Hemorrhagic Stroke

Sudden bleeding in the brain can cause a hemorrhagic stroke. The bleeding causes swelling of the brain and increased pressure in the skull. The swelling and pressure damage brain cells and tissues.

Examples of conditions that can cause a hemorrhagic stroke include high blood pressure, aneurysms, and arteriovenous malformations (AVMs).

Blood pressure is the force of blood pushing against the walls of the arteries as the heart pumps blood. If blood pressure rises and stays high over time, it can damage the body in many ways.

Aneurysms are balloon-like bulges in an artery that can stretch and burst. AVMs are tangles of faulty arteries and veins that can rupture within the brain. High blood pressure can increase the risk of hemorrhagic stroke in people who have aneurysms or AVMs.

Risk Factors for a Stroke

Certain traits, conditions, and habits can raise your risk of having a stroke or transient ischemic attack. These traits, conditions, and habits are known as "risk factors."

The more risk factors you have, the more likely you are to have a stroke. You can treat or control some risk factors, such as high blood pressure and smoking. Other risk factors, such as your age and sex, you cannot control.

The major risk factors for stroke include:

- **High blood pressure.** High blood pressure is the main risk factor for stroke. Blood pressure is considered high if it stays at or above 140/90 millimeters of mercury (mmHg) over time. If you have diabetes or chronic kidney disease (CKD), high blood pressure is defined as 130/80 mmHg or higher.

- **Diabetes.** Diabetes is a disease in which the blood sugar level is high because the body does not make enough insulin or does not use its insulin properly. Insulin is a hormone that helps move blood sugar into cells where it is used for energy.

- **Heart diseases.** Ischemic heart disease, cardiomyopathy, heart failure, and atrial fibrillation can cause blood clots that can lead to a stroke.

- **Smoking.** Smoking can damage blood vessels and raise blood pressure. Smoking also may reduce the amount of oxygen that reaches your body's tissues. Exposure to secondhand smoke also can damage the blood vessels.

- **Age and sex.** Your risk of stroke increases as you get older. At younger ages, men are more likely than women to have strokes. However, women are more likely to die from strokes. Women who take birth control pills (BCPs) also are at slightly higher risk of stroke.

- **Race and ethnicity.** Strokes occur more often in African American, Alaska Native, and American Indian adults than in White, Hispanic, or Asian American adults.

- **Personal or family history of stroke or TIA.** If you have had a stroke, you are at a higher risk for another one. Your risk of having a repeat stroke is the highest right after a stroke. A TIA also increases your risk of having a stroke, as does having a family history of stroke.

- **Brain aneurysms or arteriovenous malformations.** Aneurysms are balloon-like bulges in an artery that can stretch and burst. AVMs are tangles of faulty arteries and veins that can rupture within the brain. AVMs may be present at birth but often are not diagnosed until they rupture.

Other risk factors for stroke, many of which of you can control, include:

- Alcohol and illegal drug use, including cocaine, amphetamines, and other drugs

- Certain medical conditions, such as sickle cell disease (SCD), vasculitis (inflammation of the blood vessels), and bleeding disorders

- Lack of physical activity

- Being overweight or obese

- Stress and depression

- Unhealthy cholesterol levels

- Unhealthy diet

- Use of nonsteroidal anti-inflammatory drugs (NSAIDs), but not aspirin, may increase the risk of heart attack or stroke, particularly in patients who have had a heart attack or cardiac bypass surgery. The risk may increase the longer NSAIDs are used. Common NSAIDs include ibuprofen and naproxen.

Following a heart-healthy lifestyle can lower the risk of stroke. Some people also may need to take medicines to lower their risk. Sometimes, strokes can occur in people who do not have any known risk factors.

Screening and Prevention of Strokes

Taking action to control your risk factors can help prevent or delay a stroke. Talk to your doctor about whether you may benefit from aspirin primary prevention, or using aspirin to help prevent your first stroke. The following heart-healthy lifestyle changes can help prevent your first stroke and help prevent you from having another one.

Be physically active. Physical activity can improve your fitness level and health. Talk to your doctor about what types and amounts of activity are safe for you.

Do not smoke, or if you smoke or use tobacco, quit. Smoking can damage and tighten blood vessels and raise your risk of stroke. Talk to your doctor about programs and products that can help you quit. Also, secondhand smoke can damage the blood vessels.

Aim for a healthy weight. If you are overweight or obese, work with your doctor to create a reasonable weight-loss plan. Controlling your weight helps you control risk factors for stroke.

Make heart-healthy eating choices. Heart-healthy eating can help lower your risk or prevent a stroke.

Manage stress. Use techniques to lower your stress levels.

If you or someone in your family has had a stroke, be sure to tell your doctor. By knowing your family history of stroke, you may be able to lower your risk factors and prevent or delay a stroke. If you have had a transient ischemic attack, do not ignore it. TIAs are warnings, and it is important for your doctor to find the cause of the TIA so you can take steps to prevent a stroke.

Signs, Symptoms, and Complications of Stroke

The signs and symptoms of a stroke often develop quickly. However, they can develop over hours or even days.

The type of symptoms depends on the type of stroke and the area of the brain that is affected. How long symptoms last and how severe they vary among different people.

Signs and symptoms of a stroke may include:

- Sudden weakness

- Paralysis or numbness of the face, arms, or legs, especially on one side of the body

- Confusion

- Trouble speaking or understanding speech

- Trouble seeing in one or both eyes

- Problems breathing

- Dizziness, trouble walking, loss of balance or coordination, and unexplained falls

- Loss of consciousness

- Sudden and severe headache

A transient ischemic attack has the same signs and symptoms as a stroke. However, TIA symptoms usually last less than 1 to 2 hours (although, they may last up to 24 hours). A TIA may occur only once in a person's lifetime or more often.

At first, it may not be possible to tell whether someone is having a TIA or stroke. All stroke-like symptoms require medical care.

If you think you or someone else is having a TIA or stroke, call 911 right away. Do not drive to the hospital or let someone else drive you. Call an ambulance so that medical personnel can begin life-saving treatment on the way to the emergency room. During a stroke, every minute counts.

Stroke Complications

After you have had a stroke, you may develop other complications, such as:

- **Blood clots and muscle weakness.** Being immobile (unable to move around) for a long time can raise your risk of developing blood clots in the deep veins of the legs. Being immobile also can lead to muscle weakness and decreased muscle flexibility.

- **Problems swallowing and pneumonia.** If a stroke affects the muscles used for swallowing, you may have a hard time eating or drinking. You also may be at risk of inhaling food or drink into your lungs. If this happens, you may develop pneumonia.

- **Loss of bladder control.** Some strokes affect the muscles used to urinate. You may need a urinary catheter (a tube placed into the bladder) until you can urinate on your own. Use of these catheters can lead to urinary tract infections (UTIs). Loss of bowel control or constipation also may occur after a stroke.

Life after a Stroke

The time it takes to recover from a stroke varies—it can take weeks, months, or even years. Some people recover fully, while others have long-term or lifelong disabilities.

Ongoing care, rehabilitation, and emotional support can help you recover and may even help prevent another stroke.

If you have had a stroke, you are at risk of having another one. Know the warning signs and what to do if a stroke or transient ischemic attack occurs. Call 911 as soon as symptoms start.

Do not drive to the hospital or let someone else drive you. By calling an ambulance, medical personnel can begin life-saving treatment on the way to the emergency room. During a stroke, every minute counts.

Chapter 34

Renal Artery Stenosis

What Are Renal Artery Stenosis and Renovascular Hypertension?

Renal artery stenosis (RAS) is the narrowing of one or both renal arteries. "Renal" means "kidney," and "stenosis" means "narrowing." The renal arteries are blood vessels that carry blood to the kidneys from the aorta—the main blood vessel that carries blood from the heart to arteries throughout the body.

Renovascular hypertension (RVH) is high blood pressure caused by RAS. Blood pressure is written with two numbers separated by a slash, 120/80, and is said as "120 over 80." The top number is called the "systolic pressure" and represents the pressure as the heart beats and pushes blood through the blood vessels. The bottom number is called the "diastolic pressure" and represents the pressure as blood vessels relax between heartbeats. A person's blood pressure is considered normal if it stays at or below 120/80. High blood pressure is a systolic pressure of 140 or above or a diastolic pressure of 90 or above.

What Causes Renal Artery Stenosis

About 90 percent of RAS is caused by atherosclerosis—the clogging, narrowing, and hardening of the renal arteries. In these cases, RAS

This chapter includes text excerpted from "Renal Artery Stenosis," National Institute of Diabetes and Digestive and Kidney Diseases (NIDDK), July 2014. Reviewed June 2019.

develops when plaque—a sticky substance made up of fat, cholesterol, calcium, and other material found in the blood—builds up on the inner wall of one or both renal arteries. Plaque buildup is what makes the artery wall hard and narrow.

Most other cases of RAS are caused by fibromuscular dysplasia (FMD)—the abnormal development or growth of cells on the renal artery walls—which can cause blood vessels to narrow. Rarely, RAS is caused by other conditions.

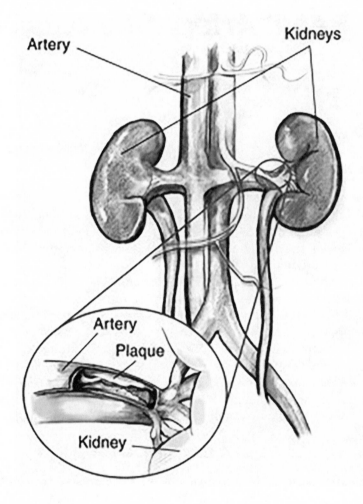

Figure 34.1. *Renal Artery Stenosis*

In most cases of RAS, plaque builds up on the inner wall of one or both renal arteries.

Who Is at Risk for Renal Artery Stenosis?

People at risk for atherosclerosis are also at risk for RAS. Risk factors for RAS caused by atherosclerosis include:

- High blood cholesterol levels
- High blood pressure
- Smoking
- Insulin resistance
- Diabetes
- Being overweight or obese
- Lack of physical activity
- A diet high in fat, cholesterol, sodium, and sugar
- Being a man older than 45 years of age or a woman older than 55 years of age
- A family history of early heart disease

The risk factors for RAS caused by FMD are unknown, but FMD is most common in people between the ages of 25 and 50. FMD can affect more than one person in a family, indicating that it may be caused by an inherited gene.

What Are the Symptoms of Renal Artery Stenosis?

In many cases, renal artery stenosis has no symptoms until it becomes severe.

The signs of renal artery stenosis are usually either high blood pressure or decreased kidney function or both, but RAS is often overlooked as a cause of high blood pressure. RAS should be considered as a cause of high blood pressure in people who:

- Are older than 50 years of age when they develop high blood pressure or have a marked increase in blood pressure
- Have no family history of high blood pressure
- Cannot be successfully treated with at least three or more different types of blood pressure medications

Symptoms of a significant decrease in kidney function include:

- Increase or decrease in urination

401

- Edema—swelling, usually in the legs, feet, or ankles and less often in the hands or face

- Drowsiness or tiredness

- Generalized itching or numbness

- Dry skin

- Headaches

- Weight loss

- Appetite loss

- Nausea

- Vomiting

- Sleep problems

- Trouble concentrating

- Darkened skin

- Muscle cramps

What Are the Possible Complications of Renal Artery Stenosis?

People with renal artery stenosis are at an increased risk for complications resulting from loss of kidney function or atherosclerosis occurring in other blood vessels, such as:

- **Chronic kidney disease (CKD)**—reduced kidney function over a period of time

- **Coronary artery disease (CAD)**—narrowing and hardening of arteries that supply blood to the heart

- **Stroke**—brain damage caused by lack of blood flow to the brain

- **Peripheral vascular disease (PVD)**—blockage of blood vessels that restricts flow of blood from the heart to other parts of the body, particularly the legs

Renal artery stenosis can lead to kidney failure, described as end-stage renal disease when treated with blood-filtering treatments called "dialysis" or a "kidney transplant," though this is uncommon in people who receive ongoing treatment for RAS.

Eating, Diet, and Nutrition

Limiting intake of fats, cholesterol, sodium, and sugar can help prevent atherosclerosis, which can lead to RAS. Most sodium in the diet comes from salt. A healthy diet that prevents people from becoming overweight or obese can also help prevent atherosclerosis. People with RAS that has caused decreased kidney function should limit their intake of protein, cholesterol, sodium, and potassium to slow the progression of kidney failure.

Chapter 35

Peripheral Vascular Disease

Chapter Contents

Section 35.1

Buerger Disease

This section includes text excerpted from "Buerger Disease," Genetic and Rare Diseases Information Center (GARD), National Center for Advancing Translational Sciences (NCATS), January 18, 2017.

What Is Buerger Disease?

Buerger disease is a disease in which small and medium-sized blood vessels in the arms and/or legs become inflamed and blocked (vasculitis). This reduces blood flow to affected areas of the body, eventually resulting in tissue damage. Symptoms of Buerger disease may include coldness, numbness, tingling or burning, and pain. Symptoms may first be felt in the fingertips or toes, and then move further up the arms or legs. Additional symptoms that may develop include changes in the texture and color of the skin, Raynaud phenomenon, painful muscle cramps, swelling (edema), skin ulcers, and gangrene. Rare complications that have been reported include transient ischemic attacks (TIAs) or stroke, and heart attack.

Buerger disease almost always occurs in people who use tobacco, but it is not known exactly how tobacco plays a role in the development of the disease. Some people may have a genetic predisposition to Buerger disease. It is also possible that Buerger disease is an autoimmune disease, as the immune system seems to play a large role in its development. More research is needed to identify the exact underlying causes.

Quitting all forms of tobacco is an essential part of stopping the progression of the disease. There are no definitive treatments, but certain therapies may improve symptoms in some people. Therapies that have been reported with varying success include medications to improve blood flow and reduce the risk of clots, pain medicines, compression of the arms and legs, spinal cord stimulation, and surgery to control pain and increase blood flow. Amputation may be necessary if gangrene or a serious infection develops.

How Common Is Buerger Disease?

Buerger disease has become less common over the past 10 years given the decrease in smoking prevalence and more strict diagnostic criteria. In 1947, it was estimated to occur in 104 out of 100,000 people. It now is estimated to occur in 12 to 20 out of 100,000 people.

What Causes Buerger Disease

Buerger disease has a strong relationship to cigarette smoking. This association may be due to direct poisoning of cells from some component of tobacco or by hypersensitivity to the same components. Many people with Buerger disease will show hypersensitivities to injection of tobacco extracts into their skin.

How Is Buerger Disease Treated?

Currently, there is not a cure for Buerger disease; however, there are treatments that can help control it. The most essential part of treatment is to avoid all tobacco and nicotine products. Even one cigarette a day can worsen the disease. A doctor can help a person with Buerger disease learn about safe medications and programs to combat smoking/nicotine addiction.

Are There Products Other than Cigarette Tobacco Associated with Buerger Disease?

Data is lacking regarding the association of Buerger disease with drugs or products other than cigarette smoking; however, there have been case reports describing Buerger disease in patients who used other products alone or in combination with tobacco. You can search for these case reports through a service called "PubMed," a searchable database of medical literature.

What Diet Is Recommended for People with Buerger Disease?

There are not any specific diet recommendations for people with Buerger disease. However, there are some online healthy diet guidelines and tools that may be of interest to you, such as:

- Choose MyPlate, from the U.S. Department of Agriculture
- Individual Dietary Assessment tools, from the U.S. Department of Agriculture
- Nutrition Basics, from the Centers for Disease Control and Prevention
- Nutrition, Diet, and Health, from Penn State University

Section 35.2

Erythromelalgia

This section contains text excerpted from the following sources:
Text beginning with the heading "What Is Erythromelalgia?" is
excerpted from "Erythromelalgia," Genetics Home Reference (GHR),
National Institutes of Health (NIH), February 2016; Text beginning
with the heading "Diagnosis of Erythromelalgia" is excerpted
from "Erythromelalgia," Genetic and Rare Diseases Information
Center (GARD), National Center for Advancing Translational
Sciences (NCATS), August 4, 2016.

What Is Erythromelalgia?

Erythromelalgia (EM) is a condition characterized by episodes of
pain, redness, and swelling in various parts of the body, particularly in
the hands and feet. These episodes are usually triggered by increased
body temperature, which may be caused by exercise or entering a warm
room. Ingesting alcohol or spicy foods may also trigger an episode.
Wearing warm socks, tight shoes, or gloves can cause a pain episode
so debilitating that it can impede everyday activities, such as wearing
shoes and walking. Pain episodes can prevent an affected person from
going to school or work regularly.

The signs and symptoms of erythromelalgia typically begin in childhood; although, mildly affected individuals may have their first pain
episode later in life. As individuals with erythromelalgia get older and
the disease progresses, the hands and feet may be constantly red, and
the affected areas can extend from the hands to the arms, shoulders,
and face, and from the feet to the entire legs.

Erythromelalgia is often considered a form of peripheral neuropathy because it affects the peripheral nervous system, which connects
the brain and spinal cord to muscles and to cells that detect sensations,
such as touch, smell, and pain.

Causes of Erythromelalgia

Mutations in the *SCN9A* gene can cause erythromelalgia. The
SCN9A gene provides instructions for making one part (the alpha
subunit) of a sodium channel called "NaV1.7." Sodium channels transport positively charged sodium atoms (sodium ions) into cells and play
a key role in a cell's ability to generate and transmit electrical signals.
NaV1.7 sodium channels are found in nerve cells called "nociceptors"
that transmit pain signals to the spinal cord and brain.

The *SCN9A* gene mutations that cause erythromelalgia result in NaV1.7 sodium channels that open more easily than usual and stays open longer than normal, increasing the flow of sodium ions into nociceptors. This increase in sodium ions enhances transmission of pain signals, leading to the signs and symptoms of erythromelalgia. It is unknown why the pain episodes associated with erythromelalgia mainly occur in the hands and feet.

An estimated 15 percent of cases of erythromelalgia are caused by mutations in the *SCN9A* gene. Other cases are thought to have a nongenetic cause or may be caused by mutations in one or more as-yet unidentified genes.

Diagnosis of Erythromelalgia

There is no specific diagnostic test for most cases of erythromelalgia, so making a diagnosis usually relies on symptoms, a clinical exam, and medical history.

Testing that may be done to support a suspected diagnosis or rule out other medical disorders includes:

- A **complete blood count (CBC)** with differential to search for evidence of a myeloproliferative disorder

- **Imaging studies,** such as X-ray of the hands and feet, which typically show no specific findings

- **Thermography**, which may reveal elevated skin temperatures in affected areas (but this is not necessary for the diagnosis)

- **Biopsy,** which may reveal characteristic findings in people with primary erythromelalgia

- *SCN9A*-**related inherited EM** can be confirmed with genetic testing of the *SCN9A* gene.

The first step to diagnosing EM is seeing your primary care doctor, who can test for some of the common causes of EM or its symptoms and refer you to a specialist to confirm a suspected diagnosis. There is not a specific type of doctor that always diagnoses and treats EM. A variety of specialists (alone or in combination) may be involved in the diagnosis and treatment. These may include dermatologists, neurologists, vascular specialists, hematologists, rheumatologists, or other types of physicians. The type of specialist that is appropriate after diagnosis may depend on the underlying cause when secondary erythromelalgia is present.

The Erythromelalgia Association (TEA) has a Patient Guide which includes helpful information about diagnosing EM. This guide can be used as an educational and awareness tool for patients, family and friends, and healthcare providers. They also have a Doctor Directory with contact information for doctors and researchers who have been suggested by TEA members over time.

Testing Resources

• The **Genetic Testing Registry (GTR)** provides information about the genetic tests for this condition. The intended audience for the GTR is healthcare providers and researchers. Patients and consumers with specific questions about a genetic test should contact a healthcare provider or a genetics professional.

• **Orphanet** lists international laboratories offering diagnostic testing for this condition.

Treatment of Erythromelalgia

No single therapy works well for every person with EM. Often, it is necessary to try different treatments or combinations of treatments until the best therapy is found. In some cases, EM may go away on its own. If EM is being caused by another medical disorder (secondary EM), treating the underlying disorder may improve or completely resolve EM symptoms.

Treatment options for EM include creams applied to the skin (topical creams), medications, certain supplements, and mind-body therapies (such as cognitive behavioral therapy or CBT). If all other treatment options have failed, epidural anesthesia, nerve blocks, or surgery may be considered depending on the severity of the pain.

Section 35.3

Peripheral Artery Disease

This section includes text excerpted from "Peripheral
Artery Disease," National Heart, Lung, and
Blood Institute (NHLBI), January 23, 2019.

What Is Peripheral Artery Disease?

Peripheral artery disease (PAD) is a disease in which plaque builds
up in the arteries that carry blood to your head, organs, and limbs.
Plaque is made up of fat, cholesterol, calcium, fibrous tissue, and other
substances in the blood.

When plaque builds up in the body's arteries, the condition is called
"atherosclerosis." Over time, plaque can harden and narrow the arteries. This limits the flow of oxygen-rich blood to your organs and other
parts of your body.

Peripheral artery disease usually affects the arteries in the legs,
but it also can affect the arteries that carry blood from your heart to
your head, arms, kidneys, and stomach. This section focuses on PAD
that affects blood flow to the legs.

Causes of Peripheral Artery Disease

The most common cause of peripheral artery disease is atherosclerosis. Atherosclerosis is a disease in which plaque builds up in your
arteries. The exact cause of atherosclerosis is not known.

The disease may start if certain factors damage the inner layers of
the arteries. These factors include:

- Smoking

- High amounts of certain fats and cholesterol in the blood

- High blood pressure

- High amounts of sugar in the blood due to insulin resistance or
  diabetes

When damage occurs, your body starts a healing process. The healing may cause plaque to build up where the arteries are damaged.

Eventually, a section of plaque can rupture (break open), causing a
blood clot to form at the site. The buildup of plaque or blood clots can

411

severely narrow or block the arteries and limit the flow of oxygen-rich blood to your body.

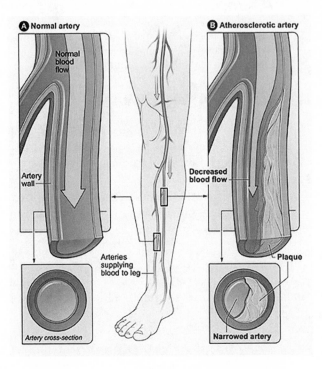

Figure 35.1. *Normal Artery and Artery with Plaque Buildup*

The illustration shows how PAD can affect arteries in the legs. Figure A shows a normal artery with normal blood flow. The inset image shows a cross-section of the normal artery. Figure B shows an artery with plaque buildup that is partially blocking blood flow. The inset image shows a cross-section of the narrowed artery.

Risk Factors of Peripheral Artery Disease

Peripheral artery disease affects millions of people in the United States. The disease is more common in Blacks than any other racial or ethnic group. The major risk factors for PAD are smoking, older age, and having certain diseases or conditions.

Smoking

Smoking is the main risk factor for PAD, and your risk increases if you smoke or have a history of smoking. Quitting smoking slows the progress of PAD. People who smoke and people who have diabetes are at the highest risk for PAD complications, such as gangrene (tissue death) in the leg from decreased blood flow.

Older Age

Older age also is a risk factor for PAD. Plaque builds up in your arteries as you age. Older age combined with other risk factors, such as smoking or diabetes, also puts you at higher risk for PAD.

Diseases and Conditions

Many diseases and conditions can raise your risk of PAD, including:

- Diabetes
- High blood pressure
- High blood cholesterol
- Ischemic heart disease
- Stroke
- Metabolic syndrome

Screening and Prevention of Peripheral Artery Disease

Taking action to control your risk factors can help prevent or delay PAD and its complications. Know your family history of health problems related to PAD. If you or someone in your family has the disease, be sure to tell your doctor. Controlling risk factors includes the following.

- Be physically active.
- Be screened for PAD. A simple office test, called an "ankle-brachial index" or "ABI," can help determine whether you have PAD.
- Follow heart-healthy eating.
- If you smoke, quit. Talk with your doctor about programs and products that can help you quit smoking.
- If you are overweight or obese, work with your doctor to create a reasonable weight-loss plan.

The lifestyle changes described above can reduce your risk of developing PAD. These changes also can help prevent and control conditions that can be associated with PAD, such as ischemic heart disease, diabetes, high blood pressure, high blood cholesterol, and stroke.

Signs, Symptoms, and Complications of Peripheral Artery Disease

Many people who have peripheral artery disease do not have any signs or symptoms.

Even if you do not have signs or symptoms, ask your doctor whether you should get checked for PAD if you are:

- 70 years of age or older

- 50 years of age or older and have a history of smoking or diabetes

- Younger than 50 years of age and have diabetes and one or more risk factors for atherosclerosis

Intermittent Claudication

People who have PAD. may have symptoms when walking or climbing stairs, which may include pain, numbness, aching, or heaviness in the leg muscles. Symptoms also may include cramping in the affected leg(s) and in the buttocks, thighs, calves, and feet. Symptoms may ease after resting. These symptoms are called "intermittent claudication."

During physical activity, your muscles need increased blood flow. If your blood vessels are narrowed or blocked, your muscles will not get enough blood, which will lead to symptoms. When resting, the muscles need less blood flow, so the symptoms will go away.

Other Signs and Symptoms

Other signs and symptoms of PAD include:

- Weak or absent pulses in the legs or feet

- Sores or wounds on the toes, feet, or legs that heal slowly, poorly, or not at all

- A pale or bluish color to the skin

- A lower temperature in one leg when compared to the other leg

- Poor nail growth on the toes and decreased hair growth on the legs

- Erectile dysfunction, especially among men who have diabetes

Living with Peripheral Artery Disease

If you have peripheral artery disease, you are more likely to also have ischemic heart disease, heart attack, stroke, and transient ischemic attack ("mini-stroke"). However, you can take steps to treat and control PAD and lower your risk for these other conditions.

Living with Peripheral Artery Disease Symptoms

If you have peripheral artery disease, you may feel pain in your calf or thigh muscles after walking. Try to take a break and allow the pain to ease before walking again. Over time, this may increase the distance that you can walk without pain.

Talk with your doctor about taking part in a supervised exercise program. This type of program has been shown to reduce PAD symptoms.

Check your feet and toes regularly for sores or possible infections. Wear comfortable shoes that fit well. Maintain good foot hygiene and have professional medical treatment for corns, bunions, or calluses.

Ongoing Healthcare Needs and Lifestyle Changes

See your doctor for checkups as she or he advises. If you have PAD without symptoms, you still should see your doctor regularly. Take all medicines as your doctor prescribes.

Heart-healthy lifestyle changes can help prevent or delay PAD and other related problems. Heart-healthy lifestyle changes include physical activity, quitting smoking, and heart-healthy eating.

Section 35.4

Raynaud Phenomenon

This section includes text excerpted from "Raynaud Phenomenon,"
National Institute of Arthritis and Musculoskeletal and Skin
Diseases (NIAMS), October 30, 2016.

What Is Raynaud Phenomenon?

Raynaud phenomenon is a condition that affects your blood vessels.
It causes some areas of your body, especially your hands and feet, to
feel numb and cold in response to cold temperatures or stress. Raynaud
phenomenon is also called "Raynaud disease" or "Raynaud syndrome."

What Happens in Raynaud Phenomenon

If you have Raynaud phenomenon, you have "attacks" when your
body does not send enough blood to your hands and feet. Attacks usually happen when you are cold or feeling stressed. During an attack,
your fingers and toes may feel very cold or numb and may change color.
These attacks are also known as "vasospasms."

Once an attack begins, you may experience three phases of skin
color changes—typically from white to blue to red—in your fingers or
toes.

- Whiteness (called "pallor") may occur in response to the collapse
  of the veins that supply the fingers and toes with blood.

- Blueness (called "cyanosis") may appear because the fingers or
  toes are not getting enough oxygen-rich blood.

- Finally, as blood returns to the fingers and toes, redness (rubor) may
  occur. During this stage, the fingers and toes may tingle or throb.

During an attack, your blood flow to the skin will remain low until
the skin is rewarmed. After warming, it usually takes 15 minutes to
recover normal blood flow to the skin.

Your prognosis often depends on what form of the disease you have
and what underlying health condition(s) you have. Many people with
Raynaud phenomenon have mild symptoms that do not cause any
blood vessel or tissue damage. These symptoms are easily managed,
often without medicines. Others have more severe symptoms. For most
people with Raynaud phenomenon, the disease is lifelong.

Who Gets Raynaud Phenomenon

Anyone can get Raynaud phenomenon, but some people are more likely to have it than others.

The primary form of Raynaud often starts between the ages of 15 and 25. It is most common in:

- Women

- People living in cold places

The secondary form of Raynaud phenomenon usually starts after the ages of 35 and 40. It is most common in people who have a disease that affects blood flow to the organs and other body tissues. This is called a "connective tissue disease." Connective tissue diseases include:

- Lupus, which causes the immune system to attack healthy tissues in the body

- Scleroderma, which causes the skin and other tissues in the body to harden

- Sjögren syndrome, which causes dryness in the mouth and eyes

Other health conditions can also increase your risk of developing Raynaud phenomenon. These include:

- Carpal tunnel syndrome, which affects nerves in the wrists

- Blood vessel disease, which causes the blood vessels in the legs, arms, and belly to narrow

Certain medicines can cause the secondary form of Raynaud phenomenon:

- Medicines used to treat high blood pressure, migraines, or cancer

- Over-the-counter (OTC) cold medicines

- Narcotics

In addition, people with certain jobs may be more likely to develop the secondary form of Raynaud phenomenon:

- People who are around certain chemicals

- People who use tools that vibrate, such as a jackhammer

Some research suggests that Raynaud phenomenon runs in certain families, but more research is needed.

Types of Raynaud Phenomenon

There are two types of Raynaud phenomenon.

- Primary Raynaud phenomenon occurs for an unknown reason. It is the more common form of Raynaud phenomenon.

- Secondary Raynaud phenomenon is caused by another health condition, such as lupus or scleroderma. Secondary Raynaud phenomenon is less common but more serious than the primary form of the disease.

Symptoms of Raynaud Phenomenon

During an attack, your body limits blood flow to the hands and feet. This makes your fingers and toes feel cold and numb. It may also cause your fingers and toes to turn white or blue. Once blood flow to the fingers and toes returns, they may turn red, tingle, and begin to hurt.

The symptoms of the primary form of Raynaud Phenomenon usually begins between the ages of 15 and 25. The symptoms of the secondary form of Raynaud Phenomenon usually start after the ages of 35 to 40.

For many people, especially those with a primary form of Raynaud phenomenon, the symptoms are mild and not very troublesome. Others have more severe symptoms.

Causes of Raynaud Phenomenon

Doctors do not know exactly what causes Raynaud phenomenon to develop, but they do know some causes of attacks.

Usually, when a person is exposed to cold, the body tries to slow the loss of heat and maintain its temperature. To do so, blood vessels in the surface of the skin move blood from veins near the skin's surface to veins deeper in the body. In people with Raynaud phenomenon, blood vessels in the hands and feet appear to overreact to cold temperatures or stress. They narrow and limit blood supply.

Living with Raynaud Phenomenon

There are steps you can take to decrease the number of Raynaud attacks you have and the severity of these attacks.

- **Keep warm.** Set your thermostat to a higher temperature. You lose a lot of body heat through your head; wear a hat. Keep your feet warm and dry. In cold weather, wear several layers of loose clothing, socks, hats, and gloves or mittens. Keep pocket warmers in your pockets if you will be outside for a long time. Use insulated drinking glasses when drinking something cold. Put on gloves before handling frozen or refrigerated foods.

- **Avoid rapidly shifting temperatures and damp climates.** Rapidly moving from 90 degrees outside to a 70-degree air-conditioned room can bring on an attack, as can damp rainy weather.

- **Avoid air conditioning.** In warm weather, air conditioning also can bring on attacks.

- **Do not smoke.** The nicotine in cigarettes causes the skin temperature to drop, which may lead to an attack.

- **Avoid medicines that bring on attacks.** Certain medicines cause the blood vessel to narrow, which can bring on an attack. These include beta-blockers, cold preparations, caffeine, narcotics, some migraine headache medications, and some chemotherapy drugs. Talk to your doctor before starting any new medicines. Do not stop any medicines you are taking without talking to your doctor first.

- **Control stress.** Because stress can bring on an attack, learning how to manage or control stress is important. Talk to your doctor about stress reduction techniques.

- **Exercise regularly.** Exercise can improve your overall well-being. In addition, it can increase your energy level, help control your weight, keep your heart healthy, and improve sleep. Talk to your doctor before starting an exercise program.

Chapter 36

Fibromuscular Dysplasia

What Is Fibromuscular Dysplasia?[1]

Fibromuscular dysplasia (FMD) is the abnormal development or growth of cells in the walls of arteries that can cause the vessels to narrow or bulge. The carotid arteries, which pass through the neck and supply blood to the brain, are commonly affected. Arteries within the brain and kidneys can also be affected. A characteristic "string of beads" pattern caused by the alternating narrowing and enlarging of the artery can block or reduce blood flow to the brain, causing a stroke or mini-stroke. Some patients experience no symptoms of the disease while others may have high blood pressure, dizziness or vertigo, chronic headache, intracranial aneurysm, ringing in the ears, weakness or numbness in the face, neck pain, or changes in vision. FMD is most often seen in persons of 25 and 50 years of age and affects women more often than men. More than one family member may be affected by the disease. The cause of FMD is unknown. An angiogram can detect the degree of narrowing or obstruction of the artery and identify changes, such as a tear (dissection) or weak area (aneurysm)

This chapter includes text excerpted from documents published by two public domain sources. Text under the headings marked 1 are excerpted from "Fibromuscular Dysplasia Information Page," National Institute of Neurological Disorders and Stroke (NINDS), March 27, 2019; Text under the headings marked 2 are excerpted from "Fibromuscular Dysplasia," Genetic and Rare Diseases Information Center (GARD), National Center for Advancing Translational Sciences (NCATS), August 9, 2016.

in the vessel wall. FMD can also be diagnosed using computed tomography, magnetic resonance imaging, or ultrasound.

Symptoms of Fibromuscular Dysplasia[2]

Table 36.1 lists symptoms that people with this disease may have. For most diseases, symptoms will vary from person to person. People with the same disease may not have all the symptoms listed. This information comes from a database called the "Human Phenotype Ontology" (HPO). The HPO collects information on symptoms that have been described in medical resources. The HPO is updated regularly.

Table 36.1. Symptoms

Medical Terms	Other Names
Aortic dissection	Tear in the inner wall of the large artery that carries blood away from the heart
Arterial fibromuscular dysplasia	
Autosomal dominant inheritance	
Intermittent claudication	
Myocardial infarction	Heart attack
Renovascular hypertension	
Stroke	

Causes of Fibromuscular Dysplasia[2]

The cause of FMD is unknown. It is likely that there are many factors that contribute to the development of this condition. These factors may include blood vessel abnormalities, tobacco use, hormone levels, and genetic predispositions.

Treatment of Fibromuscular Dysplasia[1]

There is no standard protocol to treat FMD. Any treatment to improve blood flow is based on the arteries affected and the progression and severity of the disease. The carotid arteries should be tested if FMD is found elsewhere in the body since carotid involvement is linked to an increased risk of stroke. Patients with minimal narrowing may take a daily antiplatelet, such as aspirin or an anticoagulant to thin the blood and reduce the chances that a clot might form. Medications, such as aspirin, can also be taken for headache and neck pain, which are both symptoms that can come from FMD. Patients with arterial disease who smoke should be encouraged to quit, as smoking worsens the disease. Further treatment may include angioplasty, in which a small balloon is inserted through a catheter and inflated to open the artery. Small tubes called "stents" may be inserted to keep arteries open. Surgery may be needed to treat aneurysms that have the potential to rupture and cause bleeding within the brain.

Prognosis of Fibromuscular Dysplasia[1]

Currently, there is no cure for FMD. Medicines and angioplasty can reduce the risk of initial or recurrent stroke. In rare cases, FMD-related aneurysms can burst and bleed into the brain, causing stroke, permanent nerve damage, or death.

Chapter 37

Giant Cell Arteritis

What Is Giant Cell Arteritis?

Giant cell arteritis (GCA) is a type of disorder that is marked by blood vessel inflammation.

People with giant cell arteritis often have polymyalgia rheumatica, a disorder associated with pain and stiffness in the neck, shoulder, and hip.

What Happens in Giant Cell Arteritis

Giant cell arteritis causes narrowed arteries, which reduces blood flow. The disorder mostly affects arteries located on each side of the head; although, other blood vessels can also become inflamed.

Giant cell arteritis can cause potentially serious problems if it is left untreated, including permanent vision loss and stroke. It is critical to report any symptoms to your doctor and to receive early treatment to prevent permanent tissue damage.

This chapter contains text excerpted from the following sources: Text beginning with the heading "What Is Giant Cell Arteritis?" is excerpted from "Giant Cell Arteritis," National Institute of Arthritis and Musculoskeletal and Skin Diseases (NIAMS), May 30, 2016; Text beginning with the heading "Cause of Giant Cell Arteritis" is excerpted from "Giant Cell Arteritis," Genetic and Rare Diseases Information Center (GARD), National Center for Advancing Translational Sciences (NCATS), September 21, 2018.

Who Gets Giant Cell Arteritis

Women are more likely than men to develop giant cell arteritis, but men with the disorder are more likely to suffer eye damage that could result in blindness. Giant cell arteritis mostly affects people over the age of 50, with the highest rates at 70 to 80 years of age.

What Are the Symptoms of Giant Cell Arteritis

Signs of giant cell arteritis can include:

- Flu-like symptoms early in the disease, such as tiredness, appetite loss, and fever

- Headaches

- Pain and tenderness over the temples

- Double vision or vision loss

- Dizziness

- Problems with coordination and balance

- Pain in the jaw and tongue, especially when eating

- Difficulty in opening the mouth wide

- Scalp scores (rare cases)

Cause of Giant Cell Arteritis

While the exact cause of GCA is unknown, some studies have linked genetic factors, infections with certain virus or bacteria, high doses of antibiotics, and a prior history of cardiovascular disease to the development of GCA. These associations suggest GCA is caused by an abnormal immune response, where the body's immune system attacks the arteries.

The genetic factors currently linked to the development of GCA are not thought to directly cause GCA, but they may cause a genetic predisposition to the condition. This means that a person may carry a genetic variation (or more than one genetic variation) that increases their risk to develop GCA but may also need one or more environmental triggers to develop GCA. Familial cases of GCA have been reported.

Studies have confirmed a strong association of GCA with genetic variations in the *human leukocyte antigen (HLA)* gene family, a cluster of genes on chromosome 6. The *HLA* gene family gives the body instructions to make a group of proteins known as the "HLA complex." This complex helps the immune system distinguish between the body's own proteins and those made by foreign invaders, such as viruses and bacteria. More specifically, GCA has been associated with genetic variations in the HLA class I and class II genes. HLA class I genes give the body instructions to make proteins that occur on the surface of almost all cells. HLA class II genes give instructions to make proteins that occur almost exclusively on the surface of certain immune system cells.

Variations in other genes, which are not part of the *HLA* gene family, have also been associated with an increased risk to develop GCA. These include the *PTPN22, NLRP1, IL17A, IL33*, and *LRRC32* genes. Outside of the HLA-related genes, certain variations in the *PTPN22* seem to be the most strongly associated with GCA. This gene is known as a "common susceptibility gene in autoimmunity" since different variations in the gene have been consistently associated with many autoimmune diseases.

Several additional factors are known to increase a person's risk to develop GCA. These include:

- **Age.** GCA affects older adults almost exclusively.

- **Sex.** Females are about two times more likely than males to develop GCA.

- **Ethnicity.** Higher rates of GCA occur in people with Northern European (especially Scandinavian) descent.

- **Polymyalgia rheumatica.** About 15 percent of people with polymyalgia rheumatica also have GCA.

Inheritance of Giant Cell Arteritis

While the exact cause of GCA is still being investigated, studies have linked both genetic and nongenetic factors to the development of GCA. Familial cases of GCA have been reported, and research indicates that some people with GCA may have a genetic predisposition to the condition. This means that a person may carry a genetic variation (or more than one genetic variation) that increases their risk to develop GCA, but it may not develop without environment triggers. Because GCA is thought to be caused by an interaction between several genetic and environmental factors, it is said to have multifactorial inheritance.

Treatment of Giant Cell Arteritis

Giant cell arteritis is typically treated with high doses of corticosteroids to reduce the inflammation in the arteries. Corticosteroids should be started promptly (perhaps even before the diagnosis is confirmed with a biopsy). If not treated, GCA may cause permanent vision loss or a stroke. The symptoms of GCA usually quickly disappear with treatment, but high doses of corticosteroids are typically maintained for one month. It is known that the treatment is working when the symptoms are gone and the sedimentation rate, also known as "sed rate" (a blood test that measures the level of inflammatory activity), is normal. The corticosteroid dose may gradually be reduced. Other medicines may help to reduce the doses of corticosteroids.

The U.S. Food and Drug Administration (FDA) approved the use of an under-the-skin injection (subcutaneous) of tocilizumab (brand name: Actemra) to treat adults with GCA. Remember that only your doctor can prescribe medication, so please talk to your doctor to find out if this medication may be right for you.

Prognosis of Giant Cell Arteritis

Symptoms of GCA generally improve within days of starting treatment, and blindness is now a rare complication. However, the course of GCA until full recovery can vary considerably. While the average duration of treatment is two years, some people need treatment for five years or more. The effects of steroid therapy are often worse than the symptoms of GCA. When GCA is properly treated, it rarely recurs. However, people with GCA carry a lifelong risk for the development of large vessel disease, particularly aortic aneurysms. Therefore, long-term followup is extremely important.

The outlook for people who are not treated is poor. Complications may include blindness or other eye and vision problems, death from heart attack (myocardial infarction), stroke, or dissecting aortic aneurysm. Vision damage that occurs before starting therapy is often irreversible.

Chapter 38

Vascular Birthmarks: Hemangiomas and Vascular Malformations

Vascular Birthmarks

Vascular birthmarks, also known as "vascular anomalies," affect an estimated 1 in 10 children. Birthmarks take many forms, differing in size, shape, and location on the body. The color of birthmarks varies from shades of brown or blue to red or pink. There are 2 main types of vascular birthmarks: hemangiomas and vascular malformations. About half of all birthmarks are minor and require no treatment.

Hemangiomas

Hemangiomas are noncancerous tumors that are present at birth and affect female children about 3 times as often as males. Due to their distinctive color, these birthmarks are also sometimes known as "strawberry marks" or "salmon patches." They most often appear on the head or neck but can develop anywhere on the body, including internal organs. Hemangiomas may not be visible until 1 to 4 weeks after birth. These birthmarks sometimes initially appear as faint red

"Vascular Birthmarks: Hemangiomas and Vascular Malformations," © 2016 Omnigraphics. Reviewed June 2019.

marks. Once hemangiomas appear, they change rapidly, usually growing faster than the child grows, before reaching a peak state after about 12 months. After that, hemangiomas begin to shrink and become lighter in color. This process is known as "involution" or "regression" and can last from 3 to 10 years. About 70 percent of hemangiomas disappear by the age of 7. In most cases, hemangiomas do not require treatment. Surgery may be required if the hemangioma interferes with breathing, vision, or hearing.

Vascular Malformations

Vascular malformations are noncancerous lesions that are present at birth. These birthmarks grow with the child throughout life without involution. There are four main types of vascular malformations. Port wine stains can appear anywhere on the body and are typically flat and colored pink, purple, or red. Venous birthmarks are most commonly found on the jaw, cheek, tongue, and lips. These birthmarks are soft to the touch, and their color disappears when compressed (such as by pressing on the birthmark with a finger). Lymphatic birthmarks form as a result of excess fluid in the lymphatic vessels. Arteriovenous birthmarks appear when blood pools in capillary veins.

Causes of Hemangiomas and Vascular Malformations

A tendency to develop hemangiomas and vascular malformations can be inherited, though most birthmarks of this type seem to form by chance. Hemangiomas and vascular malformations develop as a result of many different genetic syndromes, with many variables affecting the chance of a child being born with a birthmark. If 1 parent has or had a hemangioma or vascular malformation, there is a 50 percent chance that their baby will also have such a birthmark.

Treating Hemangiomas and Vascular Malformations

Some birthmarks can result in serious complications if the location of the birthmark impairs the body's critical functions, such as breathing or blood flow. Most hemangiomas do not require treatment. Treatment is usually required for hemangiomas that interfere with vision, breathing, hearing, ability to feed, or result in other medical problems. Treatment options include surgery, laser treatment, medication, or a combination of approaches.

Treatment for vascular malformations depends upon the location and type of birthmark. Venous and lymphatic malformations are typically treated by injection therapy, in which a clotting medication is used to remove excessive blood or lymphatic fluid. Capillary malfunctions, such as port wine stains are usually treated with laser surgery. Arterial malformations can be treated with a process known as "embolization," in which blood flow is block by injection of medication near the lesion. Treatments can also include oral medications, such as steroids; radiology treatment; surgery; or a combination of approaches.

References

1. "What is a Vascular Birthmark?" University of Rochester Medical Center (URMC), 2016.

2. "Vascular Malformations and Hemangiomas," Stanford Children's Health, 2016.

Chapter 39

Vasculitis

What Is Vasculitis?

Vasculitis is a condition that involves inflammation in the blood vessels. The condition occurs if your immune system attacks your blood vessels by mistake. This may happen as the result of an infection, a medicine, or another disease or condition.

"Inflammation" refers to the body's response to injury, including injury to the blood vessels. Inflammation may involve pain, redness, warmth, swelling, and loss of function in the affected tissues.

In vasculitis, inflammation can lead to serious problems. Complications depend on which blood vessels, organs, or other body systems are affected.

Overview

Vasculitis can affect any of the body's blood vessels. These include arteries, veins, and capillaries. Arteries carry blood from your heart to your body's organs. Veins carry blood from your organs and limbs back to your heart. Capillaries connect the small arteries and veins.

If a blood vessel is inflamed, it can narrow or close off. This limits or prevents blood flow through the vessel. Rarely, the blood vessel will stretch and weaken, causing it to bulge. This bulge is known as an "aneurysm."

This chapter includes text excerpted from "Vasculitis," National Heart, Lung, and Blood Institute (NHLBI), April 8, 2011. Reviewed June 2019.

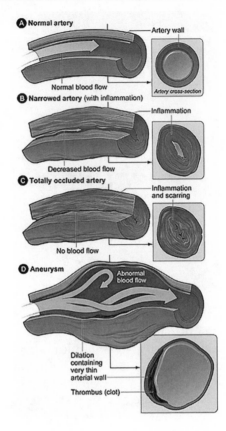

Figure 39.1. *Vasculitis*

Figure A shows a normal artery with normal blood flow. The inset image shows a cross-section of the normal artery. Figure B shows an inflamed, narrowed artery with decreased blood flow. The inset image shows a cross-section of the inflamed artery. Figure C shows an inflamed, blocked (occluded) artery and scarring on the artery wall. The inset image shows a cross-section of the blocked artery. Figure D shows an artery with an aneurysm. The inset image shows a cross-section of the artery with an aneurysm.

The disruption in blood flow caused by inflammation can damage the body's organs. Signs and symptoms depend on which organs have been damaged and the extent of the damage.

Typical symptoms of inflammation, such as fever and general aches and pains, are common among people who have vasculitis.

Outlook

There are many types of vasculitis, but the condition is rare overall. If you have vasculitis, the outlook depends on:

- The type of vasculitis you have
- Which organs are affected
- How quickly the condition worsens
- The severity of the condition

Treatment often works well if it is started early. In some cases, vasculitis may go into remission. "Remission" means the condition is not active, but it can come back, or "flare," at any time.

Sometimes vasculitis is chronic (ongoing) and never goes into remission. Long-term treatment with medicines often can control the signs and symptoms of chronic vasculitis.

Rarely, vasculitis does not respond well to treatment. This can lead to disability and even death.

Much is still unknown about vasculitis. However, researchers continue to learn more about the condition and its various types, causes, and treatments.

Types of Vasculitis

There are many types of vasculitis. Each type involves inflamed blood vessels. However, most types differ in whom they affect and the organs that are involved.

The types of vasculitis often are grouped based on the size of the blood vessels they affect.

Mostly Large Vessel Vasculitis

These types of vasculitis usually, but not always, affect the body's larger blood vessels.

Behçet Disease

Behçet disease can cause recurrent, painful ulcers (sores) in the mouth, ulcers on the genitals, acne-like skin lesions, and eye inflammation called "uveitis."

The disease occurs most often in people between the ages of 20 and 40. Men are more likely to get it, but it also can affect women. Behçet disease is more common in people of Mediterranean, Middle Eastern, and Far Eastern descent, although it rarely affects Blacks.

Researchers believe that a gene called the "*HLA-B51* gene" may play a role in Behçet disease. However, not everyone who has the gene gets the disease.

Cogan Syndrome

Cogan syndrome can occur in people who have a systemic vasculitis that affects the large blood vessels, especially the aorta and aortic valve. The aorta is the main artery that carries oxygen-rich blood from the heart to the body.

A systemic vasculitis is a type of vasculitis that affects you in a general or overall way.

Cogan syndrome can lead to eye inflammation called "interstitial keratitis." The syndrome also can cause hearing changes, including sudden deafness.

Giant Cell Arteritis

Giant cell arteritis usually affects the temporal artery, an artery on the side of your head. This condition also is called "temporal arteritis." Symptoms of this condition can include headaches, scalp tenderness, jaw pain, blurred vision, double vision, and acute (sudden) vision loss.

Giant cell arteritis is the most common form of vasculitis in adults older than 50 years of age. It is more likely to occur in people of Scandinavian origin, but it can affect people of any race.

Polymyalgia Rheumatica

Polymyalgia rheumatica, or PMR, commonly affects the large joints in the body, such as the shoulders and hips. PMR typically causes stiffness and pain in the muscles of the neck, shoulders, lower back, hips, and thighs.

Polymyalgia rheumatica usually occurs by itself, but 10–20 percent of people who have PMR also develop giant cell arteritis. Also, about half of the people who have giant cell arteritis may develop PMR.

Takayasu Arteritis

Takayasu arteritis affects medium- and large-sized arteries, particularly the aorta and its branches. The condition sometimes is called "aortic arch syndrome."

Though rare, Takayasu arteritis mainly affects teenage girls and young women. The condition is most common in Asians, but it can affect people of all races.

Takayasu arteritis is a systemic disease. A systemic disease is one that affects you in a general or overall way.

Symptoms of Takayasu arteritis may include tiredness and a sense of feeling unwell, fever, night sweats, sore joints, loss of appetite, and weight loss. These symptoms usually occur before other signs develop that point to arteritis.

Mostly Medium Vessel Vasculitis

These types of vasculitis usually, but not always, affect the body's medium-sized blood vessels.

Buerger Disease

Buerger disease, also known as "thromboangiitis obliterans," typically affects blood flow to the hands and feet. In this disease, the blood vessels in the hands and feet tighten or become blocked. As a result, less blood flows to the affected tissues, which can lead to pain and tissue damage.

Rarely, Buerger disease also can affect blood vessels in the brain, abdomen, and heart. The disease usually affects men of Asian or Eastern European descent between the ages of 20 and 40. The disease is strongly linked to cigarette smoking.

Symptoms of Buerger disease include pain in the calves or feet when walking or pain in the forearms and hands with activity. Other symptoms include blood clots in the surface veins of the limbs and Raynaud phenomenon.

In severe cases, ulcers may develop on the fingers and toes, leading to gangrene. The term "gangrene" refers to the death or decay of body tissues.

Surgical bypass of the blood vessels may help restore blood flow to some areas. Medicines generally do not work well to treat Buerger disease. The best treatment is to stop using tobacco of any kind.

Central Nervous System Vasculitis

Central nervous system (CNS) vasculitis usually occurs as a result of a systemic vasculitis. A systemic vasculitis is one that affects you in a general or overall way.

Very rarely, vasculitis affects only the brain and/or spinal cord. When it does, the condition is called "isolated vasculitis of the central nervous system" or "primary angiitis of the central nervous system."

Symptoms of CNS vasculitis include headaches; problems thinking clearly; changes in mental function; or stroke-like symptoms, such as muscle weakness and paralysis (an inability to move).

Kawasaki Disease

Kawasaki disease is a rare childhood disease in which the walls of the blood vessels throughout the body become inflamed. The disease can affect any blood vessel in the body, including arteries, veins, and capillaries.

Kawasaki disease also is known as "mucocutaneous lymph node syndrome." This is because the disease is associated with redness of the mucous membranes (tissues that line some organs and body cavities) in the eyes and mouth, redness of the skin, and enlarged lymph nodes.

Sometimes, the disease affects the coronary arteries, which carry oxygen-rich blood to the heart. As a result, a small number of children who have Kawasaki disease may have serious heart problems.

Polyarteritis Nodosa

Polyarteritis nodosa can affect many parts of the body. This disorder often affects the kidneys, the digestive tract, the nerves, and the skin.

Symptoms often include fever; a general feeling of being unwell; weight loss; and muscle and joint aches, including pain in the calf muscles that develops over weeks or months.

Other signs and symptoms include anemia (a low red blood cell count), a lace- or web-like rash, bumps under the skin, and stomach pain after eating.

Researchers believe that this type of vasculitis is very rare, although the symptoms can be similar to those of other types of vasculitis. Some cases of polyarteritis nodosa seem to be linked to hepatitis B or C infections.

Mostly Small Vessel Vasculitis

These types of vasculitis usually, but not always, affect the body's small blood vessels.

Eosinophilic Granulomatosis with Polyangiitis

Eosinophilic granulomatosis with polyangiitis, or EGPA, is a very rare disorder that causes blood vessel inflammation. The disorder is also known as "Churg-Strauss syndrome" or "allergic angiitis" and "granulomatosis."

Eosinophilic granulomatosis with polyangiitis can affect many organs, including the lungs, skin, kidneys, nervous system, and heart.

438

Symptoms can vary widely. They may include asthma, higher than normal levels of white blood cells in the blood and tissues, and abnormal lumps known as "granulomas."

Cryoglobulinemia Vasculitis

Cryoglobulinemic vasculitis occurs when abnormal immune proteins (cryoglobulins) thicken the blood and impair blood flow. This causes pain and damage to the skin, joints, peripheral nerves, kidneys, and liver.

Cryoglobulins are abnormal immune proteins in the blood that clump together and thicken the blood plasma. Cryoglobulins can be detected in the laboratory by exposing a sample of blood to cold temperature (below normal body temperature). In cold temperatures, the immune proteins form clumps; but when the blood is rewarmed, the clumps dissolve.

The cause of cryoglobulinemic vasculitis is not always known. In some cases, it is associated with other conditions, such as lymphoma, multiple myeloma, connective tissue diseases, and infection (particularly hepatitis C infection).

Immunoglobulin A Vasculitis

In immunoglobulin A (IgA) vasculitis (also known as "Henoch-Schonlein purpura"), abnormal IgA deposits develop in small blood vessels in the skin, joints, intestines, and kidneys. IgA a type of antibody (a protein) that normally helps defend the body against infections.

Symptoms of IgA vasculitis include a bruise-like, reddish-purple rash, most often seen on the buttocks, legs, and feet (but can be anywhere on the body); abdominal pain; swollen and painful joints; and blood in the urine. People with IgA vasculitis do not necessarily have all of the symptoms, but nearly all will have the characteristic rash.

IgA vasculitis is most often seen in children between 2 and 11 years of age, but it can affect people of all ages. More than 75 percent of the cases of IgA vasculitis follow an upper respiratory tract infection, a throat infection, or a gastrointestinal infection.

Most people with IgA vasculitis are well within one to two months and do not have any lasting problems. In rare cases, symptoms can last longer or come back. All IgA vasculitis patients should have a full evaluation by a medical professional.

Hypersensitivity Vasculitis

Hypersensitivity vasculitis affects the skin. This condition also is known as "allergic vasculitis," "cutaneous vasculitis," or "leukocytoclastic vasculitis."

A common symptom is red spots on the skin, usually on the lower legs. For people who are bedridden, the rash appears on the lower back.

An allergic reaction to a medicine or infection often causes this type of vasculitis. Stopping the medicine or treating the infection usually clears up the vasculitis. However, some people may need to take anti-inflammatory medicines, such as corticosteroids, for a short time. These medicines help reduce inflammation.

Microscopic Polyangiitis

Microscopic polyangiitis affects small blood vessels, particularly those in the kidneys and lungs. The disease mainly occurs in middle-aged people; it affects men slightly more often than women.

The symptoms often are not specific, and they can begin gradually with fever, weight loss, and muscle aches. Sometimes the symptoms come on suddenly and progress quickly, leading to kidney failure.

If the lungs are affected, coughing up blood may be the first symptom. Sometimes microscopic polyangiitis occurs with a vasculitis that affects the intestinal tract, the skin, and the nervous system.

The signs and symptoms of microscopic polyangiitis are similar to those of Wegener granulomatosis (another type of vasculitis). However, microscopic polyangiitis usually does not affect the nose and sinuses or cause abnormal tissue formations in the lungs and kidneys.

The results of certain blood tests can suggest inflammation. These results include a higher than normal erythrocyte sedimentation rate (ESR); lower-than-normal hemoglobin and hematocrit levels (which suggest anemia); and higher than normal white blood cell and platelet counts.

Also, more than half of the people who have microscopic polyangiitis have certain antibodies in their blood. These antibodies are called "antineutrophil cytoplasmic autoantibodies" (ANCA). ANCA also occur in people who have Wegener granulomatosis.

Testing for ANCA cannot be used to diagnose either of these two types of vasculitis. However, testing can help evaluate people who have vasculitis-like symptoms.

Causes of Vasculitis

Vasculitis occurs if your immune system attacks your blood vessels by mistake. What causes this to happen is not fully known.

A recent or chronic (ongoing) infection may prompt the attack. Your body also may attack its own blood vessels in reaction to a medicine.

Sometimes an autoimmune disorder triggers vasculitis. Autoimmune disorders occur if the immune system makes antibodies that attack and damage the body's own tissues or cells. Examples of these disorders include lupus, rheumatoid arthritis, and scleroderma. You can have these disorders for years before developing vasculitis.

Vasculitis also may be linked to certain blood cancers, such as leukemia and lymphoma.

Risk Factors of Vasculitis

Vasculitis can affect people of all ages and races and both sexes. Some types of vasculitis seem to occur more often in people who:

- Have certain medical conditions, such as chronic hepatitis B or C infection

- Have certain autoimmune diseases, such a lupus, rheumatoid arthritis, and scleroderma

- Smoke

Screening and Prevention of Vasculitis

You cannot prevent vasculitis. However, treatment can help prevent or delay the complications of vasculitis.

People who have severe vasculitis are treated with prescription medicines. Rarely, surgery may be done. People who have mild vasculitis may find relief with over-the-counter pain medicines, such as acetaminophen, aspirin, ibuprofen, or naproxen.

Signs, Symptoms, and Complications of Vasculitis

The signs and symptoms of vasculitis vary. They depend on the type of vasculitis you have, the organs involved, and the severity of the condition. Some people may have few signs and symptoms. Other people may become very sick.

Sometimes the signs and symptoms develop slowly, over months. Other times, the signs and symptoms develop quickly, over days or weeks.

441

Systemic Signs and Symptoms

Systemic signs and symptoms are those that affect you in a general or overall way. Common systemic signs and symptoms of vasculitis are:

- Fever

- Loss of appetite

- Weight loss

- Fatigue (tiredness)

- General aches and pains

Organ- or Body System-Specific Signs and Symptoms

Vasculitis can affect specific organs and body systems, causing a range of signs and symptoms.

Skin

If vasculitis affects your skin, you may notice skin changes. For example, you may have purple or red spots or bumps, clusters of small dots, splotches, bruises, or hives. Your skin also may itch.

Joints

If vasculitis affects your joints, you may ache or develop arthritis in one or more joints.

Lungs

If vasculitis affects your lungs, you may feel short of breath. You may even cough up blood. The results from a chest X-ray may show signs that suggest pneumonia, even though that may not be what you have.

Gastrointestinal Tract

If vasculitis affects your gastrointestinal tract, you may get ulcers (sores) in your mouth or have stomach pain.

In severe cases, blood flow to the intestines can be blocked. This can cause the wall of the intestines to weaken and possibly rupture (burst). A rupture can lead to serious problems or even death.

Sinuses, Nose, Throat, and Ears

If vasculitis affects your sinuses, nose, throat, and ears, you may have sinus or chronic middle ear infections. Other symptoms include ulcers in the nose and, in some cases, hearing loss.

Eyes

If vasculitis affects your eyes, you may develop red, itchy, burning eyes. Your eyes also may become sensitive to light, and your vision may blur. Rarely, certain types of vasculitis may cause blindness.

Brain

If vasculitis affects your brain, symptoms may include headaches; problems thinking clearly; changes in mental function; or stroke-like symptoms, such as muscle weakness and paralysis (an inability to move).

Nerves

If vasculitis affects your nerves, you may have numbness, tingling, and weakness in various parts of your body. You also may have a loss of feeling or strength in your hands and feet and shooting pains in your arms and legs.

Diagnosis of Vasculitis

Your doctor will diagnose vasculitis based on your signs and symptoms, your medical history, a physical exam, and test results.

Specialists Involved

Depending on the type of vasculitis you have and the organs affected, your doctor may refer you to various specialists, including:

- A rheumatologist (joint and muscle specialist)

- An infectious disease specialist

- A dermatologist (skin specialist)

- A pulmonologist (lung specialist)

- A nephrologist (kidney specialist)

- A neurologist (nervous system specialist)
- A cardiologist (heart specialist)
- An ophthalmologist (eye specialist)
- A urologist (urinary tract and urogenital system specialist)

Diagnostic Tests and Procedures

Many tests are used to diagnose vasculitis.

Blood Tests

Blood tests can show whether you have abnormal levels of certain blood cells and antibodies in your blood. These tests may look at:

- **Hemoglobin and hematocrit.** A low hemoglobin or hematocrit level suggests anemia, a complication of vasculitis. Vasculitis can interfere with the body's ability to make enough red blood cells. Vasculitis also can be linked to increased destruction of red blood cells.

- **Antineutrophil cytoplasmic antibodies (ANCA).** These antibodies are present in people who have certain types of vasculitis.

- **Erythrocyte sedimentation rate (ESR).** A high ESR may be a sign of inflammation in the body.

- The amount of **C-reactive protein (CRP)** in your blood. A high CRP level suggests inflammation.

Biopsy

A biopsy often is the best way for your doctor to make a firm diagnosis of vasculitis. During a biopsy, your doctor will take a small sample of your body tissue to study under a microscope. She or he will take the tissue sample from a blood vessel or an organ.

A pathologist will study the sample for signs of inflammation or tissue damage. A pathologist is a doctor who specializes in identifying diseases by studying cells and tissues under a microscope.

Blood Pressure

People who have vasculitis should have their blood pressure checked routinely. Vasculitis that damages the kidneys can cause high blood pressure.

Urinalysis

For this test, you will provide a urine sample for analysis. This test detects abnormal levels of protein or blood cells in the urine. Abnormal levels of these substances can be a sign of vasculitis affecting the kidneys.

Electrocardiogram

An electrocardiogram (EKG) is a simple, painless test that records the heart's electrical activity. You might have this test to show whether vasculitis is affecting your heart.

Echocardiography

Echocardiography is a painless test that uses sound waves to create a moving picture of your heart. The test gives information about the size and shape of your heart and how well your heart chambers and valves are working.

Chest X-Ray

A chest X-ray is a painless test that creates pictures of the structures inside your chest, such as your heart, lungs, and blood vessels. Abnormal chest X-ray results may show whether vasculitis is affecting your lungs or your large arteries (such as the aorta or the pulmonary arteries).

Lung Function Tests

Lung function tests measure how much air you can breathe in and out, how fast you can breathe air out, and how well your lungs deliver oxygen to your blood.

Lung function tests can help your doctor find out whether airflow into and out of your lungs is restricted or blocked.

Abdominal Ultrasound

An abdominal ultrasound uses sound waves to create a picture of the organs and structures in your abdomen. The picture may show whether vasculitis is affecting your abdominal organs.

Computed Tomography Scan

A computed tomography scan, or CT scan, is a type of X-ray that creates more detailed pictures of your internal organs than a standard X-ray. The results from this test can show whether you have a type of vasculitis that affects your abdominal organs or blood vessels.

Magnetic Resonance Imaging

A magnetic resonance imaging (MRI) test uses radio waves, magnets, and a computer to create detailed pictures of your internal organs.

Other Advanced Imaging Techniques

Several new imaging techniques are now being used to help diagnose vasculitis. Duplex ultrasonography combines an image of the structure of the blood vessel with a color image of the blood flow through that vein or artery. 18F-fluorodeoxyglucose positron emission tomography (FDG-PET) identifies areas that show higher glucose metabolism leading to problems in the blood vessels.

Angiography

Angiography is a test that uses dye and special x rays to show blood flowing through your blood vessels.

The dye is injected into your bloodstream. Special X-ray pictures are taken while the dye flows through your blood vessels. The dye helps highlight the vessels on the X-ray pictures.

Doctors use angiography to help find out whether blood vessels are narrowed, swollen, deformed, or blocked.

Treatment of Vasculitis

Treatment for vasculitis will depend on the type of vasculitis you have, which organs are affected, and the severity of the condition.

People who have severe vasculitis are treated with prescription medicines. Rarely, surgery may be done. People who have mild vasculitis may find relief with over-the-counter (OTC) pain medicines, such as acetaminophen, aspirin, ibuprofen, or naproxen.

The main goal of treating vasculitis is to reduce inflammation in the affected blood vessels. This usually is done by reducing or stopping the immune response that caused the inflammation.

Types of Treatment

Common prescription medicines used to treat vasculitis include corticosteroids and cytotoxic medicines.

Corticosteroids help reduce inflammation in your blood vessels. Examples of corticosteroids are prednisone, prednisolone, and methylprednisolone.

Doctors may prescribe cytotoxic medicines if vasculitis is severe or if corticosteroids do not work well. Cytotoxic medicines kill the cells that are causing the inflammation. Examples of these medicines are azathioprine, methotrexate, and cyclophosphamide.

Your doctor may prescribe both corticosteroids and cytotoxic medicines.

Other treatments may be used for certain types of vasculitis. For example, the standard treatment for Kawasaki disease is high-dose aspirin and immune globulin. Immune globulin is a medicine that is injected into a vein.

Certain types of vasculitis may require surgery to remove aneurysms that have formed as a result of the condition. (An aneurysm is an abnormal bulge in the wall of a blood vessel.)

Living with Vasculitis

The outcome of vasculitis is hard to predict. It will depend on the type of vasculitis you have, which organs are affected, and the severity of the condition.

If vasculitis is diagnosed early and responds well to treatment, it may go away or go into remission. "Remission" means the condition is not active, but it can come back, or "flare," at any time.

Flares can be hard to predict. You may have a flare when you stop treatment or change your treatment. Some types of vasculitis seem to flare more often than others. Also, some people have flares more often than others.

Sometimes vasculitis is chronic and never goes into remission. Long-term treatment with medicines often can control chronic vasculitis, but no cure has been found. Rarely, vasculitis does not respond well to treatment. This can lead to disability or even death.

Ongoing Care

The medicines used to treat vasculitis can have side effects. For example, long-term use of corticosteroids may lead to weight gain, diabetes, weakness, a decrease in muscle size, and osteoporosis (a bone-thinning condition). Long-term use of these medicines also may increase your risk of infection.

Your doctor may adjust the type or dose of medicine you take to lessen or prevent the side effects. If your vasculitis goes into remission, your doctor may carefully withdraw your medicines. However, she or he will still need to carefully watch you for flares.

While you are being treated for vasculitis, you will need to see your doctor regularly. Talk with your doctor about any new symptoms and other changes in your health, including side effects of your medicines.

Emotional Issues and Support

Living with a chronic condition may cause fear, anxiety, depression, and stress. Talk about how you feel with your healthcare team. Talking to a professional counselor also can help. If you are very depressed, your doctor may recommend medicines or other treatments that can improve your quality of life.

Joining a patient support group may help you adjust to living with vasculitis. You can see how other people who have the same symptoms have coped with them. Talk with your doctor about local support groups or check with an area medical center.

Support from family and friends also can help relieve stress and anxiety. Let your loved ones know how you feel and what they can do to help you.

Chapter 40

Klippel-Trénaunay Syndrome

What Is Klippel-Trénaunay Syndrome?

Klippel-Trénaunay syndrome is a condition that affects the development of blood vessels, soft tissues (such as skin and muscles), and bones. The disorder has three characteristic features: a red birthmark called a "port-wine stain" (PWS), abnormal overgrowth of soft tissues and bones, and vein malformations (VM).

Most people with Klippel-Trénaunay syndrome are born with a port-wine stain. This type of birthmark is caused by the swelling of small blood vessels near the surface of the skin. Port-wine stains are typically flat and can vary from pale pink to deep maroon in color. In people with Klippel-Trénaunay syndrome, the port-wine stain usually covers part of one limb. The affected area may become lighter or darker with age. Occasionally, port-wine stains develop small red blisters that break open and bleed easily.

Klippel-Trénaunay syndrome is also associated with overgrowth of bones and soft tissues, beginning in infancy. Usually, this abnormal growth is limited to one limb, most often one leg. However, overgrowth

This chapter contains text excerpted from the following sources: Text beginning with the heading "What Is Klippel-Trénaunay Syndrome?" is excerpted from "Klippel-Trenaunay Syndrome," Genetics Home Reference (GHR), National Institutes of Health (NIH), July 2016; Text beginning with the heading "Causes of Klippel-Trénaunay Syndrome" is excerpted from "Klippel-Trenaunay Syndrome," Genetic and Rare Diseases Information Center (GARD), National Center for Advancing Translational Sciences (NCATS), May 25, 2017.

can also affect the arms or, rarely, the torso. The abnormal growth can cause pain, a feeling of heaviness, and reduced movement in the affected area. If the overgrowth causes one leg to be longer than the other, it can also lead to problems with walking.

Malformations of veins are the third major feature of Klippel-Trénaunay syndrome. These abnormalities include varicose veins, which are swollen and twisted veins near the surface of the skin that often cause pain. Varicose veins usually occur on the sides of the upper legs and calves. Veins deep in the limbs can also be abnormal in people with Klippel-Trénaunay syndrome. Malformations of deep veins increase the risk of a type of blood clot called a "deep vein thrombosis" (DVT). If a DVT travels through the bloodstream and lodges in the lungs, it can cause a life-threatening blood clot known as a "pulmonary embolism" (PE).

Other complications of Klippel-Trénaunay syndrome can include a type of skin infection called "cellulitis," swelling caused by a buildup of fluid (lymphedema), and internal bleeding from abnormal blood vessels. Less commonly, this condition is also associated with fusion of certain fingers or toes (syndactyly) or the presence of extra digits (polydactyly).

Frequency of Klippel-Trénaunay Syndrome

Klippel-Trénaunay syndrome is estimated to affect at least 1 in 100,000 people worldwide.

Causes of Klippel-Trénaunay Syndrome

Most cases of KTS are caused by mutations in the *PIK3CA* gene. However, the mutation in the gene is not present in every cell of the body and is not inherited or passed down from either parent. The type of genetic mutation which causes KTS is called a "somatic mutation." These somatic mutations occur after conception (after the egg and sperm join together) but probably happen very early in development. Since somatic mutations are only present in some of the body's cells, the signs and symptoms of KTS usually only affect specific areas of the body. The *PIK3CA* gene provides instructions for making a protein which is part of an enzyme that is important for cell growth and division (proliferation), movement (migration) of cells, and cell survival. Mutations in the *PIK3CA* gene result in increased cell proliferation leading to abnormal growth of the bones, soft tissues, and blood vessels.

Some researchers believe all KTS is caused by somatic mutations in the *PIK3CA* gene and when a mutation cannot be found, the person may actually have a different disorder. Other researchers believe KTS can be caused by mutations in other yet to be discovered genes.

Inheritance of Klippel-Trénaunay Syndrome

Klippel-Trénaunay Syndrome is not known to be inherited. Since KTS is caused by somatic mutations and this type of mutation is not present in every cell of the body, the risk a child to be born with KTS to a parent with KTS is similar to the general population risk. In other words, children of a parent with KTS have the same risk of having KTS as someone whose parents do not have KTS. There are no confirmed reported cases of KTS being passed down to the children of a person with KTS.

Treatment of Klippel-Trénaunay Syndrome

There is no cure for KTS. Treatment is symptomatic and supportive. Conservative treatments seem most effective while limiting the chances for undesired side effects. This may include the use of elastic garments and pumps to relieve lymphedema and protect limbs from trauma or orthopedic devices for discrepancies in limb length. Laser therapy may be used to diminish or eliminate some skin lesions (port-wine stains). Surgery may be used for tissue debulking, vein repair, or to correct uneven growth in the limbs.

Chapter 41

Sepsis

What Is Sepsis?

Sepsis is a serious medical condition. It is caused by an overwhelming immune response to infection. The body releases immune chemicals into the blood to combat the infection. Those chemicals trigger widespread inflammation, which leads to blood clots and leaky blood vessels. As a result, blood flow is impaired, and that deprives organs of nutrients and oxygen, and leads to organ damage.

In severe cases, one or more organs fail. In the worst cases, blood pressure drops, the heart weakens, and the patient spirals toward septic shock. Once this happens, multiple organs—the lungs, kidneys, and liver—may quickly fail, and the patient can die.

Sepsis is a major challenge in hospitals, where it is one of the leading causes of death. It is also the main reason why people are re-admitted to the hospital. Sepsis occurs unpredictably and can progress rapidly.

What Causes Sepsis

Many types of microbes can cause sepsis, including bacteria, fungi, and viruses. However, bacteria are the most common cause. In many cases, doctors cannot identify the source of infection.

Severe cases of sepsis often result from a body-wide infection that spreads through the bloodstream. Invasive medical procedures, such

This chapter includes text excerpted from "Sepsis," National Institute of General Medical Sciences (NIGMS), January 2018.

as inserting a tube into a vein, can introduce bacteria into the blood-stream and bring on the condition. But, sepsis can also come from an infection confined to one part of the body, such as the lungs, urinary tract, skin, or abdomen (including the appendix).

Who Gets Sepsis

Anyone can get sepsis. The people at the highest risk are infants; children; the elderly; and people who have serious injuries or medical problems, such as diabetes, acquired immunodeficiency syndrome (AIDS), cancer, or liver disease.

How Many People Get Sepsis?

Severe sepsis strikes more than a million Americans every year, and 15 to 30 percent of those people die. The number of sepsis cases per year has been on the rise in the United States. This is likely due to several factors:

- There is increased awareness and tracking of sepsis.

- People with chronic diseases are living longer, and the average age in the United States is increasing. Sepsis is more common and more dangerous in the elderly and in those with chronic diseases.

- Some infections can no longer be cured with antibiotic drugs. Such antibiotic-resistant infections can lead to sepsis.

- Medical advances have made organ transplant operations more common. People are at a higher risk for sepsis if they have had an organ transplant or have undergone any other procedure that requires the use of medications to suppress the immune system.

What Are the Symptoms of Sepsis?

Common symptoms of sepsis are fever, chills, rapid breathing, and heart rate, rash, confusion, and disorientation. Many of these symptoms are also common in other conditions, making sepsis difficult to diagnose, especially in its early stages.

How Is Sepsis Diagnosed?

Doctors will start by checking for the symptoms mentioned above. They may also test the person's blood for an abnormal number of white blood cells or the presence of bacteria or other infectious agents. Doctors may also use a chest X-ray or a CT scan to locate an infection.

How Is Sepsis Treated?

Doctors typically treat people with sepsis in hospital intensive care units. Doctors try to stop the infection, protect the vital organs, and prevent a drop in blood pressure. This almost always includes the use of antibiotic medications and fluids. More seriously affected patients might need a breathing tube, kidney dialysis, or surgery to remove an infection. Despite years of research, scientists have not yet developed a medicine that specifically targets the aggressive immune response seen with sepsis.

Are There Any Long-Term Effects of Sepsis?

Many people who survive severe sepsis recover completely, and their lives return to normal. But some people, especially those with preexisting chronic diseases, may have permanent organ damage. For example, in someone who already has impaired kidneys, sepsis can lead to kidney failure that requires lifelong dialysis.

There is also some evidence that severe sepsis disrupts a person's immune system, making her or him more at risk for future infections. Studies have shown that people who have experienced sepsis have a higher risk of various medical conditions and death, even several years after the episode.

What Is the Economic Cost of Sepsis?

Sepsis treatment is expensive. It often involves a prolonged stay in the intensive care unit and complex therapies with high costs. The Agency for Healthcare Research and Quality (AHRQ) lists sepsis as the most expensive condition treated in U.S. hospitals, costing nearly $24 billion in 2013. People with sepsis are 2 to 3 times more likely to be readmitted to the hospital as people with many other conditions, including heart failure, pneumonia, and chronic obstructive pulmonary disease. Readmissions due to sepsis are also more expensive than readmissions due to any of these other conditions.

What Research Is Being Done on Sepsis?

The National Institutes of Health (NIH) supports many studies focused on sepsis, some of which are clinical trials. Some of these studies evaluate the effectiveness of potential treatments. Others seek molecular clues in patients' blood that could diagnose sepsis early, allowing doctors to treat the condition before it is too late. Still, others examine sepsis in specific populations, such as premature babies, people with traumatic injuries, or long-term survivors.

Chapter 42

Venous Disorders

Chapter Contents

Section 42.1

Arteriovenous Malformations

This section contains text excerpted from the following sources:
Text under the heading "What Are Arteriovenous Malformations?"
is excerpted from "Arteriovenous Malformation Information Page,"
National Institute of Neurological Disorders and Stroke (NINDS),
March 27, 2019; Text beginning with the heading "What Are the
Symptoms?" is excerpted from "Arteriovenous Malformations and Other
Vascular Lesions of the Central Nervous System Fact Sheet," National
Institute of Neurological Disorders and Stroke (NINDS), July 6, 2018.

What Are Arteriovenous Malformations?

Arteriovenous malformations (AVMs) are abnormal, snarled tangles
of blood vessels that cause multiple irregular connections between
the arteries and veins. These malformations most often occur in the
spinal cord and in any part of the brain or on its surface, but they can
develop elsewhere in the body. AVMs can damage the brain and spinal
cord by reducing the amount of oxygen reaching neurological tissues,
bleeding into surrounding tissue (hemorrhage) that can cause stroke
or brain damage, and by compressing or displacing parts of the brain
or spinal cord. Many people with an AVM experience few, if any, significant symptoms, which can include headache; weakness; seizures;
pain; and problems with speech, vision, or movement. Most often,
AVMs are congenital, but they can appear sporadically. In some cases,
the AVM may be inherited, but it is more likely that other inherited
conditions increase the risk of having an AVM. The malformations
tend to be discovered only incidentally, usually during treatment for
an unrelated disorder or at autopsy.

What Are the Symptoms?

Symptoms can vary greatly in severity; in some people, the severity
of symptoms becomes debilitating or even life-threatening.

Seizures and headaches that may be severe are the most generalized symptoms of AVMs, but no particular type of seizure or headache pattern has been identified. Seizures can be focal (meaning they
involve a small part of the brain) or generalized (widespread), involving
convulsions, a loss of control over movement, or a change in a person's
level of consciousness. Headaches can vary greatly in frequency, duration, and intensity, sometimes becoming as severe as migraines. Pain

may be on either one side of the head or on both sides. Sometimes, a headache consistently affecting one side of the head may be closely linked to the site of an AVM. Most often, the location of the pain is not specific to the malformation and may encompass most of the head.

AVMs also can cause a wide range of more specific neurological symptoms that vary from person to person, depending primarily upon the location of the AVM. Such symptoms may include:

- Muscle weakness or paralysis in one part of the body

- A loss of coordination (ataxia) that can lead to such problems as gait disturbances

- Difficulties carrying out tasks that require planning (apraxia)

- Back pain or weakness in the lower extremities caused by a spinal AVM

- Dizziness

- Visual problems, such as a loss of part of the visual field, inability to control eye movement, or swelling of a part of the optic nerve

- Difficulty speaking or understanding language (aphasia)

- Abnormal sensations, such as numbness, tingling, or spontaneous pain

- Memory deficits

- Confusion, hallucinations, or dementia

Arteriovenous malformations may also cause subtle learning or behavioral disorders in some people during their childhood or adolescence, long before more obvious symptoms become evident.

Symptoms caused by AVMs can appear at any age. Because the abnormalities tend to result from a slow buildup of neurological damage over time, they are most often noticed when people are in their twenties or older. If AVMs do not become symptomatic by the time people reach their late forties or early fifties, they tend to remain stable and are less likely to produce symptoms. Some pregnant women may experience a sudden onset or worsening of symptoms due to accompanying cardiovascular changes, especially increases in blood volume and blood pressure.

Although most neurological AVMs have very few, if any, significant symptoms, one particularly severe type of AVM causes symptoms to appear at, or very soon after, birth. Called a "vein of Galen defect" after the major blood vessel involved, this lesion is located deep inside the brain. It is frequently associated with hydrocephalus (an accumulation of fluid within certain spaces in the brain, often with visible enlargement of the head), swollen veins visible on the scalp, seizures, failure to thrive, and congestive heart failure. Children born with this condition who survive past infancy often remain developmentally impaired.

How Do Arteriovenous Malformations Damage the Brain and Spinal Cord?

Arteriovenous malformations damage the brain or spinal cord through three basic mechanisms: by reducing the amount of oxygen reaching neurological tissues; by causing bleeding (hemorrhage) into surrounding tissues; and by compressing or displacing parts of the brain or spinal cord.

- Arteriovenous malformations affect oxygen delivery to the brain or spinal cord by altering normal patterns of blood flow using the arteries, veins, and capillaries. In AVMs, arteries pump blood directly into veins through a passageway called a "fistula." Since the network of capillaries is bypassed, the rate of blood flow is uncontrolled and too rapid to allow oxygen to be dispersed to surrounding tissues. As a result, the cells that make up these tissues become oxygen-depleted and begin to deteriorate, sometimes dying off completely.

- This abnormally rapid rate of blood flow frequently causes blood pressure inside the vessels located in the central portion of an AVM directly adjacent to the fistula—an area doctors refer to as the nidus—to rise to dangerously high levels. The arteries feeding blood into the AVM often become swollen and distorted; the veins that drain blood away from it often become abnormally constricted (a condition called "stenosis"). Also, the walls of the involved arteries and veins are often abnormally thin and weak. Aneurysms—balloon-like bulges in blood vessel walls that are susceptible to rupture—may develop in association with approximately half of all neurological AVMs due to this structural weakness.

- Bleeding into the brain, called "intracranial hemorrhage," can result from the combination of high internal pressure and vessel wall weakness. Such hemorrhages are often microscopic in size (called "microbleeds"), causing limited damage and few significant symptoms. (Generally, microbleeds do not have short-term consequences on brain function, but microbleeds over time can lead to an increased risk of dementia and cognitive disruption.) Even many nonsymptomatic AVMs show evidence of past bleeding. But, massive hemorrhages can occur if the physical stresses caused by extremely high blood pressure, rapid blood flow rates, and vessel wall weakness are great enough. If a large enough volume of blood escapes from a ruptured AVM into the surrounding brain, the result can be a catastrophic stroke. AVMs account for approximately two percent of all hemorrhagic strokes that occur each year.

- Even in the absence of bleeding or significant oxygen depletion, large AVMs can damage the brain or spinal cord simply by their presence. They can range in size from a fraction of an inch to more than two and a half inches in diameter, depending on the number and size of the blood vessels making up the lesion. The larger the lesion, the greater the amount of pressure it exerts on surrounding brain or spinal cord structures. The largest lesions may compress several inches of the spinal cord or distort the shape of an entire hemisphere of the brain. Such massive AVMs can constrict the flow of cerebrospinal fluid (CSF)—a clear liquid that normally nourishes and protects the brain and spinal cord—by distorting or closing the passageways and open chambers (ventricles) inside the brain that allow this fluid to circulate freely. As cerebrospinal fluid accumulates, hydrocephalus results. This fluid buildup further increases the amount of pressure on fragile neurological structures, adding to the damage caused by the AVM itself.

Where Do Neurological Arteriovenous Malformations Tend to Form?

Arteriovenous malformations can form virtually anywhere in the brain or spinal cord—wherever arteries and veins exist. Some are formed from blood vessels located in the dura mater or in the pia mater, the outermost and innermost, respectively, of the three membranes surrounding the brain and spinal cord. (The third membrane, called the "arachnoid," lacks blood vessels.) AVMs of the dura mater affect the function of the spinal cord by transmitting excess pressure to the venous system of the spinal cord. AVMs of the spinal cord affect the function of the spinal cord by hemorrhage, by reducing blood flow to the spinal cord, or by causing excess venous pressure. Spinal AVMs frequently cause attacks of sudden, severe back pain, often concentrated at the roots of nerve fibers where they exit the vertebrae, with pain that is similar to that caused by a slipped disk. These lesions also can cause sensory disturbances, muscle weakness, or paralysis in the parts of the body served by the spinal cord or the damaged nerve fibers. A spinal cord AVM can lead to degeneration of the nerve fibers within the spinal cord below the level of the lesion, causing widespread paralysis in parts of the body controlled by those nerve fibers.

Arteriovenous malformations on the surface of the cerebral hemispheres—the uppermost portions of the brain—exert pressure on the cerebral cortex, the brain's "gray matter." Depending on their location, these AVMs may damage portions of the cerebral cortex involved with thinking, speaking, understanding language, hearing, taste, touch, or initiating and controlling voluntary movements.

Arteriovenous malformations located on the frontal lobe close to the optic nerve or on the occipital lobe (the rear portion of the cerebrum where images are processed) may cause a variety of visual disturbances.

Arteriovenous malformations also can form from blood vessels located deep inside the interior of the cerebrum (the main portion of the brain). These AVMs may compromise the functions of three vital structures: the thalamus, which transmits nerve signals between the spinal cord and upper regions of the brain; the basal ganglia surrounding the thalamus, which coordinates complex movements and plays a role in learning and memory; and the hippocampus, which plays a major role in memory.

Arteriovenous malformations can affect other parts of the brain besides the cerebrum. The hindbrain is formed from two major structures: the cerebellum, which is nestled under the rear portion of the cerebrum, and the brain stem, which serves as the bridge linking the upper portions of the brain with the spinal cord. These structures control finely coordinated movements, maintain balance, and regulate some functions of internal organs, including those of the heart and lungs. AVM damage to these parts of the hindbrain can result in dizziness; giddiness; vomiting; a loss of the ability to coordinate complex movements, such as walking; or uncontrollable muscle tremors.

What Are the Health Consequences of Arteriovenous Malformations?

The greatest potential danger posed by AVMs is hemorrhage. Most episodes of bleeding remain undetected at the time they occur because they are not severe enough to cause significant neurological damage. But massive, even fatal, bleeding episodes do occur. Whenever an AVM is detected, the individual should be carefully and consistently monitored for any signs of instability that may indicate an increased risk of hemorrhage.

A few physical characteristics appear to indicate a greater-than-usual likelihood of clinically significant hemorrhage:

- Smaller AVMs have a greater likelihood of bleeding than larger ones.

- Impaired drainage by unusually narrow or deeply situated veins increases the chances of hemorrhage.

- Pregnancy appears to increase the likelihood of clinically significant hemorrhage, mainly because of increases in blood pressure and blood volume.

- Arteriovenous malformations that have hemorrhaged once are about nine times more likely to bleed again during the first year after the initial hemorrhage than are lesions that have never bled.

The damaging effects of a hemorrhage are related to lesion location. Bleeding from AVMs located deep inside the interior tissues, or parenchyma, of the brain typically causes more severe neurological damage than hemorrhage by lesions that have formed in the dural or pial membranes or on the surface of the brain or spinal cord. (Deeply located bleeding is usually referred to as an "intracerebral hemorrhage" or a "parenchymal hemorrhage"; bleeding within the membranes or on the surface of the brain is known as "subdural" or "subarachnoid hemorrhage" (SAH).) Therefore, location is an important factor to consider when weighing the relative risks surgery to treat AVMs.

Section 42.2

Chronic Venous Insufficiency

What Is Chronic Venous Insufficiency?

Chronic venous insufficiency, also known as "phlebitis," "postthrombotic syndrome," or "venous leg ulcer," is a fairly common medical condition in which blood pools in the legs, resulting in increased pressure on blood vessel walls. This condition occurs most often in women, especially after multiple pregnancies, and people who are middle-aged or older. Chronic venous insufficiency affects an estimated 40 percent of people.

Symptoms of Chronic Venous Insufficiency

Chronic venous insufficiency can be painful, sometimes interfering with a person's ability to walk. The most common symptoms of chronic venous insufficiency mimic the symptoms of other medical conditions, sometimes making the disorder difficult to diagnose.

Symptoms of chronic venous insufficiency can include:

- Pain or swelling in the legs or ankles

- Cramps or muscle spasms in the legs

- Tight feeling in the calves

- Itchy or restless feeling in the legs

- Pain when walking that stops when resting

- Brown discoloration of skin on the legs or ankles

- Varicose veins, enlarged or twisted veins close to the skin surface

- Leg ulcers

Causes of Chronic Venous Insufficiency

Chronic venous insufficiency can be an inherited condition. It can also develop due to certain medical conditions, such as deep vein thrombosis or a blood clot in a deep vein. Factors that increase the chances of developing chronic venous insufficiency include obesity, pregnancy, traumatic leg injury, history of blood clots, high blood pressure, extended periods of sitting, lack of exercise, and smoking.

Diagnosis of Chronic Venous Insufficiency

Chronic venous insufficiency is diagnosed through a medical history interview, physical exam, and imaging tests that examine the structure and flow of blood in the veins in the legs.

Treatment of Chronic Venous Insufficiency

Treatment of chronic venous insufficiency varies according to a person's medical history, age, overall health, and the nature and prognosis of the individual case. Treatment options can include simple recommendations, such as wearing compression stockings, elevating (raising) the legs, and exercises to reduce swelling and encourage increased blood flow. Medication is sometimes used to treat chronic venous insufficiency. Therapeutic procedures, such as endovenous laser ablation or radiofrequency ablation, introduce heat into the affected vein, closing the vein and reducing the amount of blood that pools in the leg. Sclerotherapy treatment introduces chemicals to the affected veins by injection, ending the vein's ability to carry blood. Surgical treatments include ligation, in which affected veins are tied off to end blood flow, and a process known as "vein stripping," in which affected veins are removed from the body.

Chronic venous insufficiency can recur even after successful treatments. Long-term treatment plans often focus on maintaining a healthy weight, exercising regularly, wearing compression stockings, and taking prescribed medications regularly.

References

1. "Chronic Venous Insufficiency," University of Rochester Medical Center (URMC), 2016.

2. Henke, Dr. Peter K. "Chronic Venous Insufficiency," Society for Vascular Surgery (SVS), n.d.

Section 42.3

Varicose Veins and Spider Veins

This section includes text excerpted from "Varicose Veins and Spider Veins," Office on Women's Health (OWH), U.S. Department of Health and Human Services (HHS), March 1, 2019.

What Are Varicose Veins?

Varicose veins are twisted veins that can be blue, red, or skin-colored. The larger veins may appear rope-like and make the skin bulge out.

Varicose veins are often on the thighs; the backs and fronts of the calves; or the inside of the legs, near the ankles and feet. During pregnancy, varicose veins can happen around the inner thigh, lower pelvic area, and buttocks.

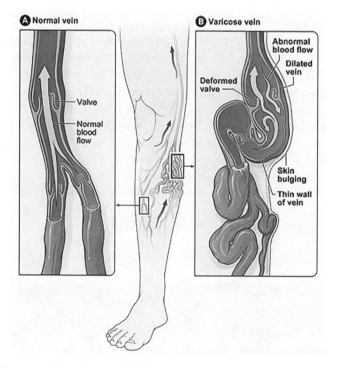

Figure 42.1. *Normal Vein and Varicose Vein*

Figure A shows a normal vein with a working valve and normal blood flow. Figure B shows a varicose vein with a deformed valve, abnormal blood flow, and thin, stretched walls. The middle image shows where varicose veins might appear in a leg.

What Are Spider Veins?

Spider veins, or thread veins, are smaller than varicose veins. They are usually red. They may look like tree branches or spider webs. Spider veins can usually be seen under the skin, but they do not make the skin bulge out as varicose veins do.

Spider veins are usually found on the legs or the face.

Who Gets Varicose Veins and Spider Veins

Varicose veins affect almost twice as many women as men and are more common in older women. Spider veins may affect more than half of women.

What Are the Symptoms of Varicose Veins and Spider Veins?

Some women do not have any symptoms with varicose veins and spider veins. If you do have symptoms, your legs may feel extremely tired, heavy, or achy. Your symptoms may get worse after sitting or standing for long periods of time. Your symptoms may get better after resting and putting your legs up.

Other symptoms that may be more common with varicose veins include:

- Throbbing or cramping
- Swelling
- Itching

Changing hormone levels may affect your symptoms. Because of this, you may notice more symptoms during certain times in your menstrual cycle or during pregnancy or menopause.

What Causes Varicose Veins and Spider Veins

Problems in the valves in your veins can prevent blood from flowing normally and cause varicose veins or spider veins.

Your heart pumps blood filled with oxygen and nutrients through your arteries to your whole body. Veins then carry the blood from different parts of your body back to your heart. Normally, your veins have valves that act as one-way flaps. But, if the valves do not close correctly, blood can leak back into the lower part of the vein rather

467

than going toward the heart. Over time, more blood gets stuck in the vein, building pressure that weakens the walls of the vein. This causes the vein to grow larger.

Are Some Women More at Risk of Varicose Veins and Spider Veins?

Yes. Varicose veins and spider veins are caused by damaged valves in the veins that prevent blood from flowing normally. Many things can damage your valves, but your risk of varicose veins and spider veins may be higher if you:

- **Have a family or personal history of varicose veins or spider veins.** In one small study, more than half of women with varicose veins had a parent with varicose veins too.

- **Sit or stand for long periods.** Sitting or standing for a long time, especially for more than four hours at a time, may make your veins work harder against gravity to pump blood to your heart.

- **Are overweight or obese.** Being overweight or obese can put extra pressure on your veins. Women who are obese are more likely to get varicose veins than women at a healthy weight.

- **Are pregnant.** During pregnancy, the amount of blood pumping through your body increases to support the fetus. The extra blood causes your veins to swell. Your growing uterus (womb) also puts pressure on your veins. Varicose veins may go away within a few months after childbirth, or they may remain and continue to cause symptoms. More varicose veins and spider veins may appear with each additional pregnancy.

- **Are older.** As you get older, the valves in your veins may weaken and not work as well. Your calf muscles also weaken as you age. Your calf muscles normally help squeeze veins and send blood back toward the heart as you walk.

- **Use hormonal birth control or menopausal hormone therapy (MHT).** The hormone estrogen may weaken vein valves and lead to varicose veins. Using hormonal birth control, including the pill or a patch, shot, vaginal ring, or intrauterine device (IUD), with estrogen and progesterone, or taking menopausal hormone therapy, may raise your risk of varicose or spider veins.

- **Have a condition that damaged the valves.** Blood clots in the legs or scarring of the veins can damage the valves.

Why Do Varicose Veins and Spider Veins Usually Appear in the Legs?

Varicose veins and spider veins appear most often in the legs. This is because the veins in your legs carry blood to your heart against gravity and for the longest distance of anywhere in the body.

Should I Call My Doctor or Nurse If I Have Varicose Veins or Spider Veins?

Maybe. If you think you have varicose veins or spider veins and they cause you pain or discomfort, talk to your doctor or nurse. Varicose veins and spider veins usually do not cause symptoms. But, you may want to remove or close varicose veins or spider veins if you have symptoms or if you do not like the way they look.

Talk to your doctor or nurse if varicose veins or spider veins cause you pain or if:

- The vein has become swollen, red, or very tender or warm to the touch, which can be a sign of a blood clot.
- You have sores or a rash on your leg or near your ankle.
- The skin on your ankle or calf changes color.
- One of the varicose veins begins to bleed.
- Your symptoms keep you from doing daily activities.

Will I Get Varicose Veins during Pregnancy?

Maybe. During pregnancy, you have more blood pumping through your body to support the fetus. The extra blood can cause your veins to get larger. Your growing uterus also puts pressure on the veins. Varicose veins may appear around the vagina and buttocks.

For some women, varicose veins shrink or disappear after childbirth. For others, varicose veins stay after childbirth, and symptoms continue to get worse. Women may also get more varicose veins or spider veins with each additional pregnancy.

Chapter 43

Aneurysm

Chapter Contents

Section 43.1

Aortic Aneurysm

This section includes text excerpted from "Aortic
Aneurysm Fact Sheet," Centers for Disease Control
and Prevention (CDC), June 16, 2016.

What Is Aortic Aneurysm?

An aortic aneurysm is a balloon-like bulge in the aorta, the large
artery that carries blood from the heart through the chest and torso.

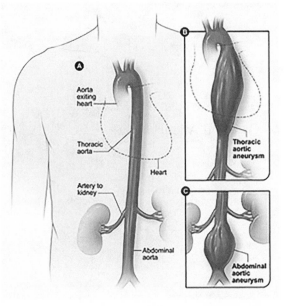

Figure 43.1. *Normal Aorta, Thoracic Aortic Aneurysm, and Abdominal
Aortic Aneurysm* (Source: National Heart, Lung, and Blood Institute
(NHLBI).)

*Figure A shows a normal aorta. Figure B shows a thoracic aortic aneurysm located
behind the heart. Figure C shows an abdominal aortic aneurysm located below the
arteries that supply blood to the kidneys.*

Aortic aneurysms work in two ways:

• The force of the blood pumping can split the layers of the artery
wall, allowing blood to leak in between them. This process is
called "dissection."

- The aneurysm can burst completely, causing bleeding inside the body. This is called a "rupture."

- Dissections and ruptures are the cause of most deaths from aortic aneurysms.

Aortic aneurysms were the primary cause of 9,863 deaths in 2014 and a contributing cause in more than 17,215 deaths in the United States in 2009.

About two-thirds of people who have an aortic dissection are male.

The U.S. Preventive Services Task Force (USPSTF) recommends that men between the ages of 65 and 75 who have smoked should get an ultrasound screening for abdominal aortic aneurysms (AAA), even if they have no symptoms.

Types of Aortic Aneurysm
Thoracic Aortic Aneurysms

A thoracic aortic aneurysm occurs in the chest. Men and women are equally likely to get thoracic aortic aneurysms, which become more common as you age.

Thoracic aortic aneurysms are usually caused by high blood pressure or sudden injury. Sometimes, people with inherited connective tissue disorders, such as Marfan syndrome (MFS) and Ehlers-Danlos syndrome (EDS), get thoracic aortic aneurysms.

Signs and symptoms of a thoracic aortic aneurysm can include:

- Sharp, sudden pain in the chest or upper back

- Shortness of breath

- Trouble breathing or swallowing

Abdominal Aortic Aneurysms

An abdominal aortic aneurysm occurs below the chest. Abdominal aortic aneurysms happen more often than thoracic aortic aneurysms.

Abdominal aortic aneurysms are more common in men and among people 65 years of age and older. Abdominal aortic aneurysms are less common among Blacks when compared to Whites.

Abdominal aortic aneurysms are usually caused by atherosclerosis (hardened arteries), but infection or injury can also cause them.

Abdominal aortic aneurysms often do not have any symptoms. If an individual does have symptoms, they can include:

- Throbbing or deep pain in your back or side

- Pain in the buttocks, groin, or legs

Other Types of Aneurysms

Aneurysms can occur in other parts of your body. A ruptured aneurysm in the brain can cause a stroke. Peripheral aneurysms—those found in arteries other than the aorta—can occur in the neck, in the groin, or behind the knees. These aneurysms are less likely to rupture or dissect than aortic aneurysms, but they can form blood clots. These clots can break away and block blood flow through the artery.

Risk Factors for Aortic Aneurysm

Diseases that damage your heart and blood vessels also increase your risk for an aortic aneurysm. These diseases include:

- High blood pressure

- High cholesterol

- Atherosclerosis

- Smoking

Some inherited connective tissue disorders, such as MFS and EDS, can also increase your risk for an aortic aneurysm. Your family may also have a history of aortic aneurysms that can increase your risk.

Unhealthy behaviors can also increase your risk for aortic aneurysm, especially for people who have one of the diseases listed above. Tobacco use is the most important behavior related to an aortic aneurysm. People who have a history of smoking are three to five times more likely to develop an abdominal aortic aneurysm.

Section 43.2

Cerebral Aneurysm

This section includes text excerpted from "Cerebral
Aneurysms Fact Sheet," National Institute of
Neurological Disorders and Stroke (NINDS), July 6, 2018.

What Is a Cerebral Aneurysm?

A cerebral aneurysm (also known as a "brain aneurysm") is a weak
or thin spot on an artery in the brain that balloons or bulges out and
fills with blood. The bulging aneurysm can put pressure on the nerves
or brain tissue. It may also burst or rupture, spilling blood into the
surrounding tissue (called a "hemorrhage"). A ruptured aneurysm
can cause serious health problems, such as hemorrhagic stroke, brain
damage, coma, and even death.

Some cerebral aneurysms, particularly those that are very small,
do not bleed or cause other problems. These types of aneurysms are
usually detected during imaging tests for other medical conditions.
Cerebral aneurysms can occur anywhere in the brain, but most form
in the major arteries along the base of the skull.

Brain aneurysms can occur in anyone and at any age. They are
most common in adults between the ages of 30 and 60 and are more
common in women than in men. People with certain inherited disorders are also at a higher risk.

All cerebral aneurysms have the potential to rupture and cause
bleeding within the brain or surrounding area. Approximately 30,000
Americans per year suffer a brain aneurysm rupture. Much less is
known about how many people have cerebral aneurysms, since they
do not always cause symptoms.

What Are the Symptoms?
Unruptured Aneurysm

Most cerebral aneurysms do not show symptoms until they either
become very large or rupture. Small unchanging aneurysms generally
will not produce symptoms.

A larger aneurysm that is steadily growing may press on tissues
and nerves causing:

- Pain above and behind the eye

- Numbness

- Weakness

- Paralysis on one side of the face

- A dilated pupil

- Vision changes or double vision

Ruptured Aneurysm

When an aneurysm ruptures, one always experiences a sudden and extremely severe headache and may also develop:

- Double vision

- Nausea

- Vomiting

- Stiff neck

- Sensitivity to light

- Seizures

- Loss of consciousness (this may happen briefly or may be prolonged)

- Cardiac arrest

Leaking Aneurysm

Sometimes, an aneurysm may leak a small amount of blood into the brain (called a "sentinel bleed"). Sentinel or warning headaches may result from an aneurysm that suffers a tiny leak, days or weeks prior to a significant rupture. However, only a minority of individuals have a sentinel headache prior to rupture.

If you experience a sudden, severe headache, especially when it is combined with any other symptoms, you should seek immediate medical attention.

How Are Aneurysms Classified?
Type

There are three types of cerebral aneurysms:

- **Saccular aneurysm.** A saccular aneurysm is a rounded sac containing blood that is attached to the main artery or one of its branches. Also known as a "berry aneurysm" (because it resembles a berry hanging from a vine), this is the most common form of cerebral aneurysm. It is typically found on arteries at the base of the brain. Saccular aneurysms occur most often in adults and are found in about two to three percent of the population.

- **Fusiform aneurysm.** A fusiform aneurysm balloons or bulges out on all sides of the artery.

- **Mycotic aneurysm.** A mycotic aneurysm occurs as the result of an infection that can sometimes affect the arteries in the brain. The infection weakens the artery wall, causing a bulging aneurysm to form.

Size

Aneurysms are also classified by size: small, large, and giant.

- Small aneurysms are less than 11 millimeters in diameter (about the size of a large pencil eraser).

- Large aneurysms are 11 to 25 millimeters (about the width of a dime).

- Giant aneurysms are greater than 25 millimeters in diameter (more than the width of a quarter).

What Causes a Cerebral Aneurysm

Cerebral aneurysms form when the walls of the arteries in the brain become thin and weaken. Aneurysms typically form at branch points in arteries because these sections are the weakest. Occasionally, cerebral aneurysms may be present from birth, usually resulting from an abnormality in an artery wall.

Risk Factors for Developing an Aneurysm

Sometimes, cerebral aneurysms are the result of inherited risk factors, including:

- Genetic connective tissue disorders that weaken artery walls

- Polycystic kidney disease (PKD) (in which numerous cysts form in the kidneys)

- Arteriovenous malformations (AVMs) (snarled tangles of arteries and veins in the brain that disrupt blood flow. Some AVMs develop sporadically, or on their own.)

- History of aneurysm in a first-degree family member (child, sibling, or parent)

Other risk factors develop over time and include:

- Untreated high blood pressure

- Cigarette smoking

- Drug abuse, especially cocaine or amphetamines, which raise your blood pressure to dangerous levels. Intravenous (IV) drug abuse is a cause of infectious mycotic aneurysms.

- Being older than 40 years of age

Less common risk factors include:

- Head trauma

- A brain tumor

- An infection in the arterial wall (mycotic aneurysm)

Additionally, high blood pressure, cigarette smoking, diabetes, and high cholesterol puts one at risk of atherosclerosis (a blood vessel disease in which fats buildup on the inside of artery walls), which can increase the risk of developing a fusiform aneurysm.

Risk Factors for an Aneurysm to Rupture

Not all aneurysms will rupture. Aneurysm characteristics, such as size, location, and growth during follow-up evaluation, may affect the risk of an aneurysm rupture. In addition, medical conditions may influence aneurysm rupture.

Risk factors include:

- **Smoking.** Smoking is linked to both the development and rupture of cerebral aneurysms. Smoking may even cause multiple aneurysms to form in the brain.

- **High blood pressure.** High blood pressure damages and weakens arteries, making them more likely to form and to rupture.

- **Size.** The largest aneurysms are the ones most likely to rupture in a person who previously did not show symptoms.

- **Location.** Aneurysms located on the posterior communicating arteries (a pair of arteries in the back part of the brain) and possibly those on the anterior communicating artery (a single artery in the front of the brain) have a higher risk of rupturing than those at other locations in the brain.

- **Growth.** Aneurysms that grow, even if they are small, are at an increased risk of rupture.

- **Family history.** A family history of aneurysm rupture suggests a higher risk of rupture for aneurysms detected in family members.

- The greatest risk occurs in individuals with multiple aneurysms who have already suffered a previous rupture or sentinel bleed.

What Are the Complications of a Ruptured Cerebral Aneurysm?

Aneurysms may rupture and bleed into the space between the skull and the brain (subarachnoid hemorrhage) and sometimes into the brain tissue (intracerebral hemorrhage). These are forms of stroke called "hemorrhagic stroke." The bleeding into the brain can cause a wide spectrum of symptoms, from a mild headache to permanent damage to the brain, or even death.

After an aneurysm has ruptured, it may cause serious complications such as:

- **Rebleeding.** Once it has ruptured, an aneurysm may rupture again before it is treated, leading to further bleeding into the brain and causing more damage or death.

- **Change in sodium level.** Bleeding in the brain can disrupt the balance of sodium in the blood supply and cause swelling in brain cells. This can result in permanent brain damage.

- **Hydrocephalus.** Subarachnoid hemorrhage can cause hydrocephalus. Hydrocephalus is a buildup of too much cerebrospinal fluid in the brain, which causes pressure that can lead to permanent brain damage or death. Hydrocephalus occurs frequently after subarachnoid hemorrhage because the blood blocks the normal flow of cerebrospinal fluid. If left untreated, increased pressure inside the head can cause coma or death.

- **Vasospasm.** This occurs frequently after subarachnoid hemorrhage when the bleeding causes the arteries in the brain to contract and limit blood flow to vital areas of the brain. This can cause strokes from a lack of adequate blood flow to parts of the brain.

- **Seizures.** Aneurysm bleeding can cause seizures (convulsions), either at the time of bleeding or in the immediate aftermath. While most seizures are evident, on occasion, they may only be seen by sophisticated brain testing. Untreated seizures or those that do not respond to treatment can cause brain damage.

What Is the Prognosis?

An unruptured aneurysm may go unnoticed throughout a person's lifetime and not cause symptoms.

After an aneurysm bursts, the person's prognosis largely depends on:

- Age and general health
- Preexisting neurological conditions
- Location of the aneurysm
- The extent of bleeding (and rebleeding)
- The time between rupture and medical attention
- Successful treatment of the aneurysm.

About 25 percent of individuals whose cerebral aneurysm has ruptured do not survive the first 24 hours; another 25 percent die from complications within 6 months. People who experience subarachnoid hemorrhage may have permanent neurological damage. Other individuals recover with little or no disability. Diagnosing and treating a cerebral aneurysm as soon as possible will help increase the chances of making a full recovery.

Recovery from treatment or rupture may take weeks to months.

Chapter 44

Atherosclerosis

What Is Atherosclerosis?

Atherosclerosis is a disease in which plaque builds up inside your arteries. Arteries are blood vessels that carry oxygen-rich blood to your heart and other parts of your body.

Plaque is made up of fat, cholesterol, calcium, and other substances found in the blood. Over time, plaque hardens and narrows your arteries. This limits the flow of oxygen-rich blood to your organs and other parts of your body.

Atherosclerosis can lead to serious problems, including heart attack, stroke, or even death.

Atherosclerosis-Related Diseases

Atherosclerosis can affect any artery in the body, including arteries in the heart, brain, arms, legs, pelvis, and kidneys. As a result, different diseases may develop based on which arteries are affected.

Ischemic Heart Disease

Ischemic heart disease happens when the arteries of the heart cannot deliver enough oxygen-rich blood to the tissues of the heart when it is needed during periods of stress or physical effort.

This chapter includes text excerpted from "Atherosclerosis," National Heart, Lung, and Blood Institute (NHLBI), February 5, 2019.

Coronary heart disease, also called "coronary artery disease," is a type of ischemic heart disease caused by the buildup of plaque in the coronary arteries that supply oxygen-rich blood to your heart.

This buildup can partially or totally block blood flow in the large arteries of the heart. If blood flow to your heart muscle is reduced or blocked, you may have angina (chest pain or discomfort) or a heart attack.

Coronary microvascular disease is another type of ischemic heart disease. It occurs when the heart's tiny arteries do not function normally.

Carotid Artery Disease

Carotid artery disease occurs if plaque builds up in the arteries on each side of your neck (the carotid arteries). These arteries supply oxygen-rich blood to your brain. If blood flow to your brain is reduced or blocked, you may have a stroke.

Peripheral Artery Disease

Peripheral artery disease (PAD) occurs if plaque builds up in the major arteries that supply oxygen-rich blood to your legs, arms, and pelvis.

If blood flow to these parts of your body is reduced or blocked, you may have numbness, pain, and, sometimes, dangerous infections.

Chronic Kidney Disease

Chronic kidney disease can occur if plaque builds up in the renal arteries. These arteries supply oxygen-rich blood to your kidneys.

Over time, chronic kidney disease causes a slow loss of kidney function. The main function of the kidneys is to remove waste and extra water from the body.

Causes of Atherosclerosis

The exact cause of atherosclerosis is not known. However, studies show that atherosclerosis is a slow, complex disease that may start in childhood. It develops faster as you age.

Atherosclerosis may start when certain factors damage the inner layers of the arteries. These factors include:

- Smoking

- High amounts of certain fats and cholesterol in the blood

- High blood pressure

- High amounts of sugar in the blood due to insulin resistance or diabetes

Plaque may begin to build up to where the arteries are damaged. Over time, plaque hardens and narrows the arteries. Eventually, an area of plaque can rupture (break open).

When this happens, blood cell fragments called "platelets" stick to the site of the injury. They may clump together to form blood clots. Clots narrow the arteries even more, limiting the flow of oxygen-rich blood to your body.

Depending on which arteries are affected, blood clots can worsen angina or cause a heart attack or stroke.

Researchers continue to look for the causes of atherosclerosis. They hope to find answers to questions such as:

- Why and how do the arteries become damaged?

- How does plaque develop and change over time?

- Why does plaque rupture and lead to blood clots?

Risk Factors of Atherosclerosis

The exact cause of atherosclerosis is not known. However, certain traits, conditions, or habits may raise your risk for the disease. These conditions are known as "risk factors." The more risk factors you have, the more likely it is that you will develop atherosclerosis.

You can control most risk factors and help prevent or delay atherosclerosis. Other risk factors cannot be controlled.

Major Risk Factors

- **Unhealthy blood cholesterol levels.** This includes high low-density lipoprotein (LDL) cholesterol (sometimes called "bad" cholesterol) and low high-density lipoprotein (HDL) cholesterol (sometimes called "good" cholesterol).

- **High blood pressure.** Blood pressure is considered high if it stays at or above 140/90 mmHg over time. If you have diabetes or chronic kidney disease, high blood pressure is defined as 130/80 mmHg or higher. (The mmHg is millimeters of mercury—the units used to measure blood pressure.)

- **Smoking.** Smoking can damage and tighten blood vessels, raise cholesterol levels, and raise blood pressure. Smoking also does not allow enough oxygen to reach the body's tissues.

- **Insulin resistance.** This condition occurs if the body cannot use its insulin properly. Insulin is a hormone that helps move blood sugar into cells where it is used as an energy source. Insulin resistance may lead to diabetes.

- **Diabetes.** With this disease, the body's blood sugar level is too high because the body does not make enough insulin or does not use its insulin properly.

- **Being overweight or obese.** The terms "overweight" and "obesity" refer to body weight that is greater than what is considered healthy for a certain height.

- **Lack of physical activity.** A lack of physical activity can worsen other risk factors for atherosclerosis, such as unhealthy blood cholesterol levels, high blood pressure, diabetes, and being overweight or obese.

- **Unhealthy diet.** An unhealthy diet can raise your risk for atherosclerosis. Foods that are high in saturated and trans fats, cholesterol, sodium (salt), and sugar can worsen other atherosclerosis risk factors.

- **Older age.** As you get older, your risk for atherosclerosis increases. Genetic or lifestyle factors cause plaque to build up in your arteries as you age. By the time you are middle-aged or older, enough plaque has built up to cause signs or symptoms. In men, the risk increases after the age of 45. In women, the risk increases after the age of 55.

- **Family history of early heart disease.** Your risk for atherosclerosis increases if your father or a brother was diagnosed with heart disease before 55 years of age, or if your mother or a sister was diagnosed with heart disease before 65 years of age.

Although age and a family history of early heart disease are risk factors, it does not mean that you will develop atherosclerosis if you have one or both. Controlling other risk factors often can lessen genetic influences and prevent atherosclerosis, even in older adults.

Studies show that an increasing number of children and youth are at risk for atherosclerosis. This is due to a number of causes, including rising childhood obesity rates.

Emerging Risk Factors

Scientists continue to study other possible risk factors for atherosclerosis.

High levels of a protein called "C-reactive protein" (CRP) in the blood may raise the risk for atherosclerosis and heart attack. High levels of CRP are a sign of inflammation in the body.

Inflammation is the body's response to injury or infection. Damage to the arteries' inner walls seems to trigger inflammation and help plaque grow.

People who have low CRP levels may develop atherosclerosis at a slower rate than people who have high CRP levels. Research is to find out whether reducing inflammation and lowering CRP levels also can reduce the risk for atherosclerosis.

High levels of triglycerides in the blood also may raise the risk for atherosclerosis, especially in women. Triglycerides are a type of fat.

Studies are underway to find out whether genetics may play a role in atherosclerosis risk.

Other Factors That Affect Atherosclerosis

Other factors also may raise your risk for atherosclerosis, such as:

- **Sleep apnea.** Sleep apnea is a disorder that causes one or more pauses in breathing or shallow breaths while you sleep. Untreated sleep apnea can raise your risk for high blood pressure, diabetes, and even a heart attack or stroke.

- **Stress.** Research shows that the most commonly reported trigger for a heart attack is an emotionally upsetting event, especially one involving anger.

- **Alcohol.** Heavy drinking can damage the heart muscle and worsen other risk factors for atherosclerosis. Men should have no more than two drinks containing alcohol a day. Women should have no more than one drink containing alcohol a day.

Screening and Prevention of Atherosclerosis

Taking action to control your risk factors can help prevent or delay atherosclerosis and its related diseases. Your risk for atherosclerosis increases with the number of risk factors you have.

One step you can take is to adopt a healthy lifestyle, which can include:

- **Heart-healthy eating.** Adopt heart-healthy eating habits, which include eating different fruits and vegetables (including beans and peas), whole grains, lean meats, poultry without skin, seafood, and fat-free or low-fat milk and dairy products. A heart-healthy diet is low in sodium, added sugar, solid fats, and refined grains. Following a heart-healthy diet is an important part of a healthy lifestyle.

- **Physical activity.** Be as physically active as you can. Physical activity can improve your fitness level and your health. Ask your doctor what types and amounts of activity are safe for you.

- **Quit smoking.** If you smoke, quit. Smoking can damage and tighten blood vessels and raise your risk for atherosclerosis. Talk with your doctor about programs and products that can help you quit. Also, try to avoid secondhand smoke.

- **Weight control.** If you are overweight or obese, work with your doctor to create a reasonable weight-loss plan. Controlling your weight helps you control risk factors for atherosclerosis.

Other steps that can prevent or delay atherosclerosis include knowing your family history of atherosclerosis. If you or someone in your family has an atherosclerosis-related disease, be sure to tell your doctor.

If lifestyle changes are not enough, your doctor may prescribe medicines to control your atherosclerosis risk factors. Take all of your medicines as your doctor advises.

Taking action to control your risk factors can help prevent or delay atherosclerosis and its related diseases. Your risk for atherosclerosis increases with the number of risk factors you have.

Signs, Symptoms, and Complications of Atherosclerosis

Atherosclerosis usually does not cause signs and symptoms until it severely narrows or totally blocks an artery. Many people do not know they have the disease until they have a medical emergency, such as a heart attack or stroke.

Some people may have signs and symptoms of the disease. Signs and symptoms will depend on which arteries are affected.

Coronary Arteries

The coronary arteries supply oxygen-rich blood to your heart. If plaque narrows or blocks these arteries (causing a disease called "ischemic heart disease"), a common symptom is angina. Angina is chest pain or discomfort that occurs when your heart muscle does not get enough oxygen-rich blood.

Angina may feel like pressure or squeezing in your chest. You also may feel it in your shoulders, arms, neck, jaw, or back. Angina pain may even feel like indigestion. The pain tends to get worse with activity and go away with rest. Emotional stress also can trigger the pain.

Other symptoms of ischemic heart disease are shortness of breath and arrhythmias. Arrhythmias are problems with the rate or rhythm of the heartbeat.

Plaque also can form in the heart's smallest arteries. This disease is called "coronary microvascular disease" (MVD). Symptoms of coronary MVD include angina, shortness of breath, sleep problems, fatigue (tiredness), and lack of energy.

Carotid Arteries

The carotid arteries supply oxygen-rich blood to your brain. If plaque narrows or blocks these arteries (a disease called "carotid artery disease"), you may have symptoms of a stroke. These symptoms may include:

- Sudden weakness

- Paralysis (an inability to move) or numbness of the face, arms, or legs, especially on one side of the body

- Confusion

- Trouble speaking or understanding speech

- Trouble seeing in one or both eyes

- Problems breathing

- Dizziness, trouble walking, loss of balance or coordination, and unexplained falls

- Loss of consciousness

- Sudden and severe headache

Peripheral Arteries

Plaque also can build up in the major arteries that supply oxygen-rich blood to the legs, arms, and pelvis (a disease called "peripheral artery disease").

If these major arteries are narrowed or blocked, you may have numbness, pain, and, sometimes, dangerous infections.

Renal Arteries

The renal arteries supply oxygen-rich blood to your kidneys. If plaque builds up in these arteries, you may develop chronic kidney disease. Over time, chronic kidney disease causes a slow loss of kidney function.

Early kidney disease often has no signs or symptoms. As the disease gets worse, it can cause tiredness, changes in how you urinate (more often or less often), loss of appetite, nausea, swelling in the hands or feet, itchiness or numbness, and trouble concentrating.

Living with Atherosclerosis

Improved treatments have reduced the number of deaths from atherosclerosis-related diseases. These treatments also have improved the quality of life for people who have these diseases.

Adopting a healthy lifestyle may help you prevent or delay atherosclerosis and the problems it can cause. This, along with ongoing medical care, can help you avoid the problems of atherosclerosis and live a long, healthy life.

Researchers continue to look for ways to improve the health of people who have atherosclerosis or may develop it.

Ongoing Care

If you have atherosclerosis, work closely with your doctor and other healthcare providers to avoid serious problems, such as heart attack and stroke.

Follow your treatment plan, and take all of your medicines as your doctor prescribes. Your doctor will let you know how often you should schedule office visits or blood tests. Be sure to let your doctor know if you have new or worsening symptoms.

Emotional Issues and Support

Having an atherosclerosis-related disease may cause fear, anxiety, depression, and stress. Talk about how you feel with your doctor.

Talking to a professional counselor also can help. If you are very depressed, your doctor may recommend medicines or other treatments that can improve your quality of life.

Community resources are available to help you learn more about atherosclerosis. Contact your local public health departments, hospitals, and local chapters of national health organizations to learn more about available resources in your area.

Talk about your lifestyle changes with your family and friends— whoever can provide support or needs to understand why you are changing your habits.

Family and friends may be able to help you make lifestyle changes. For example, they can help you plan healthier meals. Because atherosclerosis tends to run in families, your lifestyle changes may help many of your family members too.

Part Five

Diagnosing and Treating Blood and Circulatory Disorders

Chapter 45

Blood Tests

Chapter Contents

Section 45.1

Blood Tests: An Overview

This section includes text excerpted from "Blood Tests,"
National Heart, Lung, and Blood Institute (NHLBI),
August 4, 2015. Reviewed June 2019.

What Are Blood Tests?

Blood tests help doctors check for certain diseases and conditions. They also help check the function of your organs and show how well treatments are working.

Specifically, blood tests can help doctors:

- Evaluate how well organs—such as the kidneys, liver, thyroid, and heart—are working

- Diagnose diseases and conditions, such as cancer, human immunodeficiency virus (HIV)/acquired immunodeficiency syndrome (AIDS), diabetes, anemia, and coronary heart disease

- Find out whether you have risk factors for heart disease

- Check whether medicines you are taking are working

- Assess how well your blood is clotting

Types of Blood Tests

Some of the most common blood tests are:

- A complete blood count (CBC)

- Blood chemistry tests

- Blood enzyme tests

- Blood tests to assess heart disease risk

Complete Blood Count

The complete blood count is one of the most common blood tests. It is often done as part of a routine checkup.

The complete blood count can help detect blood diseases and disorders, such as anemia, infections, clotting problems, blood cancers, and immune system disorders. This test measures many different parts of your blood, as discussed in the following paragraphs.

Red Blood Cells

Red blood cells (RBCs) carry oxygen from your lungs to the rest of your body. Abnormal red blood cell levels may be a sign of anemia, dehydration (too little fluid in the body), bleeding, or another disorder.

White Blood Cells

White blood cells (WBCs) are part of your immune system, which fights infections and diseases. Abnormal white blood cell levels may be a sign of infection, blood cancer, or an immune system disorder.

A complete blood count measures the overall number of white blood cells in your blood. A CBC with differential looks at the amounts of different types of white blood cells in your blood.

Platelets

Platelets are blood cell fragments that help your blood clot. They stick together to seal cuts or breaks on blood vessel walls and to stop bleeding.

Abnormal platelet levels may be a sign of a bleeding disorder (not enough clotting) or a thrombotic disorder (too much clotting).

Hemoglobin

Hemoglobin is an iron-rich protein in red blood cells that carries oxygen. Abnormal hemoglobin levels may be a sign of anemia, sickle cell anemia, thalassemia, or other blood disorders.

If you have diabetes, excess glucose in your blood can attach to hemoglobin and raise the level of hemoglobin A1c.

Hematocrit

Hematocrit is a measure of how much space red blood cells take up in your blood. A high hematocrit level might mean that you are dehydrated. A low hematocrit level might mean that you have anemia. Abnormal hematocrit levels also may be a sign of a blood or bone marrow disorder.

Mean Corpuscular Volume

Mean corpuscular volume (MCV) is a measure of the average size of your red blood cells. Abnormal MCV levels may be a sign of anemia or thalassemia.

Blood Chemistry Tests / Basic Metabolic Panel

The basic metabolic panel (BMP) is a group of tests that measures different chemicals in the blood. These tests usually are done on the fluid (plasma) part of blood. The tests can give doctors information about your muscles (including the heart); bones; and organs, such as the kidneys and liver.

The basic metabolic panel includes blood glucose, calcium, and electrolyte tests, as well as blood tests that measure kidney function. Some of these tests require you to fast (not eat any food) before the test, and others do not. Your doctor will tell you how to prepare for the test(s) you are having.

Blood Glucose

Glucose is a type of sugar that the body uses for energy. Abnormal glucose levels in your blood may be a sign of diabetes.

For some blood glucose tests, you have to fast before your blood is drawn. Other blood glucose tests are done after a meal or at any time with no preparation.

Calcium

Calcium is an important mineral in the body. Abnormal calcium levels in the blood may be a sign of kidney problems, bone disease, thyroid disease, cancer, malnutrition, or another disorder.

Electrolytes

Electrolytes are minerals that help maintain fluid levels and acid-base balance in the body. They include sodium, potassium, bicarbonate, and chloride.

Abnormal electrolyte levels may be a sign of dehydration, kidney disease, liver disease, heart failure, high blood pressure, or other disorders.

Kidneys

Blood tests for kidney function measure levels of blood urea nitrogen (BUN) and creatinine. Both of these are waste products that the kidneys filter out of the body. Abnormal BUN and creatinine levels may be signs of a kidney disease or disorder.

Blood Enzyme Tests

Enzymes are chemicals that help control chemical reactions in your body. There are many blood enzyme tests. This section focuses on blood enzyme tests used to check for heart attack. These include troponin and creatine kinase (CK) tests.

Troponin

Troponin is a muscle protein that helps your muscles contract. When muscle or heart cells are injured, troponin leaks out, and its levels in your blood rise.

For example, blood levels of troponin rise when you have a heart attack. For this reason, doctors often order troponin tests when patients have chest pain or other heart attack signs and symptoms.

Creatine Kinase

A blood product called "CK-MB" is released when the heart muscle is damaged. High levels of CK-MB in the blood can mean that you have had a heart attack.

Blood Tests to Assess Heart Disease Risk

A lipoprotein panel is a blood test that can help show whether you are at risk for coronary heart disease (CHD). This test looks at substances in your blood that carry cholesterol.

A lipoprotein panel gives information about your:

- Total cholesterol
- Low-density lipoprotein (LDL) ("bad") cholesterol. This is the main source of cholesterol buildup and blockages in the arteries.
- High-density lipoprotein (HDL) ("good") cholesterol. This type of cholesterol helps decrease blockages in the arteries.
- Triglycerides. Triglycerides are a type of fat in your blood.

A lipoprotein panel measures the levels of LDL and HDL cholesterol and triglycerides in your blood. Abnormal cholesterol and triglyceride levels may be signs of increased risk for CHD.

Most people will need to fast for 9 to 12 hours before a lipoprotein panel.

497

Blood Clotting Tests

Blood clotting tests are sometimes called a "coagulation panel." These tests check proteins in your blood that affect the blood clotting process. Abnormal test results might suggest that you are at risk of bleeding or developing clots in your blood vessels.

Your doctor may recommend these tests if she or he thinks you have a disorder or disease related to blood clotting.

Blood clotting tests also are used to monitor people who are taking medicines to lower the risk of blood clots. Warfarin and heparin are two examples of such medicines.

What to Expect with Blood Tests

What to Expect before Blood Tests

Many blood tests do not require any special preparation and take only a few minutes.

Other blood tests require fasting for 8 to 12 hours before the test. Your doctor will tell you how to prepare for your blood test(s).

What to Expect during Blood Tests

Blood is usually drawn from a vein in your arm or other part of your body using a needle. It also can be drawn using a finger prick.

The person who draws your blood might tie a band around the upper part of your arm or ask you to make a fist. Doing this can make the veins in your arm stick out more, which makes it easier to insert the needle.

The needle that goes into your vein is attached to a small test tube. The person who draws your blood removes the tube when it is full, and the tube seals on its own. The needle is then removed from your vein. If you are getting a few blood tests, more than one test tube may be attached to the needle before it is withdrawn.

Some people get nervous about blood tests because they are afraid of needles. Others may not want to see blood leaving their bodies.

If you are nervous or scared, it can help to look away or talk to someone to distract yourself. You might feel a slight sting when the needle goes in or comes out.

Drawing blood usually takes less than three minutes.

What to Expect after Blood Tests

Once the needle is withdrawn, you will be asked to apply gentle pressure with a piece of gauze or bandage to the place where the needle was inserted. This helps stop bleeding. It also helps prevent swelling and bruising.

Most of the time, you can remove the pressure after a minute or two. You may want to keep a bandage on for a few hours.

Usually, you do not need to do anything else after a blood test. Results can take anywhere from a few minutes to a few weeks to come back. Your doctor should get the results. It is important that you follow up with your doctor to discuss your test results.

What Are the Risks of Blood Tests?

The main risks of blood tests are discomfort and bruising at the site where the needle goes in. These complications usually are minor and go away shortly after the tests are done.

What Do Blood Tests Show?

Blood tests show whether the levels of different substances in your blood fall within a normal range.

For many blood substances, the normal range is the range of levels seen in 95 percent of healthy people in a certain group. For many tests, normal ranges vary depending on your age, sex, race, and other factors.

Your blood test results may fall outside the normal range for many reasons. Abnormal results might be a sign of a disorder or disease. Other factors—such as diet, menstrual cycle, physical activity level, alcohol intake, and medicines (both prescription and over-the-counter)—also can cause abnormal results.

Your doctor should discuss any unusual or abnormal blood test results with you. These results may or may not suggest a health problem.

Many diseases and medical problems cannot be diagnosed with blood tests alone. However, blood tests can help you and your doctor learn more about your health. Blood tests also can help find potential problems early, when treatments or lifestyle changes may work best.

Result Ranges for Common Blood Tests

This section presents the result ranges for some of the most common blood tests.

NOTE: *All values in this section are for adults only. They do not apply to children. Talk to your child's doctor about values on blood tests for children.*

Complete Blood Count

The table below shows some normal ranges for different parts of the complete blood count test. Some of the normal ranges differ between men and women. Other factors, such as age and race, also may affect normal ranges.

Your doctor should discuss your results with you. She or he will advise you further if your results are outside the normal range for your group.

Table 45.1. Complete Blood Count

Test	Normal Range Results*
Red blood cell (varies with altitude)	Male: 5 to 6 million cells/mcL
	Female: 4 to 5 million cells/mcL
White blood cell	4,500 to 10,000 cells/mcL
Platelets	140,000 to 450,000 cells/mcL
Hemoglobin (varies with altitude)	Male: 14 to 17 gm/dL
	Female: 12 to 15 gm/dL
Hematocrit (varies with altitude)	Male: 41% to 50%
	Female: 36% to 44%
Mean corpuscular volume	80 to 95 femtoliter†

Cells/mcL = cells per microliter; gm/dL = grams per deciliter.
†*A femtoliter is a measure of volume.*

Blood Glucose

The table below shows the ranges for blood glucose levels after 8 to 12 hours of fasting. It shows the normal range and the abnormal ranges that are a sign of prediabetes or diabetes.

Table 45.2. Blood Glucose

Plasma Glucose Results (mg/dL)*	Diagnosis
70 to 99	Normal
100 to 125	Prediabetes
126 and above	Diabetes†

mg/dL = milligrams per deciliter.
†*The test is repeated on another day to confirm the results.*

Lipoprotein Panel

The table below shows ranges for total cholesterol, LDL cholesterol, and HDL cholesterol levels after 9 to 12 hours of fasting. High blood cholesterol is a risk factor for coronary heart disease.

Your doctor should discuss your results with you. She or he will advise you further if your results are outside the desirable range.

Table 45.3. Lipoprotein Panel

Total Cholesterol Level	Total Cholesterol Category
Less than 200 mg/dL	Desirable
200–239 mg/dL	Borderline high
240 mg/dL and above	High

LDL Cholesterol Level	LDL Cholesterol Category
Less than 100 mg/dL	Optimal
100–129 mg/dL	Near optimal/above optimal
130–159 mg/dL	Borderline high
160–189 mg/dL	High
190 mg/dL and above	Very high

HDL Cholesterol Level	HDL Cholesterol Category
Less than 40 mg/dL	A major risk factor for heart disease
40–59 mg/dL	The higher, the better
60 mg/dL and above	Considered protective against heart disease

Section 45.2

Blood Typing

"Blood Typing," © 2016 Omnigraphics.
Reviewed June 2019.

Blood typing is a classification system used to sort human blood according to the kinds of antigens (blood proteins) found on red blood cells. There are four primary types of blood: A, B, AB, and O. Each blood type is further classified by an Rh positive or negative designation. Rh refers to Rhesus factor and indicates the presence (positive) or absence (negative) of a specific protein found on the surface of red blood cells. Blood type is an inherited trait.

Blood typing is important because not all blood types are compatible with each other. Giving the wrong blood type to a person through a blood transfusion can result in serious complications and even death. Blood typing is especially important for pregnant women. If the expectant mother is Rh-negative and the expectant father is Rh-positive, the mother will need to receive treatment to help protect the fetus from complications that could arise from a mix of incompatible blood types.

Testing Blood Type

Blood type tests are performed for a variety of reasons. Some of the most common include:

- Classification of donated blood

- Preparation for a blood transfusion or any surgery

- Preparation for organ transplant

- When a woman is pregnant or plans to become pregnant

- Identification of individuals (for example, determining blood relations)

The two most common blood typing tests are the ABO and the Rh tests.

The ABO test examines red blood cells in order to classify the blood as A, B, AB, or O. Blood that is type A contains the A antigen, and type B contains the B antigen. These two blood types are incompatible. Each contains antibodies that will attack and destroy the cells of the other. Type AB blood contains both A and B antigens, meaning that it is compatible with both A and B blood types. People with type AB blood can receive blood from anyone of any blood type, making type AB the "universal recipient." Type O blood contains no antigens and can be given to anyone of any blood type. For this reason, type O blood is known as the "universal donor."

To test for blood type, a small amount of blood is mixed with serum containing blood antibodies and observed to see if the sample blood cells agglutinate (stick together). Blood cells that stick together when mixed with Anti-A serum is classified as type A. Type B blood cells stick together when mixed with Anti-B serum. Type AB blood cells stick together when mixed with both Anti-A and Anti-B serums. Blood cells that do not stick together when mixed with Anti-A or Anti-B serums is classified as type O.

A second blood type test is performed to verify the results of the first test. In the second test, known as "back-typing," a small amount of the blood being tested is mixed with a small amount of blood that has already been classified as type A or type B and observed for agglutination. If the sample blood cells stick together when mixed with type B blood, the sample is identified as type A. Conversely, if the sample blood cells stick together when mixed with type A blood, the sample is identified as type B. If the sample blood cells stick together when mixed with either type A or type B blood, the sample is identified as type O. If the sample blood cells do not stick together when mixed with type A or type B blood, the sample is identified as type AB.

The Rh test is performed by mixing a small blood sample with a serum that contains anti-Rh serum. If the sample blood cells stick together when mixed with anti-Rh serum, the blood is Rh-positive. If the sample blood cells do not stick together when mixed with anti-Rh serum, the blood is Rh-negative. People with Rh-negative blood can only receive Rh-negative blood; people with Rh-positive blood can receive either Rh-positive or Rh-negative blood.

The results of both kinds of blood type testing are used for complete identification of blood type. For example, type A blood that is Rh-positive is A-positive, type B blood that is Rh-negative is B-negative, and so on.

Blood Type Compatibility

- A person with A-negative blood can receive types A-negative and O-negative blood.
- A person with A-positive blood can receive types A-negative, A-positive, O-negative, and O-positive blood.

- A person with B-negative blood can receive types B-negative and O-negative blood.

- A person with B-positive blood can receive types B-negative, B-positive, O-negative, and O-positive blood.

- A person with AB-negative blood can receive types AB-negative and O-negative blood.

- A person with AB-positive blood can receive any type of blood.

- A person with O-negative blood can only receive type O-negative blood.

- A person with O-positive blood can receive O-negative or O-positive blood.

References

1. Gersten, Todd. "Blood Typing," MedlinePlus, National Institutes of Health (NIH), February 24, 2014.

2. "Blood Type Test," WebMD, September 9, 2014.

Section 45.3

Complete Blood Count

This section includes text excerpted from "Complete Blood Count (CBC)," MedlinePlus, National Institutes of Health (NIH), May 25, 2017.

What Is a Complete Blood Count?

A complete blood count or CBC is a blood test that measures many different parts and features of your blood, including:

- Red blood cells (RBCs), which carry oxygen from your lungs to the rest of your body

- White blood cells (WBCs), which fight infection. There are five major types of white blood cells. A CBC test measures the total number of white cells in your blood. A test called a "CBC with differential" also measures the number of each type of these white blood cells.

- Platelets, which help your blood to clot and stop bleeding

- Hemoglobin, a protein in red blood cells that carries oxygen from your lungs and to the rest of your body

- Hematocrit, a measurement of how much of your blood is made up of red blood

A complete blood count may also include measurements of chemicals and other substances in your blood. These results can give your healthcare provider important information about your overall health and risk for certain diseases.

Other names for a complete blood count include a "full blood count" and a "blood cell count."

What Is It Used For?

A complete blood count is a commonly performed blood test that is often included as part of a routine checkup. Complete blood counts can be used to help detect a variety of disorders, including infections, anemia, diseases of the immune system, and blood cancers.

Why Do I Need a Complete Blood Count?

Your healthcare provider may have ordered a complete blood count as part of your checkup or to monitor your overall health. In addition, the test may be used to:

- Diagnose a blood disease, infection, immune system disorder, or other medical conditions

- Keep track of an existing blood disorder

What Happens during a Complete Blood Count

A healthcare professional will take a blood sample from a vein in your arm, using a small needle. After the needle is inserted, a small amount of blood will be collected into a test tube or vial. You may feel a little sting when the needle goes in or out. This usually takes less than five minutes.

Will I Need to Do Anything to Prepare for the Test?

You do not need any special preparations for a complete blood count. If your healthcare provider has also ordered other blood tests, you may need to fast (not eat or drink) for several hours before the test. Your healthcare provider will let you know if there are any special instructions to follow.

Are There Any Risks to the Test?

There is very little risk to having a blood test. You may have slight pain or bruising at the spot where the needle was put in, but most symptoms go away quickly.

What Do the Results Mean?

A complete blood count counts the cells and measures the levels of different substances in your blood. There are many reasons your levels may fall outside the normal range. For instance:

- Abnormal red blood cell, hemoglobin, or hematocrit levels may indicate anemia, iron deficiency, or heart disease.

- Low white cell count may indicate an autoimmune disorder, bone marrow disorder, or cancer.

- High white cell count may indicate an infection or reaction to medication.

If any of your levels are abnormal, it does not necessarily indicate a medical problem needing treatment. Diet, activity level, medications, a women's menstrual cycle, and other considerations can affect the results. Talk to your healthcare provider to learn what your results mean.

Is There Anything Else I Need to Know about a Complete Blood Count?

A complete blood count is only one tool your healthcare provider uses to learn about your health. Your medical history, symptoms, and other factors will be considered before a diagnosis. Additional testing and follow-up care may also be recommended.

Section 45.4

Fibrinogen Test

A fibrinogen test, also known as a "Factor I," measures the level of fibrinogen in a person's blood. Fibrinogen is a blood plasma protein that is produced by the liver. It is one of 13 blood elements that help to form blood clots to stop bleeding after an injury. Low fibrinogen affects the body's ability to form blood clots, which can result in excessive bleeding.

Fibrinogen tests are usually performed on people who experience problems with blood clotting, excessive bleeding, or excessive bruising after an injury. Fibrinogen tests are also performed on people who experience blood in their urine or stool, or have had a ruptured spleen or gastrointestinal tract hemorrhage. The test is an important tool in the diagnosis of disseminated intravascular coagulation, a condition in which small blood clots form inside the blood vessels throughout the body.

Testing for elevated levels of fibrinogen is also used to help diagnose or determine the risk of cardiovascular disease (heart disease) or brain aneurysm (stroke). Elevated fibrinogen levels can result from certain health conditions, including acute infections, cancer, coronary heart disease, heart attack, stroke, rheumatoid arthritis, kidney disease, liver disease, peripheral artery disease, and pregnancy. Receiving a blood transfusion, taking certain drugs, and smoking can also cause elevated fibrinogen levels in the body.

Methods

Fibrinogen tests can be conducted using one of four methods. In the Clauss method, plasma drawn from the person being tested is mixed with concentrated thrombin (an enzyme in blood plasma) and analyzed. The time it takes for the blood clot to form is noted and compared against standard measures. Automated equipment senses when the blood clot has formed based on the optical density of the plasma/thrombin mixture.

In PT-derived fibrinogen tests, a baseline measurement for known fibrinogen levels in various diluted plasma samples (the control group) is compared to the fibrinogen levels found in equivalent plasma dilutions created from the blood plasma being tested.

Immunological fibrinogen tests are conducted to measure the fibrinogen protein concentration in blood, rather than fibrinogen function.

Gravimetric fibrinogen tests are used to measure the weight of a clot produced using the Clauss method, instead of measuring the optical density of the clot. Another type of gravimetric fibrinogen test measures the amount of fibrinogen protein present in a blood clot created using the Clauss method.

Results

A normal fibrinogen blood level is typically between 1.5 to 3.0 grams per liter.

Normal reference ranges are usually as follows:

- **Adult:** 200 mg/dl–400 mg/dl

- **Newborn:** 125 mg/dl–300 mg/dl

Fibrinogen levels are considered abnormal if the level is higher or lower than the normal range. An abnormal result may be due to an inherited or acquired conditions, such as:

- **Afibrinogenemia**—absence of fibrinogen in the body

- **Disseminated intravascular coagulation**—too much fibrinogen used by the body

- **Dysfibrinogenemia**—fibrinogen performance malfunction

- **Fibrinolysis**—excessive breakdown of fibrinogen in the body

- **Hemorrhage**—excessive bleeding

- **Hypofibrinogenemia**—too little fibrinogen in the body

- **Placenta abruptio**—the placenta separates from the uterus wall during pregnancy

Spontaneous bleeding will occur when the fibrinogen level falls below 100mg/dl.

Treatment

Fibrinogen deficiency is treatable through the use of blood products that act as a replacement or substitute for the fibrinogen protein in the body. Fibrinogen concentrate may be used to prevent excessive bleeding in people during surgery, during or after childbirth, before dental surgery, or after traumatic injury.

References

1. Chen, Yi-Bin. "Fibrinogen Blood Test," MedlinePlus, National Institutes of Health (NIH), January 27, 2015.

2. Underwood, Corinna. "Fibrinogen," HealthLine, January 4, 2016.

3. "Fibrinogen," Lab Tests Online, April 10, 2014.

4. "Fibrinogen Assays," Practical-Haemostasis.com, n.d.

Chapter 46

Bone Marrow Tests

What Are Bone Marrow Tests?

Bone marrow is a soft, spongy tissue found in the center of most bones. Bone marrow makes different types of blood cells. These include:

- Red blood cells (RBCs), also called "erythrocytes," which carry oxygen from your lungs to every cell in your body

- White blood cells (WBCs), also called "leukocytes," which help you fight infections

- Platelets, which help with blood clotting

Bone marrow tests check to see if your bone marrow is working correctly and making normal amounts of blood cells. The tests can help diagnose and monitor various bone marrow disorders, blood disorders, and certain types of cancer. There are two types of bone marrow tests:

- Bone marrow aspiration, which removes a small amount of bone marrow fluid

- Bone marrow biopsy, which removes a small amount of bone marrow tissue

Bone marrow aspiration and bone marrow biopsy tests are usually performed at the same time.

This chapter includes text excerpted from "Bone Marrow Tests," MedlinePlus, National Institutes of Health (NIH), March 20, 2018.

What Are They Used For?

Bone marrow tests are used to:

- Find out the cause of problems with red blood cells, white blood cells, or platelets

- Diagnose and monitor blood disorders, such as anemia, polycythemia vera, and thrombocytopenia

- Diagnose bone marrow disorders

- Diagnose and monitor certain types of cancers, including leukemia, multiple myeloma, and lymphoma

- Diagnose infections that may have started or spread to the bone marrow

Why Do I Need a Bone Marrow Test?

Your healthcare provider may order a bone marrow aspiration and a bone marrow biopsy if other blood tests show that your levels of red blood cells, white blood cells, or platelets are not normal. Too many or too few of these cells may mean that you have a medical disorder, such as cancer that starts in your blood or bone marrow. If you are being treated for another type of cancer, these tests can find out if the cancer has spread to your bone marrow.

What Happens during a Bone Marrow Test

Bone marrow aspiration and bone marrow biopsy tests are usually given at the same time. A doctor or other healthcare provider will perform the tests. Before the tests, the provider may ask you to put on a hospital gown. The provider will check your blood pressure, heart rate, and temperature. You may be given a mild sedative, a medicine that will help you relax. During the test:

- You will lie down on your side or your stomach, depending on which bone will be used for testing. Most bone marrow tests are taken from the hip bone.

- Your body will be covered with cloth, so that only the area around the testing site is showing.

- The site will be cleaned with an antiseptic.

- You will get an injection of a numbing solution. It may sting.

- Once the area is numb, the healthcare provider will take the sample. You will need to lie very still during the tests.

  - For a bone marrow aspiration, which is usually performed first, the healthcare provider will insert a needle through the bone and pull out bone marrow fluid and cells. You may feel a sharp but brief pain when the needle is inserted.

  - For a bone marrow biopsy, the healthcare provider will use a special tool that twists into the bone to take out a sample of bone marrow tissue. You may feel some pressure on the site while the sample is being taken.

- It takes about 10 minutes to perform both tests.

- After the test, the healthcare provider will cover the site with a bandage.

- Plan to have someone drive you home, since you may be given a sedative before the tests, which may make you drowsy.

Will I Need to Do Anything to Prepare for the Test?

You will be asked to sign a form that gives permission to perform bone marrow tests. Be sure to ask your provider any questions you have about the procedure.

Are There Any Risks to the Test?

Many people feel a little uncomfortable after bone marrow aspiration and bone marrow biopsy testing. After the test, you may feel stiff or sore at the injection site. This usually goes away in a few days. Your healthcare provider may recommend or prescribe a pain reliever to help. Serious symptoms are very rare, but may include:

- Long-lasting pain or discomfort around the injection site

- Redness, swelling, or excessive bleeding at the site

- Fever

If you have any of these symptoms, call your healthcare provider.

What Do the Results Mean?

It may take several days or even several weeks to get your bone marrow test results. The results may show whether you have a bone marrow disease, a blood disorder, or cancer. If you are being treated for cancer, the results may show:

- Whether your treatment is working

- How advanced your disease is

If your results are not normal, your healthcare provider will likely order more tests or discuss treatment options. If you have questions about your results, talk to your healthcare provider.

Chapter 47

Bleeding and Clotting Tests

Chapter Contents

Section 47.1

Bleeding Time

When a person is injured and begins to bleed, blood platelets immediately begin forming clots to seal the wound and prevent further blood loss. This process is known as "hemostasis." A bleeding time test measures platelet function during hemostasis, or the amount of time it takes to stop bleeding after an injury. This test is performed to help diagnose problems with bleeding and blood clotting. Bleeding time tests are most often performed on people who experience excessive bleeding, particularly after minor injuries, such as small cuts or punctures. A bleeding time test may also be performed on people who have a family history of bleeding disorders. It is sometimes performed before surgery to assess a person's risk of excessive bleeding during or after surgery.

To conduct a bleeding time test, a health professional inflates a blood pressure cuff around a person's upper arm. With the cuff inflated, the health professional makes two small cuts on the person's lower arm. These cuts are superficial, similar to a scratch, and just deep enough to cause a very small amount of bleeding. After the cuts are made, the blood pressure cuff is deflated. Special blotting paper is pressed on the cuts every 30 seconds until no more blood is absorbed by the paper, indicating that bleeding has stopped. The health professional notes the length of time it takes for the person to stop bleeding.

Results

During a bleeding time test, healthy people typically stop bleeding within one to nine minutes. A longer bleeding time can indicate blood platelet malfunction. This can mean either the body is producing too many or too few platelets, or the blood platelets may not be working properly. A longer bleeding time can also indicate a blood vessel defect, meaning that there may be a problem in the body's ability to deliver blood throughout the body.

Bleeding time tests are important tools in the diagnosis of certain blood disorders, such as hemophilia, thrombocythemia, and Von Willebrand's disease. Hemophilia is a genetic platelet malfunction that is present at birth. People who live with hemophilia experience excessive bleeding after injury because their bodies have difficulty forming blood clots in deep tissue (for example, in joints and muscles). Von Willebrand's disease is an inherited condition affecting the body's ability to form blood clots after injuries to skin or mucous membranes (for example, inside the nose, mouth, and intestines). Thrombocythemia is a condition in which the body produces too few blood platelets. Some people develop platelet malfunction due to chronic illness.

References

1. Chen, Yi-Bin. "Bleeding Time," MedlinePlus, National Institutes of Health (NIH), January 2, 2015.

2. Krans, Brian. "Bleeding Time Test," HealthLine, December 21, 2015.

Section 47.2

Coagulation Factor Tests

This section includes text excerpted from "Coagulation Factor Tests," MedlinePlus, National Institutes of Health (NIH), April 15, 2019.

What Are Coagulation Factor Tests?

Coagulation factors are proteins in the blood that help control bleeding. You have several different coagulation factors in your blood. When you get a cut or other injury that causes bleeding, your coagulation factors work together to form a blood clot. The clot stops you from losing too much blood. This process is called the "coagulation cascade."

Coagulation factor tests are blood tests that check the function of one or more of your coagulation factors. Coagulation factors are known by Roman numerals (I, II, VIII, etc.) or by name (fibrinogen, prothrombin, hemophilia A, etc.). If any of your factors are missing or defective, it can lead to heavy, uncontrolled bleeding after an injury.

What Is It Used For?

A coagulation factor test is used to find out if you have a problem with any of your coagulation factors. If a problem is found, you likely have a condition known as a "bleeding disorder." There are different types of bleeding disorders. Bleeding disorders are very rare. The most well-known bleeding disorder is hemophilia. Hemophilia is caused when coagulation factors VIII or IX are missing or defective.

You may be tested for one or more factors at a time.

Why Do I Need a Coagulation Factor Test?

You may need this test if you have a family history of bleeding disorders. Most bleeding disorders are inherited, meaning that it is passed down from one or both of your parents.

You may also need this test if your healthcare provider thinks you have a bleeding disorder that is not inherited. Although uncommon, other causes of bleeding disorders include:

• Liver disease

• Vitamin K deficiency

• Blood-thinning medicines

In addition, you may need a coagulation factor test if you have symptoms of a bleeding disorder. These include:

• Heavy bleeding after an injury

• Easy bruising

• Swelling

• Pain and stiffness

• An unexplained blood clot. In some bleeding disorders, the blood clots too much rather than too little. This can be dangerous because when a blood clot travels in your body, it can cause a heart attack, stroke, or other life-threatening conditions.

What Happens during a Coagulation Factor Test

A healthcare professional will take a blood sample from a vein in your arm, using a small needle. After the needle is inserted, a small amount of blood will be collected into a test tube or vial. You may feel a little sting when the needle goes in or out. This usually takes less than five minutes.

Will I Need to Do Anything to Prepare for the Test?

You do not need any special preparations for a coagulation factor test.

Are There Any Risks to the Test?

There is very little risk to having a blood test. You may have slight pain or bruising at the spot where the needle was put in, but most symptoms go away quickly.

What Do the Results Mean?

If your results show one of your coagulation factors is missing or not working right, you probably have some kind of bleeding disorder. The type of disorder depends on which factor is affected. While there is no cure for inherited bleeding disorders, there are treatments available that can manage your condition.

Section 47.3

Partial Thromboplastin Time

This section includes text excerpted from "Partial Thromboplastin Time (PTT) Test," MedlinePlus, National Institutes of Health (NIH), February 4, 2019.

What Is a Partial Thromboplastin Time Test?

A partial thromboplastin time (PTT) test measures the time it takes for a blood clot to form. Normally, when you get a cut or injury that causes bleeding, proteins in your blood called "coagulation factors" work together to form a blood clot. The clot stops you from losing too much blood.

You have several coagulation factors in your blood. If any factors are missing or defective, it can take longer than normal for blood to clot. In some cases, this causes heavy, uncontrolled bleeding. A PTT test checks the function of specific coagulation factors. These include factors known as "factor VIII," "factor IX," "factor X1," and "factor XII."

What Is It Used For?

A partial thromboplastin time test is used to:

- Check the function of specific coagulation factors. If any of these factors are missing or defective, it can mean that you have a bleeding disorder. Bleeding disorders are a group of rare conditions in which blood does not clot normally. The most well-known bleeding disorder is hemophilia.

- Find out if there is another reason for excessive bleeding or other clotting problems. These include certain autoimmune diseases that cause the immune system to attack coagulation factors.

- Monitor people taking heparin, a type of medicine that prevents clotting. In some bleeding disorders, the blood clots too much rather than too little. This can cause heart attacks, strokes, and other life-threatening conditions. But, taking too much heparin can cause excessive and dangerous bleeding.

Why Do I Need a Partial Thromboplastin Time Test?

You may need a PTT test if you:

- Have unexplained heavy bleeding

- Bruise easily

- Have a blood clot in a vein or artery

- Have liver disease, which can sometimes cause problems with blood clotting

- Will be getting surgery. Surgery can cause blood loss, so it is important to know if you have a clotting problem.

- Have had multiple miscarriages

- Are taking heparin

What Happens during a Partial Thromboplastin Time Test

A healthcare professional will take a blood sample from a vein in your arm, using a small needle. After the needle is inserted, a small amount of blood will be collected into a test tube or vial. You may feel a little sting when the needle goes in or out. This usually takes less than five minutes.

Will I Need to Do Anything to Prepare for the Test?

You do not need any special preparations for a PTT test.

Are There Any Risks to the Test?

There is very little risk to having a blood test. You may have slight pain or bruising at the spot where the needle was put in, but most symptoms go away quickly.

What Do the Results Mean?

Your partial thromboplastin time test results will show how much time it took for your blood to clot. Results are usually given as a number of seconds. If your results show that your blood took a longer-than-normal time to clot, it may mean that you have:

- A bleeding disorder, such as hemophilia or von Willebrand disease (VWD). Von Willebrand disease is the most common bleeding disorder, but it usually causes milder symptoms than other bleeding disorders.

- Liver disease

- Antiphospholipid antibody syndrome (APS) or lupus anticoagulant syndrome. These are autoimmune diseases that cause your immune system to attack your coagulation factors.

- Vitamin K deficiency. Vitamin K plays an important role in forming coagulation factors.

If you are taking heparin, your results can help show whether you are taking the right dose. You will probably be tested on a regular basis to make sure your dosage stays at the right level.

If you are diagnosed with a bleeding disorder, talk to your healthcare provider. While there is no cure for most bleeding disorders, there are treatments available that can help manage your condition.

Is There Anything Else I Need to Know about a Partial Thromboplastin Time Test?

A partial thromboplastin time test is often ordered along with another blood test called "prothrombin time." A prothrombin time test is another way to measure clotting ability.

Chapter 48

Tests Used in the Assessment of Vascular Disease

Chapter Contents

Section 48.1

Coronary Calcium Scan

This section includes text excerpted from "Coronary Calcium Scan," National Heart, Lung, and Blood Institute (NHLBI), February 6, 2013. Reviewed June 2019.

A buildup of calcium, or calcifications, are a sign of atherosclerosis or ischemic heart disease.

A coronary calcium scan may be performed in a medical imaging facility or hospital. The test does not use contrast dye and will take about 10 to 15 minutes to complete. A coronary calcium scan uses a special scanner, such as an electron beam computed tomography (CT) machine or a multidetector computed tomography (MDCT) machine. An MDCT machine is a much faster CT scanner that makes high-quality pictures of the beating heart. A coronary calcium scan will determine an Agatston score that reflects the amount of calcium found in your coronary arteries. A score of zero is normal. In general, the higher your score, the more likely you are to have heart disease. If your score is high, your doctor may recommend more tests.

A coronary calcium scan has few risks. There is a slight risk of cancer, particularly in people younger than 40 years of age. However, the amount of radiation from one test is similar to the amount of radiation you are naturally exposed to over one year. Talk to your doctor and the technicians performing the test about whether you are or could be pregnant. If the test is not urgent, they may have you wait to do the test until after your pregnancy. If it is urgent, the technicians will take extra steps to protect the fetus during this test.

Section 48.2

Cardiac Catheterization

This section includes text excerpted from "Cardiac Catheterization," National Heart, Lung, and Blood Institute (NHLBI), October 31, 2016.

Cardiac catheterization is a medical procedure used to diagnose and treat some heart conditions. It lets doctors take a close look at the heart to identify problems and perform other tests or procedures on your heart.

Your doctor may recommend cardiac catheterization to find out the cause of symptoms, such as chest pain or irregular heartbeat, or to find out whether you have ischemic heart disease due to blockages in the coronary arteries. Before the procedure, your doctor may need to do diagnostic tests, such as blood tests, heart imaging tests, or a stress test, to determine how well your heart is working and to help guide the procedure.

During cardiac catheterization, a long, thin, flexible tube called a "catheter" is put into a blood vessel in your arm, groin or upper thigh, or neck. The catheter is then threaded to your heart. Your doctor may use it to examine your heart valves or to take samples of blood or heart muscle. Your doctor also may use ultrasound or inject a dye into your coronary arteries to see whether your arteries are narrowed or blocked. Cardiac catheterization may also be used instead of some heart surgeries to repair heart defects and replace heart valves.

Cardiac catheterization is safe for most people. Complications are rare but can include bleeding and blood clots. Your doctor will monitor your condition and may recommend medicines to prevent blood clots.

Who Needs Cardiac Catheterization

Your doctor may recommend cardiac catheterization to find out what is causing signs or symptoms of a heart problem or to treat or repair a heart problem. Cardiac catheterization is safe for most people.

When Is Cardiac Catheterization Recommended?

Your doctor may recommend cardiac catheterization to help with diagnoses or to plan treatment. It can be useful when your doctor wants to do any of the following:

- Better understand the results from other tests and procedures, such as echocardiography (echo), cardiac magnetic resonance imaging (MRI), and a cardiac computed tomography (CT) scan, especially if other studies could not define the problem or if the results from other studies differ from what your doctor finds when examining you

- Diagnose the cause of your chest pain, arrhythmia, or other signs and symptoms of a heart problem or evaluate you during an emergency, such as a heart attack. The procedure may help your doctor diagnose heart conditions, such as pulmonary hypertension (PH); cardiomyopathy; ischemic heart disease; and heart valve diseases, such as aortic stenosis and mitral regurgitation.

- Evaluate you before a possible heart transplant

- Look at the pulmonary arteries for conditions, including pulmonary embolism, that can occur as a result of venous thromboembolism. The pulmonary arteries are the blood vessels that carry blood from your heart to your lungs, where the blood receives oxygen.

- Measure oxygen levels and pressures of the blood in your heart, such as in your ventricles, atria, and pulmonary arteries

Your doctor may perform additional procedures to diagnose or treat your condition during cardiac catheterization. Some of these procedures include:

- **Biopsies** to take small samples of the heart tissue for further laboratory testing. Biopsies can be used for genetic testing or to check for myocarditis, a type of heart inflammation, or transplant rejection.

- **Coronary angiography** to look at the heart or blood vessels by injecting dye through the catheter

- **Minor heart surgery** to treat congenital heart defects and replace or widen narrowed heart valves

- **Percutaneous coronary intervention (PCI)** to open narrowed or blocked areas of the coronary arteries. PCI may include balloon dilation, or angioplasty, or stent placement. Most people who have heart attacks or underlying ischemic heart diseases have narrowed or blocked coronary arteries.

Who Should Not Have Cardiac Catheterization?

Your doctor may wait to do the procedure or recommend that you do not have cardiac catheterization if you have one of the following conditions:

- Abnormal electrolyte levels in your blood

- Acute gastrointestinal bleeding

- Acute kidney failure, or severe kidney disease that is not being treated with dialysis

- Acute stroke

- Blood that is too thin from medicines, such as warfarin, or other causes

- High blood levels of a heart medicine called "digoxin"

- Previous severe allergic reaction to the dye that is used during cardiac catheterization

- Severe anemia, which is a lower-than-normal red blood cell (RBC) count or hemoglobin

- Unexplained fever

- Untreated infection

What to Expect before Cardiac Catheterization

Before cardiac catheterization, you will meet with your cardiologist, a doctor who specializes in the heart. The doctor will ask you about your medical history, including what medicines you are taking and any allergies you may have, and do a physical exam. Your doctor will also give you instructions on how to prepare for the procedure.

Diagnostic Tests and Procedures

You may have some of the following tests before your catheterization procedure:

- **Electrocardiogram (ECG or EKG)** to look at your heart's rhythm and other electrical activity of your heart. It can show arrhythmias, heart attacks, and other problems with the heart.

- **A chest X-ray** to look at your lungs, your heart, your major blood vessels, and other structures in the chest

- An **echocardiogram (echo)** to look at the structure and function of your heart

- A **stress test** to look at how well your heart works during physical stress. The stress may be physical exercise, such as walking on a treadmill, or it may be a medicine given to have the same effect.

- **Cardiac CT scan** to look for narrowing of your heart's blood vessels, and problems with the heart, larger blood vessels, and heart valves. These pictures also may help your doctor plan for procedures to open the coronary arteries.

- **Cardiac MRI** to provide information on the structure and function of your heart, as well as the type and severity of heart disease

- **Blood tests,** including a complete blood count (CBC) to check your hemoglobin and platelet levels, blood chemistry tests to check how well your liver and kidneys are working, and tests to check your blood's ability to clot

Preparing for the Procedure

Talk to your doctor about your medical history, including any medicines you take; other surgical procedures you have had; and any medical conditions you have, such as diabetes or kidney disease.

Your doctor will talk to you about how to prepare for the procedure, including:

- When to arrive at the hospital and where to go

- When you should stop eating or drinking

- If and when you should start or stop taking medicines

- How long you should expect to stay

- What happens during the procedure

- What to expect after the procedure, including potential complications, such as bleeding or soreness

- Instructions to follow after the procedure, including what medicines to take

What to Expect during Cardiac Catheterization

Cardiac catheterization takes place in a catheterization laboratory, or cath lab, which is similar to a small operating room. The procedure is often done in a hospital, but you may be able to have the procedure in a catheterization laboratory located in a medical clinic, depending on the reason you are having the procedure and the risk for complications.

How Is Cardiac Catheterization Done?

Before cardiac catheterization, an intravenous line (IV) will be placed in a vein in your arm. Through this IV, you will get a medicine to either help you relax or make you sleep during the procedure.

You will get numbing medicine, or local anesthesia, at the site where the doctor will insert the catheter. This site is called the "access site" and may be in the upper thigh, arm, neck, or under the collarbone. The doctor places a needle into a blood vessel at the access site. A guidewire is inserted into the needle, and the needle is taken out. Then the doctor places a small tube called a "sheath" in the blood vessel around the guidewire. The guidewire is removed. The catheter is then inserted through the sheath. Your doctor watches X-ray images to see where to place the tip of the catheter.

Once the catheter is in place, your doctor may use it to perform tests or treatments on your heart. For example, she or he may inject a dye into the catheter to look at blood flow in the heart. The dye will enter your blood vessels and make your coronary arteries visible in X-ray pictures.

Possible Risks and Complications

Cardiac catheterization is a relatively safe procedure, and complications are rare. Possible complications include the following:

- **Allergic reaction to the dye used.** This reaction may be hives or a more serious reaction.

- **Arrhythmias**

- **Bleeding** at the access site or inside your abdomen

- **Blood clot** formation at the access site, inside your abdomen, in a blood vessel, or in your heart

- **Collapsed lung**, called "pneumothorax," resulting in air in the space between your lung and chest wall

- **Damage to blood vessels**, heart valves, or your heart

- **Heart attack**

- **Hypothermia**, especially in small children

- **Infection**

- **Low blood pressure** from bleeding or as a reaction to the procedure

- **Need for blood transfusion**

- **Need for emergency surgery** to repair a tear in the aorta or coronary artery, and to restore blood flow to the heart. This may be done using a coronary artery bypass graft (CABG).

- **Side effects of general anesthesia**, if used. These can include nausea, vomiting, confusion, or an allergic reaction.

- **Stroke**

Although not an immediate risk, repeated radiation exposure from X-rays used to place the catheter in the heart, especially with children, may increase the risk of cancer and leukemia, damage to skin, and cataracts later in life.

What to Expect after Cardiac Catheterization

After the procedure, your doctor will remove the catheters, sheath, and guidewire. A dressing, accompanied by pressure, is applied to the site where the catheter was inserted to stop the bleeding. The pressure may be held by hand or with a sandbag or other device. You will be moved to a recovery room, where you will lie in bed. Your heartbeat and blood pressure will be monitored.

Depending on your health before the cardiac catheterization and what additional procedures were done during the cardiac catheterization, you may have to spend the night in the hospital. You should follow your doctor's instructions on what medicines to take and when to resume activity.

Life after Cardiac Catheterization

If you have had cardiac catheterization, it is important that you receive follow-up care, know about the possible complications that may occur after the procedure, and follow the treatment plan that your doctor recommends for your condition.

Receive Follow-Up Care

It is important to get routine follow-up care after you have cardiac catheterization. Talk with your doctor about how often you should schedule office visits.

- Adopt a heart-healthy lifestyle, especially if your cardiac catheterization was needed because of ischemic heart disease or heart attack.

- Follow any instructions for when to resume physical activity and lifting and at what levels.

- Follow instructions on how to care for the site where the doctor accessed your blood vessel, including when you can take a bath or swim.

- Keep any follow-up appointments or tests.

- Take any medicines as directed by your doctor.

- Talk to your doctor about any blood tests you may need if you were placed on blood thinners after your procedure.

Learn the Warning Signs of Complications and Have a Plan

Complications from cardiac catheterization are rare but can be serious. A small bruise and tenderness at the access site is normal. Call your doctor immediately if you experience any of the following, as they may be signs of serious complications.

- Bleeding from the access site that cannot be stopped with firm pressure

- Chest pain or shortness of breath

- Dizziness

- Fever

- Increased pain, redness, or bruising at the access site

- Irregular, very slow, or fast heartbeat

- Swelling at the access site

- Yellow or green discharge draining from the access site

- Your leg or arm that was used for access becoming numb or weak, or any part of it turning cold or blue

Other serious complications after catheterization, although rare, include heart attack and stroke. If you think that you are or someone else is having the following symptoms, call 911 immediately.

Heart attack signs and symptoms include:

- **Chest pain or discomfort** in the center of the chest or upper abdomen that lasts for more than a few minutes or goes away and comes back. It can feel like pressure, squeezing, fullness, heartburn, or indigestion.

- **Nausea, vomiting, light-headedness or fainting, or breaking out in a cold sweat**. These symptoms of a heart attack are more common in women.

- **Shortness of breath,** which may occur with or before chest discomfort

- **Upper body discomfort** in one or both arms or the back, neck, jaw, or upper part of the stomach

If you think someone may be having a stroke, act F.A.S.T. and perform the following simple test.

- **F—Face:** Ask the person to smile. Does one side of the face droop?

- **A—Arms:** Ask the person to raise both arms. Does one arm drift downward?

- **S—Speech:** Ask the person to repeat a simple phrase. Is their speech slurred or strange?

- **T—Time:** If you observe any of these signs, call for help immediately. Early treatment is essential.

Section 48.3

Cardiac Magnetic Resonance Imaging

This section includes text excerpted from "Cardiac
MRI," National Heart, Lung, and Blood Institute (NHLBI),
April 26, 2013. Reviewed June 2019.

What Is Cardiac Magnetic Resonance Imaging?

Cardiac magnetic resonance imaging (MRI) is a painless imaging
test that uses radio waves, magnets, and a computer to create detailed
pictures of your heart. Cardiac MRI can provide detailed information
on the type and severity of heart disease to help your doctor decide
the best way to treat heart problems, such as coronary heart disease
(CHD); heart valve problems; pericarditis; cardiac tumors; or damage
from a heart attack. Cardiac MRI can help explain results from other
imaging tests, such as chest X-rays and chest computed tomography
(CT) scans.

How Is Cardiac Magnetic Resonance Imaging Done?

Cardiac MRI may be done in a medical imaging facility or hospital.
Before your procedure, a contrast dye to highlight your heart and blood
vessels may be injected into a vein in your arm. You may feel discomfort from the needle or a cool feeling as the contrast dye is injected.
The MRI machine is a large, tunnel-like machine that has a table. You
will lie still on the table, and the table will slide into the machine. You
will hear loud humming, tapping, and buzzing sounds when you are
inside the machine as pictures of your heart are being taken. You will
be able to hear from and talk to the technician performing the test
while you are inside the machine. The technician may ask you to hold
your breath for a few seconds during the test.

Risks of Cardiac Magnetic Resonance Imaging

Cardiac MRI has few risks. In rare instances, the contrast dye may
harm people who have kidney or liver disease, or it may cause an allergic reaction. Researchers are studying whether multiple contrast dye
injections, defined as four or more, may cause other adverse effects.
Talk to your doctor and the technicians performing the test about
whether you are or could be pregnant. Let your doctor know if you are

breastfeeding because the contrast dye can pass into your breast milk. If you must have the contrast dye injected, you may want to pump and save enough breast milk for one to two days after your test, or you may bottle-feed your baby for that time. Tell your doctor if you have:

- A pacemaker or other implanted device because the MRI machine can damage these devices.

- Metal inside your body from previous surgeries because it can interfere with the MRI machine.

- Metal on your body from piercings, jewelry, or some transdermal skin patches because they can interfere with the MRI machine or cause skin burns. Tattoos may cause a problem because older tattoo inks may contain small amounts of metal.

Section 48.4

Chest X-Ray

This section includes text excerpted from "Chest X-Ray," National Heart, Lung, and Blood Institute (NHLBI), December 10, 2016.

A chest X-ray can help diagnose and monitor conditions such as pneumonia; heart failure; lung cancer; tuberculosis; sarcoidosis; and lung tissue scarring, called "fibrosis." Doctors may use chest X-rays to see how well certain treatments are working and to check for complications after certain procedures or surgeries.

The test may be done in the doctor's office, clinic, hospital, or other medical facility. Before having a chest X-ray, you will undress from the waist up, wear a gown, and remove jewelry and objects that could interfere with the test. You will stand, sit, or lie still for the test. A lead apron may be worn to protect your reproductive organs from the X-ray. The technician will operate the X-ray machine from behind a wall or in the next room. Usually, the technician takes two views, one from straight on and one from the side of your chest, but more views may be taken. A radiologist will analyze the images and send a report to your doctor.

Chest X-rays have few risks. The amount of radiation used in a chest X-ray is very small. Talk to your doctor and the technicians performing the test about whether you are or could be pregnant. If the procedure is not urgent, they may have you wait to do the test until after your pregnancy. If it is urgent, the technicians will take extra steps to protect the fetus during this test.

Section 48.5

Coronary Angiography

This section includes text excerpted from "Coronary Angiography," National Heart, Lung, and Blood Institute (NHLBI), January 31, 2013. Reviewed June 2019.

What Is Coronary Angiography?

Coronary angiography is a procedure that uses contrast dye, usually containing iodine, and X-ray pictures to detect blockages in the coronary arteries that are caused by plaque buildup.

Blockages prevent your heart from getting oxygen and important nutrients. Coronary angiography is used to diagnose ischemic heart disease after chest pain; sudden cardiac arrest (SCA); or abnormal results from tests, such as an electrocardiogram (EKG) of the heart or an exercise stress test. It is important to detect blockages because over time they can cause chest pain, especially with physical activity or stress, or a heart attack. If you are having a heart attack, coronary angiography can help your doctors plan your treatment.

What Happens during Coronary Angiography

Cardiologists, or doctors who specialize in the heart, will perform coronary angiography in a hospital or specialized laboratory. You will stay awake so you can follow your doctor's instructions, but you will get medicine to relax you during the procedure. You will lie on your back on a movable table. Often, coronary angiography is done with a cardiac catheterization procedure. For this, your doctor will clean and numb an area on the arm, groin or upper thigh, or neck before making a small hole in a blood vessel. Your doctor will insert a catheter tube into your blood vessel. Your doctor will take X-ray pictures to help place the catheter in your coronary artery. After the catheter is in place, your doctor will inject the contrast dye through the catheter to highlight blockages and take X-ray pictures of your heart. If blockages are detected, your doctor may use percutaneous coronary intervention (PCI), also known as "coronary angioplasty," to improve blood flow to your heart.

What Happens after Coronary Angiography

After coronary angiography, your doctor will remove the catheter; possibly use a closure device to close the blood vessel; and close and bandage the opening on your arm, groin, or neck. You may develop a bruise and soreness where the catheter was inserted. You will stay in the hospital for a few hours or overnight. During this time, your heart rate and blood pressure will be monitored. Your movement will be limited to prevent bleeding from the hole where the catheter was inserted. You will need a ride home after the procedure because of the medicines or anesthesia you received.

Complications Associated with Coronary Angiography

Coronary angiography is a common procedure that rarely causes serious problems. Possible complications may include bleeding, allergic reactions to the contrast dye, infection, blood vessel damage, arrhythmias, blood clots that can trigger a heart attack or stroke, kidney damage, and fluid buildup around the heart. The risk of complications is higher in people who are older or who have certain conditions, such as chronic kidney disease (CKD) or diabetes. An imaging test called "coronary computed tomography angiography," or "coronary CTA," may be preferred over coronary angiography to detect blockages in the heart. Even though coronary CTA still uses contrast dye, it does not require the invasive cardiac catheterization procedure that causes many of the complications of coronary angiography.

Section 48.6

Echocardiography

This section includes text excerpted from "Echocardiography,"
National Heart, Lung, and Blood Institute (NHLBI), November 5,
2011. Reviewed June 2019.

What Is Echocardiography?

Echocardiography, or echo, is a painless test that uses sound waves
to create moving pictures of your heart. The pictures show the size and
shape of your heart. They also show how well your heart's chambers
and valves are working.

An echo also can pinpoint areas of heart muscle that are not con-
tracting well because of poor blood flow or injury from a previous heart
attack. A type of echo called "Doppler ultrasound" shows how well
blood flows through your heart's chambers and valves.

An echo can detect possible blood clots inside the heart, fluid buildup
in the pericardium (the sac around the heart), and problems with the
aorta. The aorta is the main artery that carries oxygen-rich blood from
your heart to your body.

Doctors also use echo to detect heart problems in infants and
children.

Who Needs Echocardiography

Your doctor may recommend echocardiography if you have signs or
symptoms of heart problems.

For example, shortness of breath and swelling in the legs are possible signs of heart failure. Heart failure is a condition in which your
heart cannot pump enough oxygen-rich blood to meet your body's
needs. An echo can show how well your heart is pumping blood.

An echo also can help your doctor find the cause of abnormal heart
sounds, such as heart murmurs. Heart murmurs are extra or unusual
sounds heard during the heartbeat. Some heart murmurs are harmless, while others are signs of heart problems.

Your doctor also may use an echo to learn about:

- **The size of your heart.** An enlarged heart might be the result
  of high blood pressure (HBP), leaky heart valves, or heart
  failure. An echo also can detect the increased thickness of the

ventricles (the heart's lower chambers). Increased thickness may be due to high blood pressure, heart valve disease, or congenital heart defects.

- **Heart muscles that are weak and are not pumping well.** Damage from a heart attack may cause weak areas of heart muscle. Weakening also might mean that the area is not getting enough blood supply, a sign of coronary heart disease (CHD).

- **Heart valve problems.** An echo can show whether any of your heart valves do not open normally or close tightly.

- **Problems with your heart's structure.** An echo can detect congenital heart defects, such as holes in the heart. Congenital heart defects are structural problems present at birth. Infants and children may have echo to detect these heart defects.

- **Blood clots or tumors.** If you have had a stroke, you may have an echo to check for blood clots or tumors that could have caused the stroke.

Your doctor also might recommend an echo to see how well your heart responds to certain heart treatments, such as those used for heart failure.

Types of Echocardiography

There are several types of echocardiography—all of which use sound waves to create moving pictures of your heart. This is the same technology that allows doctors to see a fetus.

Unlike X-rays and some other tests, an echo does not involve radiation.

Transthoracic Echocardiography

Transthoracic echo is the most common type of echocardiogram test. It is painless and noninvasive. "Noninvasive" means that no surgery is done, and no instruments are inserted into your body.

This type of echo involves placing a device called a "transducer" on your chest. The device sends special sound waves, called "ultrasound," through your chest wall to your heart. The human ear cannot hear ultrasound waves.

As the ultrasound waves bounce off the structures of your heart, a computer in the echo machine converts them into pictures on a screen.

Stress Echocardiography

A stress echo is done as part of a stress test. During a stress test, you exercise or take medicine (given by your doctor) to make your heart work hard and beat fast. A technician will use echo to create pictures of your heart before you exercise and as soon as you finish.

Some heart problems, such as coronary heart disease, are easier to diagnose when the heart is working hard and beating fast.

Transesophageal Echocardiography

Your doctor may have a hard time seeing the aorta and other parts of your heart using a standard transthoracic echo. Thus, she or he may recommend a transesophageal echo, or TEE.

During this test, the transducer is attached to the end of a flexible tube. The tube is guided down your throat and into your esophagus (the passage leading from your mouth to your stomach). This allows your doctor to get more detailed pictures of your heart.

Fetal Echocardiography

Fetal echo is used to look at a fetus's heart. A doctor may recommend this test to check a fetus for heart problems. When recommended, the test is commonly done at about 18 to 22 weeks of pregnancy. For this test, the transducer is moved over the pregnant woman's belly.

Three-Dimensional Echocardiography

A three-dimensional (3-D) echo creates 3-D images of your heart. These detailed images show how your heart looks and works.

During transthoracic echo, 3-D images can be taken as part of the process used to do these types of echo.

Doctors may use 3-D echo to diagnose heart problems in children. They also may use 3-D echo for planning and overseeing heart valve surgery.

Researchers continue to study new ways to use 3-D echo.

What to Expect before Echocardiography

Echocardiography is done in a doctor's office or a hospital. No special preparations are needed for most types of echo. You usually can eat, drink, and take any medicines as you normally would.

The exception is if you are having a transesophageal echo. This test usually requires that you do not eat or drink for eight hours prior to the test.

If you are having a stress echo, you may need to take steps to prepare for the stress test. Your doctor will let you know what steps you need to take.

What to Expect during Echocardiography

Echocardiography is painless; the test usually takes less than an hour to do. For some types of echo, your doctor will need to inject saline or a special dye into one of your veins. The substance makes your heart show up more clearly on the echo pictures.

The dye used for an echo is different from the dye used during angiography (a test used to examine the body's blood vessels).

For most types of echo, you will remove your clothing from the waist up. Women will be given a gown to wear during the test. You will lie on your back or left side on an exam table or stretcher.

Soft, sticky patches called "electrodes" will be attached to your chest so an electrocardiogram (EKG) can be done. An EKG is a test that records the heart's electrical activity.

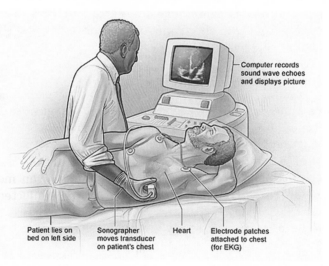

Figure 48.1. *Echocardiography*

The illustration shows a patient having echocardiography. The patient lies on his left side. A sonographer moves the transducer on the patient and chest, while viewing the echo pictures on a computer

A doctor or sonographer (a person specially trained to do ultrasounds) will apply gel to your chest. The gel helps the sound waves reach your heart. A transducer will then be moved around on your chest.

The transducer transmits ultrasound waves into your chest. A computer will convert echoes from the sound waves into pictures of your heart on a screen. During the test, the lights in the room will be dimmed so the computer screen is easier to see.

The sonographer will record pictures of various parts of your heart. She or he will put the recordings on a computer disc for a cardiologist (heart specialist) to review.

During the test, you may be asked to change positions or hold your breath for a short time. This allows the sonographer to get better pictures of your heart.

At times, the sonographer may apply a bit of pressure to your chest with the transducer. You may find this pressure a little uncomfortable, but it helps get the best picture of your heart. You should let the sonographer know if you feel too uncomfortable.

The process described above is similar to the process for a fetal echo. For that test, however, the transducer is placed over the pregnant woman's belly at the location of the fetus's heart.

Transesophageal Echocardiography

A transesophageal echo is used if your doctor needs a more detailed view of your heart. For example, your doctor may use TEE to look for blood clots in your heart. A doctor, not a sonographer, will perform this type of echo.

A transesophageal echo uses the same technology as a transthoracic echo, but the transducer is attached to the end of a flexible tube.

Your doctor will guide the tube down your throat and into your esophagus. From this angle, your doctor can get a more detailed image of the heart and major blood vessels leading to and from the heart.

For a transesophageal echo, you will likely be given medicine to help you relax during the test. The medicine will be injected into one of your veins.

Your blood pressure, the oxygen content of your blood, and other vital signs will be checked during the test. You will be given oxygen through a tube in your nose. If you wear dentures or partials, you will have to remove them.

The back of your mouth will be numbed with gel or spray. Your doctor will gently place the tube with the transducer in your throat and guide it down until it is in place behind your heart.

The pictures of your heart are then recorded as your doctor moves the transducer around in your esophagus and stomach. You should not feel any discomfort as this happens.

Although the imaging usually takes less than an hour, you may be watched for a few hours at the doctor's office or hospital after the test.

Stress Echocardiography

A stress echo is a transthoracic echo that is combined with either an exercise or pharmacological stress test.

For an exercise stress test, you will walk or run on a treadmill or pedal a stationary bike to make your heart work hard and beat fast. For a pharmacological stress test, you will be given medicine to increase your heart rate.

A technician will take pictures of your heart using echo before you exercise and as soon as you finish.

What You May See and Hear during Echocardiography

As the doctor or sonographer moves the transducer around, you will see different views of your heart on the screen of the echo machine. The structures of your heart will appear as white objects, while any fluid or blood will appear black on the screen.

Doppler ultrasound often is used during echo tests. Doppler ultrasound is a special ultrasound that shows how blood is flowing through the blood vessels.

This test allows the sonographer to see blood flowing at different speeds and in different directions. The speed and direction of blood flow appear as different colors moving within the black and white images.

The human ear is unable to hear the sound waves used in echo. If you have a Doppler ultrasound, you may be able to hear "whooshing" sounds. Your doctor can use these sounds to learn about blood flow through your heart.

What to Expect after Echocardiography

You usually can go back to your normal activities right after having echocardiography.

If you have a transesophageal echo, you may be watched for a few hours at the doctor's office or hospital after the test. Your throat might be sore for a few hours after the test.

You also may not be able to drive for a short time after having a TEE. Your doctor will let you know whether you need to arrange for a ride home.

What Does Echocardiography Show?

An echocardiography shows the size, structure, and movement of various parts of your heart. These parts include the heart valves, the septum (the wall separating the right and left heart chambers), and the walls of the heart chambers. Doppler ultrasound shows the movement of blood through your heart.

Your doctor may use echo to:

- Diagnose heart problems

- Guide or determine next steps for treatment

- Monitor changes and improvement

- Determine the need for more tests

Echo can detect many heart problems. Some might be minor and pose no risk to you. Others can be signs of serious heart disease or other heart conditions. Your doctor may use echo to learn about:

- **The size of your heart.** An enlarged heart might be the result of high blood pressure, leaky heart valves, or heart failure. Echo also can detect increased thickness of the ventricles. Increased thickness may be due to high blood pressure, heart valve disease, or congenital heart defects.

- **Heart muscles that are weak and are not pumping well.** Damage from a heart attack may cause weak areas of heart muscle. Weakening also might mean that the area is not getting enough blood supply, a sign of coronary heart disease.

- **Heart valve problems.** An echo can show whether any of your heart valves do not open normally or close tightly.

- **Problems with your heart's structure.** An echo can detect congenital heart defects, such as holes in the heart. Congenital heart defects are structural problems present at birth. Infants and children may have echo to detect these heart defects.

- **Blood clots or tumors.** If you have had a stroke, you may have echo to check for blood clots or tumors that could have caused the stroke.

What Are the Risks of Echocardiography?

Transthoracic and fetal echocardiography have no risks. These tests are safe for adults, children, and infants.

If you have a transesophageal echo, some risks are associated with the medicine given to help you relax. For example, you may have a bad reaction to the medicine, problems breathing, and nausea (feeling sick to your stomach).

Your throat also might be sore for a few hours after the test. Rarely, the tube used during TEE causes minor throat injuries.

Stress echo has some risks, but they are related to the exercise or medicine used to raise your heart rate, not the echo. Serious complications from stress tests are very uncommon.

Section 48.7

Electrocardiogram

This section includes text excerpted from "Electrocardiogram," MedlinePlus, National Institutes of Health (NIH), January 31, 2019.

What Is an Electrocardiogram Test?

An electrocardiogram (EKG) test is a simple, painless procedure that measures electrical signals in your heart. Each time your heart beats, an electrical signal travels through the heart. An EKG can show if your heart is beating at a normal rate and strength. It also helps show the size and position of your heart's chambers. An abnormal EKG can be a sign of heart disease or damage.

What Is an Electrocardiogram Test Used For?

An electrocardiogram test is used to find and/or monitor various heart disorders. These include:

- Irregular heartbeat (known as "arrhythmia")
- Blocked arteries
- Heart damage
- Heart failure

- Heart attack. EKGs are often used in the ambulance, emergency room, or other hospital rooms to diagnose a suspected heart attack.

An electrocardiogram test is sometimes included in a routine exam for middle-aged and older adults, as they have a higher risk of heart disease than younger people.

Why Do You Need an Electrocardiogram Test?

You may need an EKG test if you have symptoms of a heart disorder. These include:

- Chest pain

- Rapid heartbeat

- Arrhythmia (it may feel like your heart has skipped a beat or is fluttering)

- Shortness of breath

- Dizziness

- Fatigue

You may also need this test if you:

- Have had a heart attack or other heart problems in the past

- Have a family history of heart disease

- Are scheduled for surgery. Your healthcare provider may want to check your heart health before the procedure.

- Have a pacemaker. The EKG can show how well the device is working.

- Are taking medicine for heart disease. The EKG can show if your medicine is effective or if you need to make changes in your treatment.

What Happens during an Electrocardiogram Test

An electrocardiogram test may be done in a provider's office, outpatient clinic, or a hospital. During the procedure:

- You will lie on an exam table.

- A healthcare provider will place several electrodes (small sensors that stick to the skin) on your arms, legs, and chest. The provider may need to shave or trim excess hair before placing the electrodes.

- The electrodes are attached by wires to a computer that records your heart's electrical activity.

- The activity will be displayed on the computer's monitor and/or printed out on paper.

- The procedure only takes about three minutes.

Will You Need to Do Anything to Prepare for the Electrocardiogram Test?

You do not need any special preparations for an EKG test.

Are There Any Risks to the Test?

There is very little risk of having an EKG. You may feel a little discomfort or skin irritation after the electrodes are removed. There is no risk of electric shock. The EKG does not send any electricity to your body. It only records electricity.

What Do the Electrocardiogram Test Results Mean?

Your healthcare provider will check your EKG results for a consistent heartbeat and rhythm. If your results were not normal, it may mean you have one of the following disorders:

- Arrhythmia, a heartbeat that is too fast or too slow

- Inadequate blood supply to the heart

- A bulge in the heart's walls. This bulge is known as an "aneurysm."

- Thickening of the heart's walls

- A heart attack. (Results can show if you have had a heart attack in the past or if you are having an attack during the EKG.)

If you have questions about your results, talk to your healthcare provider.

Elektrokardiogramm versus Electrocardiogram

An electrocardiogram may be called an "EKG" or an "electrocardiogram" (ECG). Both are correct and commonly used. EKG is based on the German spelling, elektrokardiogramm. EKG may be preferred over ECG to avoid confusion with an EEG, a test that measures brain waves.

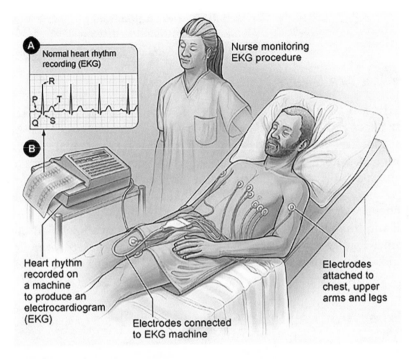

Figure 48.2. *Electrocardiogram*

The image shows the standard setup for an EKG. In figure A, a normal heart rhythm recording shows the electrical pattern of a regular heartbeat. In figure B, a patient lies in a bed with EKG electrodes attached to his chest, upper arms, and legs. A nurse monitors the painless procedure

Section 48.8

Stress Testing

This section includes text excerpted from
"Stress Tests," MedlinePlus, National Institutes of
Health (NIH), January 31, 2019.

What Are Stress Tests?

Stress tests show how well your heart handles physical activity. Your heart pumps harder and faster when you exercise. Some heart disorders are easier to find when your heart is hard at work. During a stress test, your heart will be checked while you exercise on a treadmill or stationary bicycle. If you are not healthy enough to exercise, you will be given a medicine that makes your heart beat faster and harder, as if you were actually exercising.

If you have trouble completing the stress test in a specified period of time, it may mean that there is reduced blood flow to your heart. Reduced blood flow can be caused by several different heart conditions, some of which are very serious.

What Are They Used For?

Stress tests are most often used to:

- Diagnose coronary artery disease (CAD), a condition that causes a waxy substance called "plaque" to build up in the arteries. It can cause dangerous blockages in blood flow to the heart.

- Diagnose arrhythmia, a condition that causes an irregular heartbeat

- Find out what level of exercise is safe for you

- Find out how well your treatment is working if you have already been diagnosed with heart disease

- Show if you are at risk for a heart attack or other serious heart condition

Why Do You Need a Stress Test?

You may need a stress test if you have symptoms of limited blood flow to your heart. These include:

- Angina, a type of chest pain or discomfort caused by poor blood flow to the heart

- Shortness of breath

- Rapid heartbeat

- Irregular heartbeat (arrhythmia). This may feel like a fluttering in your chest.

You may also need a stress test to check your heart health if you:

- Are planning to start an exercise program

- Have had recent heart surgery

- Are being treated for heart disease. The test can show how well your treatment is working.

- Have had a heart attack in the past

- Are at a higher risk for heart disease due to health problems, such as diabetes, family history of heart disease, and/or previous heart problems

What Happens during a Stress Test

There are three main types of stress tests: exercise stress tests, nuclear stress tests, and stress echocardiograms. All types of stress tests may be done in a healthcare provider's office, outpatient clinic, or hospital.

During an exercise stress test:

- A healthcare provider will place several electrodes (small sensors that stick to the skin) on your arms, legs, and chest. The provider may need to shave excess hair before placing the electrodes.

- The electrodes are attached by wires to an electrocardiogram (EKG) machine, which records your heart's electrical activity.

- You will then walk on a treadmill or ride a stationary bicycle, starting slowly.

- Then, you will walk or pedal faster, with the incline and resistance increasing as you go.

- You will continue walking or riding until you reach a target heart rate set by your provider. You may need to stop sooner if you develop symptoms, such as chest pain, shortness of breath, dizziness, or fatigue. The test may also be stopped if the EKG shows a problem with your heart.

- After the test, you will be monitored for 10 to 15 minutes or until your heart rate returns to normal.

Both nuclear stress tests and stress echocardiograms are imaging tests. That means that pictures will be taken of your heart during testing.

During a nuclear stress test:

- You will lie down on an exam table.

- A healthcare provider will insert an intravenous (IV) line into your arm. The IV contains a radioactive dye. The dye makes it possible for the healthcare provider to view images of your heart. It takes between 15 to 40 minutes for the heart to absorb the dye.

- A special camera will scan your heart to create the images, which show your heart at rest.

- The rest of the test is the same as an exercise stress test. You will be hooked up to an EKG machine, then walk on a treadmill or ride a stationary bicycle.

- If you are not healthy enough to exercise, you will take a medicine that makes your heart beat faster and harder.

- When your heart is working at its hardest, you will get another injection of the radioactive dye.

- You will wait for about 15 to 40 minutes for your heart to absorb the dye.

- You will resume exercising, and the special camera will take more pictures of your heart.

- Your provider will compare the two sets of images: one of your heart at rest, the other while hard at work.

- After the test, you will be monitored for 10 to 15 minutes or until your heart rate returns to normal.

- The radioactive dye will naturally leave your body through your urine. Drinking lots of water will help remove it faster.

During a stress echocardiogram:

- You will lie on an exam table.

- The provider will rub a special gel on a wand-like device called a "transducer." She or he will hold the transducer against your chest.

- This device makes sound waves, which create moving pictures of your heart.

- After these images are taken, you will exercise on a treadmill or bicycle, as in the other types of stress tests.

- If you are not healthy enough to exercise, you will take a medicine that makes your heart beat faster and harder.

- More images will be taken when your heart rate is increasing or when it is working at its hardest.

- Your provider will compare the two sets of images: one of your heart at rest, the other while hard at work.

- After the test, you will be monitored for 10 to 15 minutes or until your heart rate returns to normal.

Will You Need to Do Anything to Prepare for the Test?

You should wear comfortable shoes and loose clothing to make it easier to exercise. Your provider may ask you to not eat or drink for several hours before the test. If you have questions about how to prepare, talk to your healthcare provider.

Are There Any Risks to the Test?

Stress tests are usually safe. Sometimes, exercise or the medicine that increases your heart rate can cause symptoms, such as chest pain, dizziness, or nausea. You will be monitored closely throughout the test to reduce your risk of complications or to quickly treat any health problems. The radioactive dye used in a nuclear stress test is safe for most people. In rare cases, it may cause an allergic reaction. Also, a nuclear stress test is not recommended for pregnant women, as the dye might be harmful to the fetus.

What Do the Results Mean?

A normal test result means that no blood flow problems were found. If your test result was not normal, it can mean that there is reduced blood flow to your heart. Reasons for reduced blood flow include:

- Coronary artery disease (CAD)

- Scarring from a previous heart attack

- Your current heart treatment is not working well

- Poor physical fitness

If your exercise stress test results were not normal, your healthcare provider may order a nuclear stress test or a stress echocardiogram. These tests are more accurate than exercise stress tests, but they are also more expensive. If these imaging tests show a problem with your heart, your provider may recommend more tests and/or treatment.

If you have questions about your results, talk to your healthcare provider.

Chapter 49

Commonly Used Medications for Cardiovascular Health

Chapter Contents

Section 49.1

Aspirin

This section includes text excerpted from "Talk with Your Doctor about Taking Aspirin to Prevent Disease," Office of Disease Prevention and Health Promotion (ODPHP), U.S. Department of Health and Human Services (HHS), February 26, 2019.

The Basics

Taking low-dose aspirin (or "baby aspirin") regularly can lower your risk for heart attack, stroke, and colorectal cancer. For most people, aspirin is safe. But it is not right for everyone.

Ask your doctor about taking aspirin regularly if you are between the ages of 50 and 59, and you have any of these risk factors for heart disease:

- Smoking
- High blood pressure
- High cholesterol
- Diabetes

Talk with your doctor about your health history and ask if low-dose aspirin is right for you.

Usually, taking aspirin to prevent disease means taking it every day. Most people will need to take aspirin regularly for at least 5 to 10 years to get all of the benefits. Make sure your doctor says it is okay before you start taking aspirin every day.

What Are the Benefits of Taking Aspirin Regularly?

Taking low-dose aspirin regularly can reduce your risk of heart attack or stroke by preventing blood clots. Blood clots are clumps of thickened blood that can block blood flow to parts of the body. They can cause serious health problems or even death.

A blood clot can:

- Block blood flow to your heart and cause a heart attack
- Prevent blood from getting to your brain and cause a stroke

Taking aspirin regularly can prevent blood clots and lower your risk of heart attack or stroke. If you have already had a heart attack or stroke, aspirin can lower your risk of having another one.

Taking aspirin regularly for at least 5 to 10 years can also lower your risk of colorectal cancer, but experts are not sure why.

Can Taking Aspirin Every Day Cause Any Side Effects?

Taking aspirin regularly is not right for everyone. For some people, it may cause side effects, such as bleeding in the stomach.

Talk with your doctor before you start taking aspirin. Be sure to tell your doctor about any health conditions you have (such as stomach problems or bleeding problems).

Take Action

Take these steps to protect your health if you are at risk of heart attack or stroke.

Find Out If Daily Aspirin Is Right for You

Your doctor can help you decide if low-dose aspirin is the right choice for you. Talk with your doctor about:

- Your risk of heart attack or stroke

- What kind of aspirin to take

- How much to take

- How often to take it

- Side effects that it may cause

It is important to tell your doctor about all the other medicines you take, including vitamins, herbs, and over-the-counter (OTC) medicines (medicines you can get without a prescription). It may be dangerous to mix aspirin with other medicines.

What about Cost

Aspirin is inexpensive and sold over-the-counter. For some adults, aspirin is covered under the Affordable Care Act, the healthcare reform law passed in 2010. Check with your insurance provider to find out what is included in your plan.

Know Your Family's Health History

Your family history affects your risk for heart attack, stroke, and colorectal cancer. Use this family health history tool to keep track of your family's health. Share this information with your doctor.

Use Aspirin Safely

If you and your doctor decide that regularly taking low-dose aspirin is right for you, follow these safety tips:

- Make sure you understand how much aspirin to take and how often to take it. Most people who take aspirin to prevent disease take 81 mg every day—though your doctor may recommend you take a higher dose every other day.

- Talk with your doctor before you start taking a new medicine or vitamin. Ask if it is safe to take with aspirin.

- If you drink alcohol, drink only in moderation. This means no more than one drink a day for women and no more than two drinks a day for men. Alcohol can increase some risks of taking aspirin regularly.

- Check with your doctor first if you want to stop taking aspirin regularly.

Make It Easy to Remember

Here are a few things that may help you remember to take aspirin regularly:

- Take it at the same time every day. For example, take it after you brush your teeth or when you eat breakfast.

- Put a reminder note on your bathroom mirror where you will see it each day.

- Use a weekly pillbox to keep track of the medicines you take each day.

Take Steps to Protect Your Health

Taking low-dose aspirin regularly is just one of many ways to stay healthy.

To lower your risk of heart disease, stroke, and colorectal cancer:

- Quit smoking.

- Get active.

- Watch your weight.

Keep Your Heart Healthy

Eating healthy is another way to lower your risk of heart disease and stroke.

Get Tested for Colorectal Cancer

If you are between the ages of 50 and 75, get screened (tested) regularly for colorectal cancer. Screening can help prevent colorectal cancer or find it early, when it is easier to treat.

Section 49.2

Blood Thinner Pills

This section includes text excerpted from "Blood Thinner Pills: Your Guide to Using Them Safely," Agency for Healthcare Research and Quality (AHRQ), U.S. Department of Health and Human Services (HHS), November 2018.

About Your Blood Thinner

Your doctor has prescribed a medicine called a "blood thinner" to prevent blood clots. Blood clots can put you at risk for heart attack, stroke, and other serious medical problems. A blood thinner is a kind of drug called an "anticoagulant." "Anti" means against, and "coagulant" means to thicken into a gel or solid.

Depending on where you receive care, you may be seen by a doctor, nurse, physician's assistant, nurse practitioner, pharmacist, or other healthcare professional. The term "doctor" is used in this section to refer to the person who helps you manage your blood-thinner medicine.

You and your doctor will work together as a team to make sure that taking your blood thinner does not stop you from living well and safely. The information in this section will help you understand why you are taking a blood thinner and how to keep yourself healthy. There are different types of blood thinners. The most common blood thinner that doctors prescribe is warfarin (Coumadin®). Your doctor may also discuss using one of the newer blood thinners, depending on your individual situation.

How to Take Your Blood Thinner

Always take your blood thinner as directed. For example, some blood thinners need to be taken at the same time of day, every day.

Never skip a dose, and never take a double dose.

If you miss a dose, take it as soon as you remember. If you do not remember until the next day, call your doctor for instructions. If this happens when your doctor is not available, skip the missed dose and start again the next day. Mark the missed dose in a diary or on a calendar.

A pillbox with a slot for each day may help you keep track of your medicines.

Check Your Medicine

Check your medicine when you get it from the pharmacy.

- Does the medicine seem different from what your doctor prescribed or look different from what you expected?

- Does your pill look different from what you used before?

- Are the color, shape, and markings on the pill the same as what you were given before?

If something seems different, ask the pharmacist to double check it. Many medication errors are found by patients.

Using Other Medicines

Tell your doctor about every medicine you take. The doctor needs to know about all of your medicines, including medicines you used before you started taking a blood thinner.

Other medicines can change the way your blood thinner works. Your blood thinner can also change how other medicines work.

It is very important to talk with your doctor about all the medicines you take, including other prescription medicines, over-the-counter (OTC) medicines, vitamins, and herbal products.

Products that contain aspirin may lessen the blood's ability to form clots and may increase your risk of bleeding when you also are taking a blood thinner. **If you are taking a blood thinner, talk to your doctor before taking any medication that has aspirin in it.**

Medicines you get over-the-counter may also interact with your blood thinner. Following is a list of some common medicines that you should talk with your doctor or pharmacist about before using.

Pain relievers, cold medicines, or stomach remedies, such as:

- Advil®
- Aleve®
- Alka-Seltzer®
- Excedrin®
- ex-lax®
- Midol®
- Motrin®
- Nuprin®
- Pamprin HB®
- Pepto Bismol®
- Sine-Off®
- Tagamet HB®
- Tylenol®

Vitamins and herbal products, such as:

- Centrum®, One A Day®, or other multivitamins
- Garlic
- Ginkgo biloba
- Green tea

Talk to your doctor about every medication and over-the-counter product that you take.

Talk to Your Other Doctors

Because you take a blood thinner, you will be seen regularly by the doctor who prescribed the medicine. You may also see other doctors for different problems. When you see other doctors, it is very important that you tell them you are taking a blood thinner. You should also tell your dentist and the person who cleans your teeth.

If you use different pharmacies, make sure each pharmacist knows that you take a blood thinner.

Blood thinners can interact with medicines and treatments that other doctors might prescribe for you. If another doctor orders a new medicine for you, tell the doctor who ordered your blood thinner because dose changes for your blood thinner may be needed.

Tell all your doctors about every medication and over-the-counter product that you take.

Tell your doctor about all your medicines.

Always tell your doctor about all the medicines you are taking. Tell your doctor when you start taking new medicine, when you stop taking a medicine, and if the amount of medicine you are taking changes. When you visit your doctor, bring a list of current medicines; over-the-counter drugs, such as aspirin; and any vitamins and herbal products you take. A personal, medication wallet card can help you keep track of this list.

Possible Side Effects

When taking a blood thinner, it is important to be aware of its possible side effects. Bleeding is the most common side effect.

Call your doctor immediately if you have any of the following signs of serious bleeding:

- Menstrual bleeding that is much heavier than normal

- Red or brown urine

- Bowel movements that are red or look like tar

- Bleeding from the gums or nose that does not stop quickly

- Vomit that is brown or bright red

- Anything red in color that you cough up

- Severe pain, such as a headache or stomach ache

- Unusual bruising

- A cut that does not stop bleeding

- A serious fall or bump on the head

- Dizziness or weakness

Stay Safe While Taking Your Blood Thinner

Call your doctor and go to the hospital immediately if you have had a fall or hit your head, even if you are not bleeding. You can be bleeding but not see any blood. For example, if you fall and hit your head, bleeding can occur inside your skull. Or, if you hurt your arm during a fall and then notice a large purple bruise, this means that you are bleeding under your skin.

Because you are taking a blood thinner, you should try to not hurt yourself and cause bleeding. You need to be careful when you use knives, scissors, razors, or any sharp object that can make you bleed.

You also need to avoid activities and sports that could cause injury. Swimming and walking are safe activities. If you would like to start a new activity that will increase the amount of exercise you get every day, talk to your doctor.

You can still do many things that you enjoy. If you like to work in the yard, you still can. Just be sure to wear sturdy shoes and gloves to protect yourself. If you like to ride your bike, be sure you wear a helmet.

Tell others.

Keep a current list of all the medicines you take. Ask your doctor about whether you should wear a medical alert bracelet or necklace. If you are badly injured and unable to speak, the bracelet lets healthcare workers know that you are taking a blood thinner.

To prevent injury indoors:

- Be very careful using knives and scissors.

- Use an electric razor.

- Use a soft toothbrush.

- Use waxed dental floss.

- Do not use toothpicks.

- Wear shoes or nonskid slippers in the house.

- Be careful when you trim your toenails.

- Do not trim corns or calluses yourself.

To prevent injury outdoors:

- Always wear shoes.

- Wear gloves when using sharp tools.

- Avoid activities and sports that can easily hurt you.

- Wear gardening gloves when doing yard work.

Food and Your Blood Thinner

If your doctor has prescribed warfarin, the foods you eat can affect how well your blood thinner works for you. High amounts of vitamin K can work against warfarin. Other blood thinners are not affected by vitamin K. Ask your doctor if your diet can affect how well your blood thinner works.

If you are taking a blood thinner, you should avoid drinking alcohol.

Call your doctor if you are unable to eat for several days, for whatever reason. Also call if you have stomach problems, vomiting, or diarrhea that lasts longer than one day. These problems could affect your blood-thinner dose.

Keep your diet the same.

Do not make any major changes in your diet or start a weight-loss plan unless you talk to your doctor first.

Blood Tests

You will have to have your blood tested often if you are taking warfarin. The blood test helps your doctor decide how much medicine you need.

The international normalized ratio (INR) blood test measures how fast your blood clots and lets the doctor know if your dose needs to be changed. Testing your blood helps your doctor keep you in a safe range. If there is too much blood thinner in your body, you could bleed too much. If there is not enough, you could get a blood clot.

Regular blood tests are not needed for some of the newer blood thinners.

Important reminders:

- Take your blood thinner as directed by your doctor.

- Go for blood tests as directed.

- Never skip a dose.

- Never take a double dose.

Chapter 50

Iron Supplements for Anemia

Hemoglobin is an iron-rich protein that helps red blood cells carry oxygen from the lungs to the rest of the body. If you have anemia, your body does not get enough oxygen-rich blood. This can cause you to feel tired or weak. You may also have shortness of breath, dizziness, headaches, or an irregular heartbeat.

There are many types and causes of anemia. Mild anemia is a common and treatable condition that can occur in anyone. Some people—including women during their menstrual periods and pregnancy, and people who donate blood frequently; do not get enough iron or certain vitamins; or take certain medicines, such as chemotherapy for cancer—are at a higher risk for anemia.

Anemia may also be a sign of a more serious condition. It may result from chronic bleeding in the stomach. Chronic inflammation from an infection, kidney disease, cancer, or autoimmune disease can also cause the body to make fewer red blood cells.

Your doctor will consider your medical history, physical exam, and test results when diagnosing and treating anemia. She or he will use a simple blood test to confirm that you have low amounts of red blood

This chapter contains text excerpted from the following sources: Text in this chapter begins with excerpts from "Anemia," National Heart, Lung, and Blood Institute (NHLBI), January 18, 2019; Text beginning with the heading "What Is Iron and What Does It Do?" is excerpted from "Iron," Office of Dietary Supplements (ODS), National Institutes of Health (NIH), February 17, 2016.

cells or hemoglobin. For some types of mild to moderate anemia, your doctor may recommend over-the-counter or prescription iron supplements, certain vitamins, intravenous iron therapy, or medicines that make your body produce more red blood cells. To prevent anemia in the future, your doctor may also suggest healthy eating changes. If you have severe anemia, your doctor may recommend red blood cell transfusions.

What Is Iron and What Does It Do?

Iron is a mineral that the body needs for growth and development. Your body uses iron to make hemoglobin, a protein in red blood cells (RBCs) that carries oxygen from the lungs to all parts of the body, and myoglobin, a protein that provides oxygen to muscles. Your body also needs iron to make some hormones and connective tissue.

How Much Iron Do I Need?

The amount of iron you need each day depends on your age, your sex, and whether you consume a mostly plant-based diet. The average daily recommended amounts are listed below in milligrams (mg). Vegetarians who do not eat meat, poultry, or seafood need almost twice as much iron as listed in the table because the body does not absorb nonheme iron in plant foods as well as heme iron in animal foods.

Table 50.1. Amount of Iron in Each Stages of Life

Life Stage	Recommended Amount
Birth to 6 months	0.27 mg
Infants 7 to 12 months	11 mg
Children 1 to 3 years	7 mg
Children 4 to 8 years	10 mg
Children 9 to 13 years	8 mg
Teens boys 14 to 18 years	11 mg
Teens girls 14 to 18 years	15 mg
Adult men 19 to 50 years	8 mg
Adult women 19 to 50 years	18 mg
Adults 51 years and older	8 mg
Pregnant teens	27 mg
Pregnant women	27 mg
Breastfeeding teens	10 mg
Breastfeeding women	9 mg

What Foods Provide Iron

Iron is found naturally in many foods and is added to some fortified food products. You can get recommended amounts of iron by eating a variety of foods, including the following:

- Lean meat, seafood, and poultry

- Iron-fortified breakfast cereals and breads

- White beans, lentils, spinach, kidney beans, and peas

- Nuts and some dried fruits, such as raisins

Iron in food comes in two forms: heme iron and nonheme iron. Nonheme iron is found in plant foods and iron-fortified food products. Meat, seafood, and poultry have both heme and nonheme iron.

Your body absorbs iron from plant sources better when you eat it with meat; poultry; seafood; and foods that contain vitamin C, such as citrus fruits, strawberries, sweet peppers, tomatoes, and broccoli.

Am I Getting Enough Iron?

Most people in the United States get enough iron. However, certain groups of people are more likely than others to have trouble getting enough iron:

- Teen girls and women with heavy periods

- Pregnant women and teens

- Infants (especially if they are premature or had a low birthweight)

- Frequent blood donors

- People with cancer, gastrointestinal (GI) disorders, or heart failure

What Kinds of Iron Dietary Supplements Are Available?

Iron is available in many multivitamin-mineral supplements and in supplements that contain only iron. Iron in supplements is often in the form of ferrous sulfate, ferrous gluconate, ferric citrate, or ferric sulfate. Dietary supplements that contain iron have a statement on the label warning that they should be kept out of the reach of children. Accidental overdose of iron-containing products is a leading cause of fatal poisoning in children under six years of age.

Chapter 51

Blood Transfusion

What Is Blood Transfusion?

A blood transfusion is a safe, common procedure in which blood is given to you through an intravenous (IV) line in one of your blood vessels.

Blood transfusions are done to replace blood lost during surgery or due to a serious injury. A transfusion also may be done if your body cannot make blood properly because of an illness.

During a blood transfusion, a small needle is used to insert an IV line into one of your blood vessels. Through this line, you receive healthy blood. The procedure usually takes one to four hours, depending on how much blood you need.

Blood transfusions are very common. Each year, almost five million Americans need a blood transfusion. Most blood transfusions go well. Mild complications can occur. Very rarely, serious problems develop.

Important Information about Blood

The heart pumps blood through a network of arteries and veins throughout the body. Blood has many vital jobs. It carries oxygen and other nutrients to your body's organs and tissues. Having a healthy supply of blood is important to your overall health.

This chapter includes text excerpted from "Blood Transfusion," National Heart, Lung, and Blood Institute (NHLBI), January 18, 2019.

Blood is made up of various parts, including red blood cells (RBCs), white blood cells (WBCs), platelets, and plasma. Blood is transfused either as whole blood or, more often, as individual parts.

Blood Types

Every person has one of the following blood types: A, B, AB, or O. Also, every person's blood is either Rh-positive or Rh-negative. So, if you have type A blood, it is either A positive or A negative.

The blood used in a transfusion must work with your blood type. If it does not, antibodies (proteins) in your blood attack the new blood and make you sick.

Type O blood is safe for almost everyone. About 40 percent of the population has type O blood. People who have this blood type are called "universal donors." Type O blood is used for emergencies when there is no time to test a person's blood type.

People who have type AB blood are called "universal recipients." This means they can get any type of blood.

If you have Rh-positive blood, you can get Rh-positive or Rh-negative blood. But if you have Rh-negative blood, you should only get Rh-negative blood. Rh-negative blood is used for emergencies when there is no time to test a person's Rh type.

Blood Banks

Blood banks collect, test, and store blood. They carefully screen all donated blood for possible infectious agents, such as viruses, that could make you sick.

Blood bank staff also screen each blood donation to find out whether it is type A, B, AB, or O and whether it is Rh-positive or Rh-negative. Getting a blood type that does not work with your own blood type will make you very sick. That is why blood banks are very careful when they test the blood.

To prepare blood for a transfusion, some blood banks remove white blood cells. This process is called "white cell reduction" or "leukocyte reduction." Although rare, some people are allergic to white blood cells in donated blood. Removing these cells makes allergic reactions less likely.

Not all transfusions use blood donated from a stranger. If you are going to have surgery, you may need a blood transfusion because of blood loss during the operation. If it is surgery that you are able to schedule months in advance, your doctor may ask whether you would like to use your own blood, rather than donated blood.

If you choose to use your own blood, you will need to have blood drawn one or more times prior to the surgery. A blood bank will store your blood for your use.

Alternatives to Blood Transfusions

Researchers are trying to find ways to make blood. There is currently no human-made alternative to human blood. However, researchers have developed medicines that may help do the job of some blood parts.

For example, some people who have kidney problems can now take a medicine called "erythropoietin" that helps their bodies make more red blood cells. This means they may need fewer blood transfusions.

Surgeons try to reduce the amount of blood lost during surgery so that fewer patients need blood transfusions. Sometimes they can collect and reuse the blood for the patient.

Types of Blood Transfusion

Blood is transfused either as whole blood or, more often, as individual parts. The type of blood transfusion you need depends on your situation.

For example, if you have an illness that stops your body from properly making a part of your blood, you may need only that part to treat the illness.

Red Blood Cell Transfusions

Red blood cells are the most commonly transfused part of the blood. These cells carry oxygen from the lungs to your body's organs and tissues. They also help your body get rid of carbon dioxide and other waste products.

You may need a transfusion of red blood cells if you have lost blood due to an injury or surgery. You also may need this type of transfusion if you have severe anemia due to disease or blood loss.

Anemia is a condition in which your blood has a lower-than-normal number of red blood cells. Anemia also can occur if your red blood cells do not have enough hemoglobin.

Hemoglobin is an iron-rich protein that gives blood its red color. This protein carries oxygen from the lungs to the rest of the body.

Platelets and Clotting Factor Transfusions

Platelets and clotting factors help stop bleeding, including internal bleeding that you cannot see. Some illnesses may cause your body to not make enough platelets or clotting factors. You may need regular transfusions of these parts of your blood to stay healthy.

For example, if you have hemophilia, you may need a special clotting factor to replace the clotting factor you are lacking. Hemophilia is a rare, inherited bleeding disorder in which your blood does not clot normally.

If you have hemophilia, you may bleed for a longer time than others after an injury or accident. You also may bleed internally, especially in the joints (knees, ankles, and elbows).

Plasma Transfusions

Plasma is the liquid part of your blood. It is mainly water, but also contains proteins, clotting factors, hormones, vitamins, cholesterol, sugar, sodium, potassium, calcium, and more.

If you have been badly burned or have liver failure or a severe infection, you may need a plasma transfusion.

Who Needs a Blood Transfusion

Blood transfusions are very common. Each year, almost five million Americans need blood transfusions. This procedure is used for people of all ages.

Many people who have surgery need blood transfusions because they lose blood during their operations. For example, about one-third of all heart surgery patients have a transfusion.

Some people who have serious injuries—such as from car crashes, war, or natural disasters—need blood transfusions to replace blood lost during the injury.

Some people need blood or parts of blood because of illnesses. You may need a blood transfusion if you have:

- A severe infection or liver disease that stops your body from properly making blood or some parts of blood

- An illness that causes anemia, such as kidney disease or cancer. Medicines or radiation used to treat a medical condition also can cause anemia. There are many types of anemia, including aplastic, Fanconi, hemolytic, iron-deficiency, and sickle cell anemias and thalassemia.

- A bleeding disorder, such as hemophilia or thrombocytopenia

What to Expect before a Blood Transfusion

Before a blood transfusion, a technician tests your blood to find out what blood type you have. She or he pricks your finger with a needle to get a few drops of blood or draws blood from one of your veins.

The blood type used in your transfusion must work with your blood type. If it does not, antibodies (proteins) in your blood attack the new blood and make you sick.

Some people have allergic reactions even when the blood given does work with their own blood type. To prevent this, your doctor may prescribe a medicine to stop allergic reactions.

If you have allergies or have had an allergic reaction during a past transfusion, your doctor will make every effort to make sure you are safe.

Most people do not need to change their diets or activities before or after a blood transfusion. Your doctor will let you know whether you need to make any lifestyle changes prior to the procedure.

What to Expect during a Blood Transfusion

Blood transfusions take place in either a doctor's office or a hospital. Sometimes they are done at a person's home, but this is less common. Blood transfusions also are done during surgery and in emergency rooms.

A needle is used to insert an IV line into one of your blood vessels. Through this line, you receive healthy blood. The procedure usually takes one to four hours. The time depends on how much blood you need and what part of the blood you receive.

During the blood transfusion, a nurse carefully watches you, especially for the first 15 minutes. This is when allergic reactions are most likely to occur. The nurse continues to watch you during the rest of the procedure as well.

What to Expect after a Blood Transfusion

After a blood transfusion, your vital signs are checked (such as your temperature, blood pressure, and heart rate). The IV line is taken out. You may have some bruising or soreness for a few days at the site where the IV was inserted.

You may need blood tests that show how your body is reacting to the transfusion. Your doctor will let you know about the signs and symptoms to watch for and report.

Risk Factors

Most blood transfusions go very smoothly. However, mild problems and, very rarely, serious problems can occur.

Allergic Reactions

Some people have allergic reactions to the blood given during transfusions. This can happen even when the blood given is the right blood type.

Allergic reactions can be mild or severe. Symptoms can include:

- Anxiety
- Chest and/or back pain
- Trouble breathing
- Fever, chills, flushing, and clammy skin
- A quick pulse or low blood pressure
- Nausea (feeling sick to the stomach)

A nurse or doctor will stop the transfusion at the first signs of an allergic reaction. The healthcare team determines how mild or severe the reaction is, what treatments are needed and whether the transfusion can safely be restarted.

Viruses and Infectious Diseases

Some infectious agents, such as human immunodeficiency virus (HIV), can survive in blood and infect the person receiving the blood transfusion. To keep blood safe, blood banks carefully screen donated blood.

The risk of catching a virus from a blood transfusion is very low.

- **Human immunodeficiency virus (HIV).** Your risk of getting HIV from a blood transfusion is lower than your risk of getting killed by lightning. Only about 1 in 2 million donations might carry HIV and transmit HIV if given to a patient.

- **Hepatitis B and C.** The risk of having a donation that carries hepatitis B is about 1 in 205,000. The risk for hepatitis C is 1 in 2 million. If you receive blood during a transfusion that contains hepatitis, you will likely develop the virus.

- **Variant Creutzfeldt-Jakob disease (vCJD).** This disease is the human version of Mad Cow Disease. It is a very rare, yet fatal brain disorder. There is a possible risk of getting vCJD from a blood transfusion, although the risk is very low. Because of this, people who may have been exposed to vCJD are not eligible blood donors.

Fever

You may get a sudden fever during or within a day of your blood transfusion. This is usually your body's normal response to white blood cells in the donated blood. Over-the-counter (OTC) fever medicine usually will treat the fever.

Some blood banks remove white blood cells from whole blood or different parts of the blood. This makes it less likely that you will have a reaction after the transfusion.

Iron Overload

Getting many blood transfusions can cause too much iron to build up in your blood (iron overload). People who have a blood disorder, such as thalassemia, which requires multiple transfusions, are at risk for iron overload. Iron overload can damage your liver, heart, and other parts of your body.

If you have iron overload, you may need iron chelation therapy. For this therapy, medicine is given through an injection or as a pill to remove the extra iron from your body.

Lung Injury

Although it is unlikely, blood transfusions can damage your lungs, making it hard to breathe. This usually occurs within about six hours of the procedure.

Most patients recover. However, 5 to 25 percent of patients who develop lung injuries die from the injuries. These people usually were very ill before the transfusion.

Doctors are not completely sure why blood transfusions damage the lungs. Antibodies (proteins) that are more likely to be found in the plasma of women who have been pregnant may disrupt the normal way that lung cells work. Because of this risk, hospitals are starting to use men's and women's plasma differently.

Acute Immune Hemolytic Reaction

Acute immune hemolytic reaction is very serious, but it is also very rare. It occurs if the blood type you get during a transfusion does not match or work with your blood type. Your body attacks the new red blood cells, which then produce substances that harm your kidneys.

The symptoms include chills, fever, nausea, pain in the chest or back, and dark urine. The doctor will stop the transfusion at the first sign of this reaction.

Delayed Hemolytic Reaction

This is a much slower version of acute immune hemolytic reaction. Your body destroys red blood cells so slowly that the problem can go unnoticed until your red blood cell level is very low.

Both acute and delayed hemolytic reactions are most common in patients who have had a previous transfusion.

Graft-Versus-Host Disease

Graft-versus-host disease (GVHD) is a condition in which white blood cells in the new blood attack your tissues. GVHD usually is fatal. People who have weakened immune systems are the most likely to get GVHD.

Symptoms start within a month of the blood transfusion. They include fever, rash, and diarrhea. To protect against GVHD, people who have weakened immune systems should receive blood that has been treated so the white blood cells cannot cause GVHD.

Chapter 52

Blood-Forming Stem Cell Transplants

What Are Bone Marrow and Hematopoietic Stem Cells?

Bone marrow is the soft, sponge-like material found inside bones. It contains immature cells known as "hematopoietic" or "blood-forming stem cells." (Hematopoietic stem cells are different from embryonic stem cells. Embryonic stem cells can develop into every type of cell in the body.) Hematopoietic stem cells divide to form more blood-forming stem cells, or they mature into one of three types of blood cells: white blood cells, which fight infection; red blood cells, which carry oxygen; and platelets, which help the blood to clot. Most hematopoietic stem cells are found in the bone marrow, but some cells, called "peripheral blood stem cells" (PBSCs), are found in the bloodstream. Blood in the umbilical cord also contains hematopoietic stem cells. Cells from any of these sources can be used in transplants.

This chapter contains text excerpted from the following sources: Text beginning with the heading "What Are Bone Marrow and Hematopoietic Stem Cells?" is excerpted from "Blood-Forming Stem Cell Transplants," Centers for Disease Control and Prevention (CDC), August 12, 2013. Reviewed June 2019; Text under the heading "During and after the Transplant" is excerpted from "Blood and Bone Marrow Transplant," National Heart, Lung, and Blood Institute (NHLBI), May 19, 2015. Reviewed June 2019.

What Are Bone Marrow Transplantation and Peripheral Blood Stem Cell Transplantation?

Bone marrow transplantation (BMT) and peripheral blood stem cell transplantation (PBSCT) are procedures that restore stem cells that have been destroyed by high doses of chemotherapy and/or radiation therapy. There are three types of transplants:

- In **autologous transplants**, patients receive their own stem cells.

- In **syngeneic transplants,** patients receive stem cells from their identical twin.

- In **allogeneic transplants**, patients receive stem cells from their brother, sister, or parent. A person who is not related to the patient (an unrelated donor) also may be used.

How Are the Donor's Stem Cells Matched to the Patient's Stem Cells in Allogeneic or Syngeneic Transplantation?

To minimize potential side effects, doctors most often use transplanted stem cells that match the patient's own stem cells as closely as possible. People have different sets of proteins, called "human leukocyte-associated" (HLA) antigens, on the surface of their cells. The set of proteins, called the "HLA type," is identified by a special blood test.

In most cases, the success of allogeneic transplantation depends in part on how well the HLA antigens of the donor's stem cells match those of the recipient's stem cells. The higher the number of matching HLA antigens, the greater the chance that the patient's body will accept the donor's stem cells. In general, patients are less likely to develop a complication known as "graft-versus-host disease" (GVHD) if the stem cells of the donor and patient are closely matched.

Close relatives, especially brothers and sisters, are more likely than unrelated people to be HLA-matched. However, only 25 to 35 percent of patients have an HLA-matched sibling. The chances of obtaining HLA-matched stem cells from an unrelated donor are slightly better, approximately 50 percent. Among unrelated donors, HLA-matching is greatly improved when the donor and recipient have the same ethnic and racial background. Although the number of donors is increasing overall, individuals from certain ethnic and racial groups still have a lower chance of finding a matching donor. Large volunteer donor registries can assist in finding an appropriate unrelated donor.

Because identical twins have the same genes, they have the same set of HLA antigens. As a result, the patient's body will accept a transplant from an identical twin. However, identical twins represent a small number of all births, so syngeneic transplantation is rare.

How Is Bone Marrow Obtained for Transplantation?

The stem cells used in BMT come from the liquid center of the bone, called the "marrow." In general, the procedure for obtaining bone marrow, which is called "harvesting," is similar for all three types of BMTs. The donor is given either general anesthesia, which puts the person to sleep during the procedure, or regional anesthesia, which causes, a loss of feeling below the waist. Needles are inserted through the skin over the pelvic (hip) bone or, in rare cases, the sternum (breastbone) and into the bone marrow to draw the marrow out of the bone. Harvesting the marrow takes about an hour.

The harvested bone marrow is then processed to remove blood and bone fragments. Harvested bone marrow can be combined with a preservative and frozen to keep the stem cells alive until they are needed. This technique is known as "cryopreservation." Stem cells can be cryopreserved for many years.

How Are Peripheral Blood Stem Cells Obtained for Transplantation?

The stem cells used in PBSCT come from the bloodstream. A process called "apheresis" or "leukapheresis" is used to obtain PBSCs for transplantation. For four or five days before apheresis, the donor may be given a medication to increase the number of stem cells released into the bloodstream. In apheresis, blood is removed through a large vein in the arm or a central venous catheter (a flexible tube that is placed in a large vein in the neck, chest, or groin area). The blood goes through a machine that removes the stem cells. The blood is then returned to the donor and the collected cells are stored. Apheresis typically takes four to six hours. The stem cells are then frozen until they are given to the recipient.

How Are Umbilical Cord Stem Cells Obtained for Transplantation?

Stem cells also may be retrieved from umbilical cord blood. For this to occur, the mother must contact a cord blood bank before the baby's birth. The cord blood bank may request that she complete a questionnaire and give a small blood sample.

Cord blood banks may be public or commercial. Public cord blood banks accept donations of cord blood and may provide the donated stem cells to another matched individual in their network. In contrast, commercial cord blood banks will store the cord blood for the family in case it is needed later for the child or another family member.

After the baby is born and the umbilical cord has been cut, blood is retrieved from the umbilical cord and placenta. This process poses minimal health risk to the mother or the child. If the mother agrees, the umbilical cord blood is processed and frozen for storage by the cord blood bank. Only a small amount of blood can be retrieved from the umbilical cord and placenta, so the collected stem cells are typically used for children or small adults.

Are Any Risks Associated with Donating Bone Marrow?

Because only a small amount of bone marrow is removed, donating usually does not pose any significant problems for the donor. The most serious risk associated with donating bone marrow involves the use of anesthesia during the procedure.

The area where the bone marrow was taken out may feel stiff or sore for a few days, and the donor may feel tired. Within a few weeks, the donor's body replaces the donated marrow; however, the time required for a donor to recover varies. Some people are back to their usual routine within two or three days, while others may take up to three to four weeks to fully recover their strength.

What Are the Costs of Donating Bone Marrow, Peripheral Blood Stem Cells, or Umbilical Cord Blood?

All medical costs for the donation procedure are covered by Be The Match® or by the patient's medical insurance, as are travel expenses and other nonmedical costs. The only costs to the donor might be time taken off from work.

A woman can donate her baby's umbilical cord blood to public cord blood banks at no charge. However, commercial blood banks do charge varying fees to store umbilical cord blood for the private use of the patient or her or his family.

Where Can People Get More Information about Potential Donors and Transplant Centers?

The National Marrow Donor Program® (NMDP), a nonprofit organization, manages the world's largest registry of more than 11 million potential donors and cord blood units. The NMDP operates Be The Match®, which helps connect patients with matching donors.

During and after the Transplant

Blood or bone marrow transplants are usually performed in a hospital. Often, you must stay in the hospital for one to two weeks before the transplant to prepare. During this time, you will have a narrow tube placed in one of your large veins. You may be given medicine to make you sleepy for this procedure. You also will receive special medicines and possibly radiation to destroy your abnormal stem cells and to weaken your immune system so that it will not reject the donor cells after the transplant.

On the day of the transplant, you will be awake and may get medicine to relax you during the procedure. The stem cells will be given to you through the narrow tube in your vein. The stem cells will travel through your blood to your bone marrow, where they will begin making new healthy blood cells.

After the transplant, your doctor will check your blood counts every day to see if new blood cells have started to grow in your bone marrow. Depending on the type of transplant, you may be able to leave but stay near the hospital, or you may need to remain in the hospital for weeks or months. The length of time will depend on how your immune system is recovering and whether or not the transplanted cells stay in your body. Before you leave the hospital, the doctors will give you detailed instructions that you must follow to prevent infection and other complications. Your doctor will keep monitoring your recovery, possibly for up to one year.

Although a blood or bone marrow transplant is an effective treatment for some conditions, the procedure can cause early or late complications. The required medicines and radiation can cause nausea, vomiting, diarrhea, tiredness, mouth sores, skin rashes, hair loss, or liver damage. These treatments also can weaken your immune system and increase your risk for infection. Some people may experience a serious complication called "graft-versus-host disease" (GVHD) if the donated stem cells attack the body. Other people's bodies may reject the donor stem cells after the transplant, which can be an extremely serious complication.

Part Six

Additional Help and Information

Chapter 53

Glossary of Terms Related to Blood and Circulatory Disorders

acute lymphoblastic leukemia: A type of leukemia (blood cancer) that comes on quickly and is fast growing. In acute lymphoblastic leukemia, there are too many lymphoblasts (immature white blood cells (WBCs)) in the blood and bone marrow.

agranulocyte: A type of white blood cell. Monocytes and lymphocytes are agranulocytes.

albumin: A type of protein found in blood, egg white, milk, and other substances.

angina: A recurring pain or discomfort in the chest that happens when some part of the heart does not receive enough blood.

antibody: A protein found in the blood that is produced in response to foreign substances invading the body.

aorta: The largest artery in the body which has its origin at the heart. It gives off branches to the extremities, neck and major organs for the purpose of supplying oxygenated blood.

arteries: Blood vessels that carry oxygen and blood to the heart, brain and other parts of the body.

This glossary contains terms excerpted from documents produced by several sources deemed reliable.

B cell: A small white blood cell crucial to the immune defenses.

basophil: A white blood cell that contributes to inflammatory reactions.

bilirubin: When the hemoglobin in a person's blood breaks down, causing a yellowing of the skin and whites of the eyes.

blood banking: The process that takes place in the laboratory to ensure that donated blood, or blood products, are safe before they are used in blood transfusions and other medical procedures.

blood clot: A mass of blood that forms when blood platelets, proteins, and cells stick together.

blood plasma: The fluid part of blood that contains nutrients, glucose, proteins, minerals, enzymes, and other substances.

blood pressure: The force of blood against the walls of arteries.

blood test: A test done on a sample of blood to measure the amount of certain substances in the blood or to count different types of blood cells.

blood thinner: A substance that is used to prevent and treat blood clots in blood vessels and the heart.

blood transfusion: The transfer of blood or blood products from one person (donor) into another person's bloodstream (recipient).

blood vessel: An artery, vein, or capillary that carries blood to and from the heart and body tissues.

cardiovascular diseases: Disease of the heart and blood vessels.

chronic myelogenous leukemia: A malignant cancer of the bone marrow that causes rapid growth of the blood-forming cells in the bone marrow, peripheral blood, and body tissues.

complete blood count: A blood test that measures the following components in a sample of blood red blood cells (RBCs), WBCs, platelets, and hemoglobin.

connective tissue: The supporting or framework tissue of the body, formed of fibrous and ground substance with more or less numerous cells of various kinds.

diabetes: A disease in which blood glucose (blood sugar) levels are above normal.

diapedesis: Passage of blood cells (especially WBCs) through intact capillary walls and into the surrounding tissue.

differential: In performing the blood count, a total of 100 cells are counted. The percent of each type found in these 100 cells is the cell "differential" for each type.

erythropoietin: A glycoprotein hormone produced primarily by cells of the peritubular capillary endothelium of the kidney that is responsible for the regulation of RBC production.

Fanconi anemia: A rare, inherited blood disorder that leads to bone marrow failure. It causes your bone marrow to stop making enough new blood cells for your body to work normally.

hematocrit: The percentage of the volume of a blood sample occupied by cells, as determined by a centrifuge or device which separates the cells and other particulate elements of the blood from the plasma. The remaining fraction of the blood sample is called plasmocrit (blood plasma volume).

hemorrhage: A copious discharge of blood from the blood vessels.

heparin: A drug given directly into a vein that thins the blood when there is a danger of clotting (an anticoagulant)

immune system: The complex system in the body responsible for fighting disease.

ischemic stroke: A blockage of blood vessels supplying blood to the brain, causing a decrease in blood supply.

lymphocyte: A small white blood cell produced in the lymphoid organs and essential to immune defenses.

lymphocytopenia: An abnormally small number of lymphocytes in the circulating blood.

megakaryocyte: Very large bone marrow cells which release mature blood platelets.

myeloid: A collective term for the nonlymphocyte groups of WBCs. It includes cells from the granulocyte, monocyte, and platelet lineages.

plasma: The fluid part of blood, lymph, or milk as distinguished from suspended material.

platelet: A cellular fragment critical for blood clotting and sealing off wounds.

pleural effusion: A collection of fluid (or blood) in the pleural space (in one side of the chest cavity around the lung).

serum: The clear liquid that separates from the blood when it is allowed to clot.

sickle cell anemia: It involves problems in the red blood cells (RBCs). Normal RBCs are round and smooth and move through blood vessels easily. Sickle cells are hard and have a curved edge. These cells cannot squeeze through small blood vessels. They block the organs from getting blood. Your body destroys sickle red cells quickly, but it cannot make new RBCs fast enough—a condition called anemia.

stem cell: An immature cell from which other cells derive.

T-cells: Thymus-derived lymphocytes. T-cells are the major component of cell-mediated immunity.

thalassemia: A group of blood diseases, that are inherited, which affect a person's hemoglobin and cause anemia. Hemoglobin is a protein in RBCs that carries oxygen and nutrients to cells in the body.

transient ischemic attack: A mini-stroke where there is a short-term reduction in blood flow to the brain usually resulting in temporary stroke symptoms. Does not cause damage to the brain, but puts a person at higher risk of having a full stroke.

triglyceride: A type of fat in the bloodstream and fat tissue. High triglyceride levels can contribute to the hardening and narrowing of arteries.

vaccine: A product made from very small amounts of weak or dead germs that can cause diseases — for example, viruses, bacteria, or toxins. It prepares your body to fight the disease faster and more effectively so you won't get sick. Vaccines are administered through needle injections, by mouth, and by aerosol.

vein: A blood vessel that carries blood to the heart from the body tissues.

venous: The system or veins by which blood is returned to the lungs for oxygenation.

Waldenström macroglobulinemia: A cancer of white blood cells known as B lymphocytes.

white blood cells: Key components of the immune system and help fight infection and disease.

X-ray: A type of high-energy radiation. In low doses, X-rays are used to diagnose diseases by making pictures of the inside of the body.

yoga: A mind and body practice with origins in ancient Indian philosophy. The various styles of yoga typically combine physical postures, breathing techniques, and meditation or relaxation.

Chapter 54

Directory of Resources Related to Blood and Circulatory Disorders

General

American Society of Hematology (ASH)
2021 L. St. N.W.
Ste. 900
Washington, DC 20036
Toll-Free: 866-828-1231
Phone: 202-776-0544
Fax: 202-776-0545
Website: www.hematology.org

Iron Disorders Institute (IDI)
P.O. Box 4891
Greenville, SC 29608
Toll-Free: 888-565-IRON
(888-565-4766)
Phone: 864-292-1175
Fax: 864-292-1878
Website: www.irondisorders.org
E-mail: info@irondisorders.org

Resources in this chapter were compiled from several sources deemed reliable; all contact information was verified and updated in June 2019.

National Heart, Lung, and Blood Institute (NHLBI)
Health Information Center
(HIC)
P.O. Box 30105
Bethesda, MD 20824-0105
Phone: 301-592-8573
TTY: 240-629-3255
Website: www.nhlbi.nih.gov
E-mail: nhlbiinfo@nhlbi.nih.gov

National Institute of Arthritis and Musculoskeletal and Skin Diseases (NIAMS)
1 AMS Cir.
Bethesda, MD 20892-3675
Toll-Free: 877-22-NIAMS
(877-226-4267)
Phone: 301-495-4484
TTY: 301-565-2966
Fax: 301-718-6366
Website: www.niams.nih.gov
E-mail: NIAMSinfo@mail.nih.gov

National Institute of Diabetes and Digestive and Kidney Diseases (NIDDK)
Health Information Center
(HIC)
Toll-Free: 800-860-8747
Toll-Free TTY: 866-569-1162
Website: www.niddk.nih.gov
E-mail: healthinfo@niddk.nih.gov

National Institute of Neurological Disorders and Stroke (NINDS)
NIH Neurological Institute
P.O. Box 5801
Bethesda, MD 20824
Toll-Free: 800-352-9424
Phone: 301-496-1807
Website: www.ninds.nih.gov

National Organization for Rare Disorders (NORD)
55 Kenosia Ave.
Danbury, CT 06810
Toll-Free: 800-999-6673
Phone: 203-744-0100
Fax: 203-263-9938
Website: rarediseases.org
E-mail: orphan@rarediseases.org

The Nemours Foundation / KidsHealth®
1600 Rockland Rd.
Wilmington, DE 19803
Phone: 302-651-4046
Website: kidshealth.org
E-mail: info@KidsHealth.org

Anemia

American Sickle Cell Anemia Association (ASCAA)
DD Bldg. at the Cleveland Clinic
10900 Carnegie Ave.
Ste. DD1-201
Cleveland, OH 44106
Phone: 216-229-8600
Fax: 216-229-4500
Website: www.ascaa.org
E-mail: irabragg@ascaa.org

*The Aplastic Anemia
and MDS International
Foundation (AAMDSIF)*
4330 E. W. Hwy
Ste. 230
Bethesda, MD 20814
Toll-Free: 800-747-2820
Phone: 301-279-7202
Website: www.aamds.org
E-mail: help@aamds.org

*Diamond Blackfan Anemia
Foundation, Inc. (DBAF)*
P.O. Box 1092
Ste. 700, N. Tower
West Seneca, NY 14224
Phone: 716-674-2818
Website: dbafoundation.org
E-mail: dbafoundation@juno.com

*Fanconi Anemia (FA)
Research Fund*
1801 Willamette St.
Ste. 200
Eugene, OR 97401
Toll-Free: 888-FANCONI
(888-326-2664)
Phone: 541-687-4658
Fax: 541-687-0548
Website: www.fanconi.org
E-mail: info@fanconi.org

*National Center for
Chronic Disease Prevention
and Health Promotion
(NCCDPHP)*
Centers for Disease Control and
Prevention (CDC)
1600 Clifton Rd.
Atlanta, GA 30329-4027
Toll-Free: 800-CDC-INFO
(800-232-4636)
Toll-Free TTY: 888-232-6348
Website: www.cdc.gov/nccdphp

Aneurysms

*American Association of
Neurological Surgeons
(AANS)*
Executive Office
5550 Meadowbrook Dr.
Rolling Meadows, IL 60008-3852
Toll-Free: 888-566-AANS
(888-566-2267)
Phone: 847-378-0500
Fax: 847-378-0600
Website: www.aans.org
E-mail: info@aans.org

*American Stroke Association
(ASA)*
National Center
7272 Greenville Ave.
Dallas, TX 75231
Toll-Free: 888-4-STROKE
(888-478-7653)
Website: www.strokeassociation.
org

Brain Aneurysm Foundation (BAF)
269 Hanover St.
Bldg. 3
Hanover, MA 02339
Toll-Free: 888-BRAIN-02
(888-272-4602)
Phone: 781-826-5556
Fax: 781-826-5566
Website: bafound.org
E-mail: office@bafound.org

Brain Resources and Information Network (BRAIN)
National Institute of Neurological Disorders and Stroke (NINDS)
P.O. Box 5801
Bethesda, MD 20824
Toll-Free: 800-352-9424
Fax: 301-402-2186
Website: www.ninds.nih.
gov/Disorders/Patient-
Caregiver-Education/
Know-Your-Brain
E-mail: braininfo@ninds.nih.gov

Antiphospholipid Antibody Syndrome

APS Foundation of America, Inc. (APSFA)
P.O. Box 801
LaCrosse, WI 54602-0801
Website: apsfa.org

Bleeding and Clotting Disorders

Cure HHT
P.O. Box 329
Monkton, MD 21111
Phone: 410-357-9932
Fax: 410-472-5559
Website: curehht.org
E-mail: hhtinfo@curehht.org

Foundation for Women & Girls with Blood Disorders (FWGBD)
P.O. Box 1358
Montclair, NJ 07042
Website: www.fwgbd.org

National Blood Clot Alliance (NBCA)
8321 Old Courthouse Rd.
Ste. 255
Vienna, VA 22182
Toll-Free: 877-4-NO-CLOT
(877-466-2568)
Phone: 703-935-8845
Website: stoptheclot.org
E-mail: info@stoptheclot.org

Preeclampsia Foundation
3840 W. Eau Gallie Blvd.
Ste. 104
Melbourne, FL 32934
Toll-Free: 800-665-9341
Phone: 321-421-6957
Website: www.preeclampsia.org
E-mail: info@preeclampsia.org

Blood Donation

American Association of Blood Banks (AABB)
4550 Montgomery Ave.
Ste. 700, N. Tower
Bethesda, MD 20814
Phone: 301-907-6977
Fax: 301-907-6895
Website: www.aabb.org
E-mail: aabb@aabb.org

America's Blood Centers
1717 K. St. N.W.
Ste. 900
Washington, DC 20006
Phone: 202-393-5725
Fax: 202-899-2621
Website: www.americasblood.org
E-mail: MemberServices@
americasblood.org

The American National Red Cross
National Headquarters
431 18th St. N.W.
Washington, DC 20006
Toll-Free: 800-RED-CROSS
(800-733-2767)
Phone: 202-303-4498
Website: www.redcross.org

Bone Marrow Donation and Stem Cell Transplantation

The Center for International Blood and Marrow Transplant Research (CIBMTR)
Froedtert and the Medical
College of Wisconsin Clinical
Cancer Center
9200 W. Wisconsin Ave.
Ste. C5500
Milwaukee, WI 53226
Phone: 414-805-0700
Fax: 414-805-0714
Website: www.cibmtr.org
E-mail: contactus@cibmtr.org

International Society for Stem Cell Research (ISSCR)
5215 Old Orchard Rd.
Ste. 270
Skokie, IL 60077
Phone: 224-592-5700
Fax: 224-365-0004
Website: www.isscr.org
E-mail: isscr@isscr.org

National Marrow Donor Program (NMDP)
500 N. Fifth St.
Minneapolis, MN 55401-1206
Toll-Free: 800-MARROW-2
(800-627-7692)
Phone: 612-817-6442
Website: www.bethematch.org
E-mail: patientinfo@nmdp.org

Circulatory Disorders

American Heart Ass.ociation (AHA)
7272 Greenville Ave.
Dallas, TX 75231
Toll-Free: 800-AHA-USA-1
(800-242-8721)
Website: www.heart.org

The Erythromelalgia Association (TEA)
200 Old Castle Ln.
Wallingford, PA 19086
Phone: 610-566-0797
Website: www.erythromelalgia.
org

Fibromuscular Dysplasia Society of America (FMDSA)
26777 Lorain Rd.
Ste. 408
North Olmsted, OH 44070
Toll-Free: 888-709-7089
Phone: 216-834-2410
Website: www.fmdsa.org
E-mail: admin@fmdsa.org

UC Davis Vascular Center
Lawrence J. Ellison Ambulatory
Care Center
4860 Y. St.
Ste. 2100
Sacramento, CA 95817
Toll-Free: 800-2-UC-DAVIS
(800-282-3284)
Phone: 916-734-3800
TDD: 916-451-1974
Website: health.ucdavis.edu/
vascular

Vascular Birthmarks Foundation (VBF)
P.O. Box 106
Latham, NY 12110
Toll-Free: 877-VBF-4646
(877-823-4646)
Website: www.birthmark.org
E-mail: vbfpresident@gmail.com

Vascular Cures
274 Redwood Shores Pkwy
Ste. 717
Redwood City, CA 94065
Phone: 650-368-6022
Website: vascularcures.org

Vasculitis Foundation (VF)
P.O. Box 28660
Kansas City, MO 64188
Toll-Free: 800-277-9474
Phone: 816-436-8211
Fax: 816-656-3838
Website: www.vascularcures.org

Hemochromatosis

American Hemochromatosis Society, Inc. (AHS)
P.O. Box 950871
Lake Mary, FL 32795-0871
Toll-Free: 888-655-IRON
(888-655-4766)
Phone: 407-829-4488
Fax: 407-333-1284
Website: www.americanhs.org
E-mail: mail@americanhs.org

American Liver Foundation (ALF)
National Office
39 Bdwy.
Ste. 2700
New York, NY 10006
Toll-Free: 800-GO-LIVER
(800-465-4837)
Phone: 212-668-1000
Website: www.liverfoundation.org

Hemophilia

Children's Cancer & Blood Foundation (CCBF)
Administrative Office
466 Lexington Ave.
16th Fl.
New York, NY 10017
Phone: 212-297-4336
Fax: 212-297-4340
Website: www.childrenscbf.org

The Coalition for Hemophilia B
757 Third Ave.
20th Fl.
New York, NY 10017
Phone: 212-520-8272
Fax: 212-520-8501
Website: www.hemob.org
E-mail: contact@hemob.org

Hemophilia Federation of America (HFA)
999 N. Capitol St. N.E.
Ste. 201
Washington, DC 20002
Toll-Free: 800-230-9797
Phone: 202-675-6984
Fax: 202-675-6983
Website: www.hemophiliafed.org
E-mail: info@hemophiliafed.org

National Hemophilia Foundation (NHF)
Seven Penn Plaza
Ste. 1204
New York, NY 10001
Phone: 212-328-3700
Fax: 212-328-3777
Website: www.hemophilia.org

World Federation of Hemophilia (WFH)
1425, boul. René-Lévesque
Ouest
Bureau 1200
Montreal, Quebec H3G 1T7
Canada
Phone: 514-875-7944
Fax: 514-875-8916
Website: www.wfh.org
E-mail: wfh@wfh.org

Leukemia

American Cancer Society (ACS)
250 Williams St. N.W.
Atlanta, GA, 30303
Toll-Free: 800-227-2345
Website: www.cancer.org

Leukemia & Lymphoma Society (LLS)
Three International Dr.
Ste. 200, Rye Brook, NY 10573
Toll-Free: 888-557-7177
Website: www.lls.org

Leukemia Research Foundation (LRF)
191 Waukegan Rd.
Ste. 105
Northfield, IL 60093
Phone: 847-424-0600
Fax: 847-424-0606
Website: www.allbloodcancers.org

National Cancer Institute (NCI)
9609 Medical Center Dr.
BG 9609, MSC 9760
Bethesda, MD 20892-9760
Toll-Free: 800-4-CANCER
(800-422-6237)
Website: www.cancer.gov
E-mail: NCIinfo@nih.gov

Myeloproliferative Disorders

Myelodysplastic Syndromes (MDS) Foundation
4573 S. Broad St.
Ste. 150, Yardville, NJ 08620
Toll-Free: 800-MDS-0839
(800-637-0839)
Phone: 609-298-1035
Fax: 609-298-0590
Website: www.mds-foundation.org
E-mail: patientliaison@mds-foundation.org

MPN Research Foundation
180 N. Michigan Ave.
Ste. 1870
Chicago, IL 60601
Phone: 312-683-7247
Fax: 312-332-0840
Website: www.mpnresearchfoundation.org
E-mail: lmoore@mpnrf.org

Plasma Cell Disorders

The Amyloidosis Center
Boston University School of Medicine (BUSM)
72 E. Concord St.
K-503
Boston, MA 02118
Phone: 617-358-4750
Fax: 617-358-4735
Website: www.bu.edu/amyloid
E-mail: amyloid@bmc.org

Amyloidosis Foundation (AF)
7151 N. Main St.
Ste. 2
Clarkston, MI 48346
Toll-Free: 877-AMYLOID
(877-269-5643)
Fax: 248-922-9620
Website: www.amyloidosis.org
E-mail: info@amyloidosis.org

International Waldenstrom's Macroglobulinemia Foundation (IWMF)
6144 Clark Center Ave.
Sarasota, FL 34238
Phone: 941-927-4963
Fax: 941-927-4467
Website: www.iwmf.com

*The Multiple Myeloma
Research Foundation
(MMRF)*
383 Main Ave.
Fifth Fl.
Norwalk, CT 06851
Phone: 203-229-0464
Fax: 203-972-1259
Website: themmrf.org
E-mail: info@themmrf.org

Sickle Cell Disease

*Sickle Cell Disease Asso-
ciation of America, Inc.
(SCDAA)*
3700 Koppers St.
Ste. 570
Baltimore, MD 21227
Toll-Free: 800-421-8453
Phone: 410-528-1555
Fax: 410-528-1495
Website: www.sicklecelldisease.
org
E-mail: admin@sicklecelldisease.
org

*Sickle Cell Information
Center (SCIC)*
Emory Center for Digital
Scholarship
201 Dowman Dr.
Atlanta, GA 30322
Phone: 404-727-7857
Fax: 404-727-7880
Website: scinfo.org
E-mail: aplatt@emory.edu

White Blood Cell Disorders

*American Partnership For
Eosinophilic Disorders
(APFED)*
P.O. Box 29545
Atlanta, GA 30359
Phone: 713-493-7749
Website: www.apfed.org
E-mail: mail@apfed.org

*Campaign Urging Research
for Eosinophilic Disease
(CURED)*
P.O. Box 32
Lincolnshire, IL 60069
Website: curedfoundation.org

*Center for Pediatric
Eosinophilic Disorders
(CPED)*
Children's Hospital of
Philadelphia (CHOP)
3401 Civic Center Blvd.
Philadelphia, PA 19104
Phone: 215-590-7644
Website: www.chop.edu/centers-
programs/center-pediatric-
eosinophilic-disorders

*Neutropenia Support
Association Inc. (NSAI)*
971 Corydon Ave.
P.O. Box 243
Winnipeg, Manitoba R3M 3S7
Canada
Toll-Free: 800-6-NEUTRO
(800-663-8876)
Phone: 204-489-8454
Website: www.neutropenia.ca

Index

Index